D1635697

AN INTRODUCTION

Radiobiology

SECOND EDITION

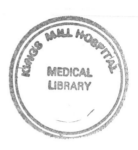

AN INTRODUCTION TO
Radiobiology
SECOND EDITION

A. H. W. NIAS
DM (Oxon), FRCR, MRCPath

Formerly Emeritus Richard Dimbleby Professor of Cancer Research, United Medical and Dental Schools, University of London, St Thomas' Hospital, London, UK

JOHN WILEY & SONS
Chichester · New York · Weinheim · Brisbane · Singapore · Toronto

Other Wiley Editorial Offices

John Wiley & Sons, Inc., 605 Third Avenue,
New York, NY 10158-0012, USA

WILEY-VCH Verlag GmbH, Pappelallee 3,
D-69469 Weinheim, Germany

Jacaranda Wiley Ltd, 33 Park Road, Milton,
Queensland 4064, Australia

John Wiley & Sons (Asia) Pte Ltd, 2 Clementi Loop #02-01,
Jin Xing Distripark, Singapore 129809

John Wiley & Sons (Canada) Ltd, 22 Worcester Road,
Rexdale, Ontario M9W 1L1, Canada

Library of Congress Cataloging-in-Publication Data

Nias, A. H. W.
    An introduction to radiobiology / A. H. W. Nias. — 2nd ed.
      p. cm.
    Includes bibliographical references and index.
    ISBN 0–471–97589–3 (hbk : alk. paper). — ISBN 0–471–97590–7 (pbk.
    : alk. paper)
    1. Radiology, Medical. 2. Radiobiology. I. Title.
    [DNLM: 1. Radiobiology. 2. Nuclear Medicine. 3. Radiation
    Effects. WN 610 N577i 1998]
    R895.N53 1998
    616.07´57—dc21
    DNLM/DLC
    for Library of Congress   97–42811
                                             CIP

British Library Cataloguing in Publication Data

A catalogue record for this book is available from the British Library

ISBN 0–471–97589–3 (cased)
ISBN 0–471–97590–7 (paper)

Typeset in 10/12pt Palatino by Dobbie Typesetting Limited, Tavistock, Devon.
Printed and bound in Great Britain by Biddles Ltd, Guildford and King's Lynn
This book is printed on acid-free paper responsibly manufactured from sustainable forestry, in which at least two trees are planted for each one used for paper production.

To Bibi, who continues to be patient

Contents

Preface

The object of this book is to provide an introduction to quantitative radiobiology and particularly to those aspects of the subject that have a practical application. Radiation is used to cure cancer but can also cause it. Radiation is also used in medical diagnosis and in nuclear power stations. In all these fields, where questions of benefit and detriment arise, the biological effects of the radiation can now be predicted. There are not many walks of life where risk estimates are so firmly founded on quantitative data. This is not only because of the precision with which radiation dose can be measured but also because of the large body of radiobiological observations that have been made since X-rays were discovered.

Given some knowledge of physics and chemistry, the reader will have no difficulty in understanding both the very fast processes that initiate the damage in irradiated tissues and the kinetic patterns in which such damage is expressed at the cellular level. These dynamic aspects of radiation biology are described in detail at a level appropriate to readers with a basic knowledge of mammalian cell biology. Standard textbooks are listed for those who need background reading.

Nearly all the figures have been taken from the radiobiological literature, not only because they provide good illustrations of scientific principles but also because they refer to useful sources of further reading. Some of them have been retained for historical interest. I am grateful to the many colleagues who have generously and willingly given permission for diagrams and illustrations from their published work to be reproduced in this book.

I am also grateful to the many radiobiologists who have offered me advice on how best to revise the first edition so as to bring my book up to date. The subject has made many advances since my first edition and they have pointed the way. Their names are listed in the Acknowledgements but, of course, they are not responsible for my text. I thank those who have reviewed my text and made many constructive comments, and also the staff of John Wiley & Sons for all their help in producing this book.

London, 1997.   A.H.W.N.

Acknowledgements

I thank all the following scientists who have made suggestions to me during the preparation of this second edition. I am lucky to have been able to telephone so many friends who responded with unstinting help.

Stan Batchelor
Richard Camplejohn
John Coggle
Dudley Goodhead
Jolyon Hendry
John Hopewell
Mike Joiner
Brian Lord
Barry Michael
Jens Overgaard
Mike Robbins
Anamaria Rojas
John Saunders
John Savage
Gordon Steel
Ian Stratford
John Thacker
Catherine West
Tom Wheldon
George Wilson
Eric Wright

PUBLISHER'S NOTE

Professor A.H.W. Nias died in October 1997 shortly after delivering the manuscript of this book to us.

1 History and Definitions

It is now more than a century since X-rays were discovered by Wilhelm Roentgen in 1895. Soon after, it was realized that the biological effect of such radiation could be either beneficial or harmful, depending on how it was used. To start with, X-rays were used for diagnostic purposes (such as the examination of injury to bones, which show up particularly well in X-ray photographs). Within 4 months of their discovery there was a report of hair loss in a radiation worker, and this led to the logical step of using X-rays in the treatment of a benign hairy tumour in 1897. Thus, within 2 years of their discovery, X-rays had been shown not only to be useful in the diagnosis and treatment of abnormal tissue but also to produce unacceptable changes in normal tissue.

At about the same time, in 1896 and 1898, respectively, Antoine Becquerel and Marie Curie discovered the radioactive properties of uranium and radium. These are natural isotopes that emit gamma rays, which are like very penetrating X-rays. Then, in 1931, Irene Curie and François Joliot discovered that such radioactivity could be induced artificially, and in 1932 James Chadwick discovered the neutron.

All these discoveries have been put to good use in medicine and industry. The medical use of X-rays continues to be the diagnosis of all forms of disease and the treatment of cancer. Artificial radioactive isotopes are also used for diagnosis and sometimes for treatment, as is the natural isotope radium. In industry, X-rays are used for quality control (e.g. the examination of welded joints) and for the sterilization of food and medical equipment (such as plastic syringes). These are all peaceful uses of ionizing radiation that arouse no public debate, although there are hazards from improper use.

The hazards of ionizing radiation that *have* aroused public interest are those concerned with the use of radioactive isotopes and neutrons for the peaceful purpose of energy production by nuclear power stations and the military purpose of nuclear weapons. These two uses are poles apart but are unfortunately linked in the public mind. Weapons involve a deliberate release of uncontrolled energy and radioactivity, while power stations are designed to control their energy output but prevent the release of radioactivity into the environment.

This book does not make any direct contribution to that nuclear debate because there is already a large amount of literature concerned with the choice of a proper balance between the benefit and detriment of nuclear energy for mankind. However, the main hazards from the peaceful uses of ionizing radiation are the carcinogenic and mutagenic effects of chronic exposure to very low dosage, and these topics will be discussed towards the end of the book (Chapters 17–20). Unlike other environmental hazards, such as toxic chemicals, ionizing radiation can be measured with great precision, even at very low dosage, owing to its physical characteristics. By contrast, the biological effects of such very low dosage are more difficult to measure. This is why most of the examples in this book are based upon the effects of higher doses of radiation.

SYNOPSIS

Although many of the basic principles of radiobiology have been studied using bacterial cells and other prokaryotes, the material in this book will be drawn from studies with mammalian cells and tissues. Chapter 2 provides a brief description of these for the benefit of readers with a limited knowledge of this branch of biology. In addition, because the most important radiobiological effect is that upon the proliferation of cells and tissues, Chapter 3 describes the kinetics of their proliferation under normal circumstances, before such cells and tissues are irradiated. Having set the biological scene, it will then be time to discuss the physics and chemistry of ionizing radiation and its primary effects (Chapter 4).

Those first four chapters should have prepared the reader for the main purpose of this book, namely to describe the biological effects of radiation. These will include biochemical effects (Chapter 5), cell lethality (Chapter 6), repair (Chapter 7) and the measurement of radiosensitivity to X-rays (Chapter 8) and to more densely ionizing radiation (Chapter 9). Experience from the treatment of cancer by radiation has shown that radiosensitivity can be influenced by the oxygen tension in a tissue (Chapter 10) as well as by radiosensitizers and radioprotectors (Chapter 11). The difference in the response to radiation of normal and malignant cells (Chapter 12), tissues (Chapter 13) and the whole body (Chapter 14) all illustrate the principles of radiobiology. One of the remaining problems of radiotherapy is to devise the optimum regime for each individual patient. This requires a knowledge of the sensitivity and proliferation kinetics of each tumour (Chapter 15) so that the most suitable fractionation regime can be devised (Chapter 16).

The remainder of the book examines the effects of radiation used either at low dose rates (Chapter 17) or at the low dose levels used in diagnosis (Chapter 18). This enables the very low levels of background radiation to be placed in perspective (Chapter 19) and guidelines to be devised for the safe use of radiation in everyday life (Chapter 20).

HISTORY

All of the foregoing comprises the science of radiobiology, which can be said to have begun with that observation in 1896 of hair loss following irradiation. The lack of a systematic system of radiation dosimetry prevented a proper scientific study of the biological effects of radiation. In those early days, the common practice of radiotherapists was to determine the 'skin erythema dose', which produced a reddening of the skin in 1 or 2 weeks after irradiation. This very crude method of dosimetry was not replaced until 1928, when the roentgen unit (R) was accepted internationally. This was based on radiation-induced ionization in air. It was about that time that the first quantitative radiobiology was conducted by Müller (1927), who measured mutation rates in the *Drosophila* fruit fly by using X-rays and demonstrated a dose–response relationship. In 1940, Gray and his colleagues described some of the biological effects of fast neutrons, and in 1953 Gray and his team went on to show the influence of oxygen concentration on the response of tissues to radiation.

Mammalian radiobiology was revolutionized in 1956 when Puck and Marcus used their newly developed quantitative cell culture technique to demonstrate the exponential radiation dose–response relationship shown in Figure 1.1 (the technique is described in Chapter 6 and the dose–response curve in Chapter 8). This really put the science of radiobiology on the map and provided the basis for all subsequent studies of the effects of radiation on proliferating cell populations and the tissues that they form.

It was at about this time that the proliferative cycle of plant cells was shown by Howard and Pelc (1953) to include a discrete central phase of DNA synthesis. Lajtha et al (1954) showed that this also applied to the mammalian cell cycle, which could thus be divided into a DNA synthetic

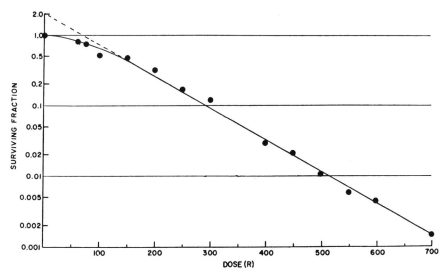

Figure 1.1. Radiation dose–response of human cancer cells. (Reproduced from Puck and Marcus, 1956, by copyright permission of The Rockefeller University Press.

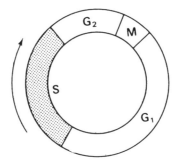

Figure 1.2. The phases of the mammalian cell cycle. (Reproduced from Aherne et al, *An Introduction to Cell Population Kinetics*, 1977, by permission of Cambridge University Press.)

(or S) phase, pre- and post-synthetic phases or 'gaps' (G_1 and G_2) and the mitotic phase (M). These phases are depicted in Figure 1.2, where the S phase is shown to be labelled as it would be by the uptake of a DNA precursor (see Chapter 3).

This discovery opened the door to another new technique of mammalian biology: cell population kinetics. By good fortune, many of the scientists involved in this work were also radiobiologists, so the two new techniques were quickly drawn together. One result was to provide an explanation for the so-called 'law' that Bergonié and Tribondeau had described in 1906. They had thought that actively dividing cell populations are more radiosensitive than non-dividing tissues. It is now realized that rapidly proliferating tissues are more 'radioresponsive' (i.e. they respond more quickly to radiation) but not necessarily more 'radiosensitive' (i.e. they may not suffer so much damage). The third important development in radiobiology also took place in the 1950s, when Elkind and Sutton (1959) showed that not all radiation damage is lethal to mammalian cells and that some repair is possible (Chapter 7). The precise mechanism of this repair can now be explained on the molecular basis of DNA repair enzymes; DNA is generally assumed to be the principal target of radiation damage (Chapter 5).

Four years later, the simultaneous discovery of the hydrated electron by Boag and Hart (1963) and by Keene (1963) led to an expansion of the technique of pulse radiolysis, allowing the study of radiation chemistry (Chapter 4) to advance. The hydrated electron has proved important in the mechanism of action of electron-affinic radiosensitizers (Chapter 11).

In the 1980s the radiation response of human tumours was correlated with their cell survival over the low dose range, and the concept of the surviving fraction after 2 Gy (SF2) was established (Chapters 8 and 12). A systematic difference was shown between the effect of dose fractionation on early and late reacting tissues (Chapter 16).

Towards the end of a century of radiobiology (Nias, 1995) there have been contributions from molecular genetics (e.g. a human gene for the repair of radiation damage). All these were important stages in the development of radiobiology, which is the scientific study of the biological effects of radiation; but what is meant by the word 'radiation'?

RADIATION

From the beginning of time, mankind has been exposed to some form of radiation. This is because radiation is the process by which a body emits radiant energy, and we are all exposed to the radiant energy emitted by the Sun. When the Sun rises each morning, the Earth receives its radiation in the form of heat and light. Life would not continue without such solar radiation, which is almost entirely beneficial to mankind. The same cannot be said of nuclear radiation, which is the subject of this book. Yet nuclear radiation is similar to solar radiation in many respects because they are both forms of electromagnetic waves. The important difference is in the wavelength of such radiations.

Figure 1.3 shows the full spectrum of electromagnetic radiations and how their wavelengths become progressively shorter, from radiowaves at the right end of the diagram to X-rays at the left. Only radiations with shorter wavelengths affect living organisms. Radio uses much longer wavelengths, which may be as long as a kilometre for the long waveband. The shorter the wavelength of the radiation, the higher is its frequency; modern radios use very high frequencies (VHF) and television uses ultrahigh frequencies (UHF). Radar uses shorter wavelengths in the range 1–10 cm, and microwave ovens use still shorter wavelengths down to 10^{-2} cm.

While the electromagnetic radiations with even shorter wavelengths affect living organisms, some are only harmful if used to excess. The infrared radiation from an electric radiator is beneficial but too much heat will burn. Visible light is very useful, but too much ultraviolet (UV) light can burn the skin. Ultraviolet radiation does not penetrate the skin, however, and only causes *excitation*, where the orbital electrons within atoms are raised to higher energy levels. At still shorter wavelengths *ionization* occurs, and then the orbital electrons are actually removed from atoms. This happens with X-rays and gamma rays, which is why they are the most damaging forms of electromagnetic radiation (Figure 1.3). It is because of their very high frequency and very short wavelength that X-rays ionize any molecules in their path and can sometimes penetrate the whole body. This certainly happens with gamma rays at the extreme end of the spectrum of electromagnetic radiations.

Although one cannot see X-rays, they still behave in many ways like the light that we can see, the heat that we can feel and the radiowaves with

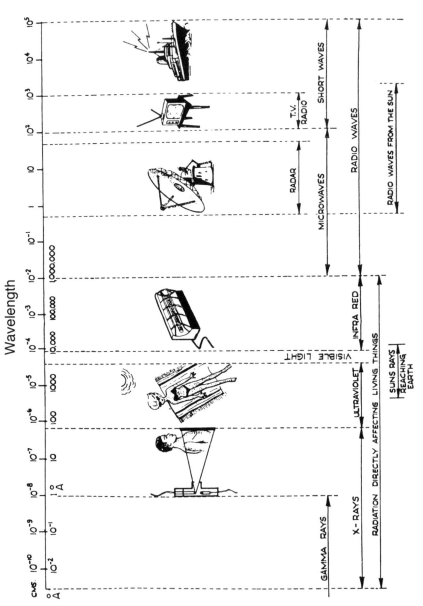

Figure 1.3. Electromagnetic radiations. (Reproduced from *Radiation, Part of Life*, 1965, by permission of Which? Ltd (Consumers' Association).)

which we communicate. All these electromagnetic radiations travel in straight lines and the intensity of the radiation falls off with distance travelled. This is because of the inverse square law: e.g. a beam of light is only a quarter as bright after it has travelled twice the distance from its source. The inverse square law applies to a beam of X-rays, which is why one of the best ways to protect oneself against nuclear radiation is to retire to a safe distance. Another way is to stand behind a protective wall made of a radio-opaque substance that will shield the radiation, just as a beam of light is shielded by a lamp-shade. The important difference is that a very dense material, such as a sheet of lead or a concrete wall, is needed to shield X-rays.

Man-made X-rays are produced when a beam of fast electrons is stopped in a block of metal, such as tungsten, in an X-ray tube. However, only 14% of the nuclear radiation received by man comes from medical uses (Figure 1.4). Over 85% comes from the natural background that we are all exposed to, whether we like it or not. The largest proportion of this is from exposure to natural radioactivity in the air, from radon. Gamma radiation comes from radioactivity in the ground and there is internal radiation from some food and drink. Then there is cosmic radiation from outer space. These various forms of radiation only amount to a comparatively low dose of radiation to the average person (Chapter 19). Despite this relatively low exposure, radiobiologists have to try to measure the biological effects of this form of

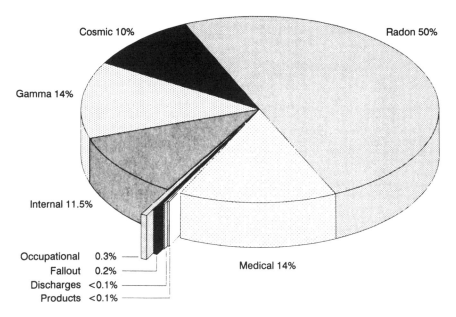

Figure 1.4. Relative contribution of sources of radiation to the UK population. (Reproduced from Hughes and O'Riordan, 1993, by permission of NRPB/SO.)

electromagnetic radiation in order to guide the authorities when they issue guidelines for radiation protection (Chapter 20). To do this, various techniques have to be used, and these depend on the time scale of the events induced in the mammalian cell populations exposed to radiation.

TIME SCALE

The techniques that can provide information about the processes peculiar to each time interval following irradiation are listed in Figure 1.5. Initially, the absorption of the electromagnetic radiation is a physical process (lasting 10^{-18} s) involving excitation, but particularly ionization in the tracks of the X-ray photons (or nuclear particles). This will be described in Chapter 4, together with the subsequent radiation chemical events. These involve rapid free-radical processes that can occur within the tracks directly and the diffusion-controlled free-radical reactions that then occur indirectly (lasting 10^{-12} s). Over this time scale, the pulse radiolysis technique is essential in detecting the various free-radical ions, such as OH·, e^-_{aq} and H·, produced by the radiolysis of water. The relatively slower, but still rapid, mix technique is needed to examine the processes (lasting 10^{-6} s) that result in the decay of radicals in target molecules, particularly those that can result in altered chemical structures.

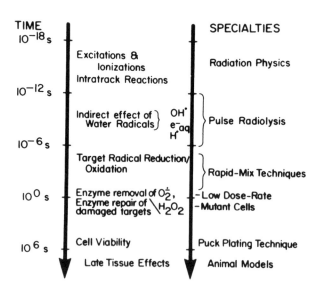

Figure 1.5. Time scale of radiation-induced events in mammalian cells. (Reproduced from Chapman, 1980, by permission of Lippincott-Raven Publishers.)

The subsequent events involve biochemical mechanisms, which will be described in Chapter 5. These include enzymatic processes that can remove toxic radiation products and repair damaged molecules (Chapter 7). Although these biochemical events may only take seconds, this represents a much longer time scale in comparison with the earlier physical and chemical processes. Low dose-rate radiation, mutant cells and molecular biological techniques are used to analyse these phenomena.

Finally, we come to the biological and physiological mechanisms whereby altered cell molecules result in cell death and the loss of proliferative capacity. This can be analysed by the Puck and Marcus (1956) technique (used for Figure 1.1) over a period of 1–2 weeks. After considerable cell death, whole tissues will show damage, which may be detected within a few days but may also develop much later, some months after the radiation dose was delivered. The extent of such damage will always depend upon the size of the dose. Radiation dosimetry will be described in Chapter 4 but it is useful to mention the units of radiation dose in this chapter.

RADIATION UNITS

Before 1928, radiation dosimetry was very crude. There was the pastille unit, estimated by a change in colour – a chemical process. There was also the skin erythema dose, a biological endpoint used in radiotherapy. The roentgen unit (R) was then accepted internationally as a measure of ionization in air. This was defined as the quantity of X- or γ-radiation such that the associated secondary electrons emitted produce ions of either sign carrying a negative or positive charge of 2.58×10^{-4} coulombs per kilogram of air. The use of the roentgen was restricted to X-rays below 3 MeV in energy, because of the difficulty of measuring the ionizations in air of more energetic secondary electrons. The R unit was a unit of exposure, i.e. the amount of radiation directed at the material. It did not indicate the amount of dose actually absorbed by the material.

The need for a unit of absorbed dose was recognized by the International Commission on Radiological Units (ICRU) in 1956 when they adopted the rad (radiation absorbed dose) unit. One rad was defined as the absorption of 10^{-2} joules of radiation energy per kilogram of material (0.01 J kg^{-1}).

Fortunately, the energy absorbed in tissue following exposure to 1 R is 0.0095 J kg^{-1}. Thus, a tissue exposed to a dose of 1 R will receive an absorbed dose of 0.95 rad. Therefore, for most purposes the R and the rad units can be regarded as equivalent in radiobiology, and this is convenient for comparing the doses in older radiobiological work, such as the dose–response in Figure 1.1 for which the R unit was used.

Nowadays, SI units are used in science (Table 1.1) and the unit of absorbed dose is the gray (Gy), defined as 1 J kg^{-1}, i.e. it is 100 times larger than the rad (1 Gy = 100 rad). For some purposes, like radiotherapy, it has been found convenient to use the centigray (cGy), which, being exactly the same as the rad, avoids the necessity (and sometimes even the danger) of multiplying or dividing by 100. There is no SI unit for the exposure dose and so the R unit is being phased out altogether.

For most of the data presented in this book, the radiation doses will be based on the gray, the unit of absorbed radiation dose. Many of the diagrams will use centigrays (cGy). A few will use R units when they are historical examples of the radiobiological literature (e.g. Figures 1.1 and 16.10). For most purposes the cGy, the rad and the R can be accepted as equivalent in radiation dose, so the biological effect can be considered to be comparable.

However, in Chapter 20, where the problems of radiation protection are discussed, the unit of dose equivalence has to be used. The old unit was the rem (or rad equivalent man) and, just as the new gray unit equals 100 rad, so the new unit for radiation protection purposes, the sievert (Sv), equals 100 rem for conventional X-rays. Where different types of radiation, such as neutrons and other more densely ionizing radiations are concerned, a radiation weighting factor has to be used to take into account the increased radiobiological effectiveness of those types of radiation (see Table 9.1, Chapter 9). This may increase the sievert dose by as much as 20 times.

Finally, mention should be made of the unit for measuring the dose from radioactive isotopes, which decay in radioactivity with a half-life that is unique for each isotope (Chapter 4). The old unit was the curie (Ci), which was based on the fact that 1 g of radium undergoes 3.7×10^{10} disintegrations per second. The new unit is the becquerel (Bq), which is defined as one disintegration per second and so $1 \text{ Ci} = 3.7 \times 10^{10}$ Bq. In practice, the becquerel is far too small a unit for measuring the radioactivity of those isotopes in common use, and so the megabecquerel (MBq = 10^6 Bq) is often used.

Table 1.1. International system of radiological units

Quantity	SI unit	Other SI units	Old unit	Conversion factor
Exposure	–	$C \text{ kg}^{-1}$	roentgen (R)	$1 \text{ C kg}^{-1} \sim 3876 \text{ R}$
Absorbed dose	gray (Gy)	$J \text{ kg}^{-1}$	rad (rad)	$1 \text{ Gy} = 100 \text{ rad}$
Dose equivalent	sievert (Sv)	$J \text{ kg}^{-1}$	rem (rem)	$1 \text{ Sv} = 100 \text{ rem}$
Activity	becquerel (Bq)	s^{-1}	curie (Ci)	$1 \text{ Bq} \sim 2.7 \times 10^{-11} \text{ Ci}$

Reproduced from Hughes and O'Riordan, 1993, by permission of NRPB/SO.

SUMMARY OF CONCLUSIONS

(1) Since X-rays were discovered in 1895, their beneficial and harmful effects have been studied in great detail. The history is summarized in this chapter.

(2) X-rays are a type of electromagnetic radiation with such a short wavelength that they can ionize biological molecules and damage mammalian cells.

(3) Ionizing radiation is beneficial in medicine and can be used safely in the nuclear power industry. There is a low level of radiation in the environment that is unavoidable.

(4) Because radiation is a physical agent, the doses received by the cells and tissues of the body can be measured with great accuracy.

(5) The time scale of the biological effects of radiation follows a predictable sequence, which is described in this book.

REFERENCES

Aherne, W. A., Camplejohn, R. S. and Wright, N. A., 1977. *An Introduction to Cell Population Kinetics*. Cambridge University Press.

Bergonié, J. and Tribondeau, L. (1906). Actions des rayons x sur le testicle. *Archives d'electricité medicale*, **14**, 779–791 and 911–927.

Boag, J. W. and Hart, E. J. (1963). Absorption spectra of 'hydrated' electron. *Nature*, **197**, 45–47.

Chapman, J. D. (1980). Biological models of mammalian cell inactivation by radiation. In *Radiation Biology in Cancer Research*, edited by R. E. Meyn and H. R. Withers. Lippincott-Raven Publishers, New York, pp. 21–32.

Consumers' Association, 1965. *Radiation, Part of Life*. Consumers' Association, London.

Elkind, M. M. and Sutton, H. (1959). Radiation response of mammalian cells grown in culture. 1. Repair of X-ray damage in surviving Chinese hamster cells. *Radiation Research*, **13**, 556–593.

Gray, L. H., Mottram, J. C., Read, J. and Spear, F. G., 1940. Some experiments upon biological effects of fast neutrons. *British Journal of Radiology*, **13**, 371–375.

Gray, L. H., Conger, A. D., Ebert, M., Hornsey, S. and Scott, O. C. A., 1953. The concentrations of oxygen in dissolved tissues at the time of irradiation as a factor in radiotherapy. *British Journal of Radiology*, **26**, 638–648.

Howard, A. and Pelc, S. R., 1953. Synthesis of deoxyribonucleic acid in normal and irradiated cells and its relationship to chromosome breakage. *Heredity Supplement*, **6**, 261–273.

Hughes, J. S. and O'Riordan, M. C., 1993. *Radiation Exposure of the UK Population – 1993 Review*. National Radiological Protection Board, HMSO, London.

Keene, J. P., 1963. Optical absorptions in irradiated water. *Nature*, **197**, 47–48.

Lajtha, L. G., Oliver, R. and Ellis, F., 1954. Incorporation of ^{32}P and Adenine ^{14}C into DNA by human bone marrow cells *in vitro*. *British Journal of Cancer*, **8**, 367–379.

Müller, H. J., 1927. Artificial transmutation of the gene. *Science*, **66**, 84–87.

Nias, A. H. W., 1995. 100 years of radiobiology. In *The Invisible Light*, edited by A. M. K. Thomas, Blackwell Science, Oxford.

Puck, T. T. and Marcus, P. I., 1956. Action of X-rays on mammalian cells. *Journal of Experimental Medicine*, **103**, 653–666.

2 Cells and Tissues

If a standard man weighs 70 kg, his body will consist of approximately 7×10^{13} cells. Each of these cells will contain the structures shown in Figure 2.1. Such cells are the 'building bricks' of animal life. They are the basic unit of biological existence. Although cells may exist as independent units when they are bacteria and protozoans, this book is concerned with the metazoa: the subkingdom of animals in which the body is composed of many cells grouped into tissues and coordinated by a nervous system. Metazoa comprise both vertebrates and invertebrates but this book will only deal with the mammalian class of vertebrates.

The cells group in patterns that are recognizable as tissues, the tissues form organs and the whole animal consists of an orderly arrangement of such organs and connective tissues. The destruction of any one of the vital organs in an animal will result in its death. This book will describe how

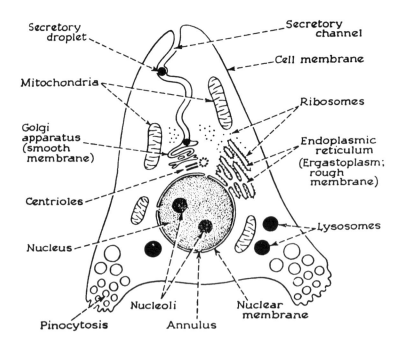

Figure 2.1. Schematic diagram of a mammalian cell. (Reproduced from Paul, 1975, by permission of Churchill Livingstone.)

ionizing radiation can produce effects ranging from a quasi-threshold of negligible damage at the cellular level, through tissue damage from which the animal may survive, to whole-body effects that may be lethal. In order to explain the basis for this broad range of radiation effect, it is necessary to describe the cellular organization of the tissues of the body.

All mammalian cells have certain common features of internal organization. They all have a functional *nucleus* containing DNA, which is embedded in the main body, or *cytoplasm*. This nucleus functions as the control centre for the cell. It is surrounded by a *nuclear membrane*, which contains many pores for the exchange of material between the nucleus and the cytoplasm. When the nucleus is not dividing, the genetic material is dispersed as chromatin and *nucleoli* are present. During cell division, the chromatin is condensed into chromosomes and the nucleoli disappear. Nucleoli contain ribosomal RNA.

CYTOPLASMIC ORGANELLES

In the surrounding cytoplasm are a number of structures of variable importance:

(1) *Mitochondria* are sausage-shaped structures bounded by two membranes, the inner one being folded into finger-like projections. They carry out aerobic respiration, and are the site of the Krebs cycle and electron transport chains. They are responsible for energy production in the cell and are most numerous in cells with a high level of metabolic activity.

(2) *Ribosomes* are small spherical bodies that are the site of protein synthesis and consist of ribosomal RNA and protein. Most cells have a number of ribosomes either attached to the endoplasmic reticulum or free in the cytoplasm. During protein synthesis, they are associated with messenger RNA in the process of translation.

(3) *The Golgi apparatus* is an assembly of vesicles and folded membranes that stores and transports secretory products (such as enzymes and hormones) and plays a role in the formation of the cell wall.

(4) *Lysosomes* are membrane-bound sacs that contain enzymes responsible for the digestion of material in food vacuoles (formed by pinocytosis of liquid and phagocytosis of solid material). They are responsible for the dissolution of foreign particles entering the cell (such as bacteria) and, on the death of the cell, the breakdown of cell structures.

(5) *Centrioles* occur in pairs and are cylindrical structures that have a role in cell division, during which they move to opposite ends of the nucleus to form the ends of the mitotic spindle. This is formed of bundles of minute protein filaments called microtubules, which also function as a

cytoskeleton, helping the cell to maintain its shape. Surrounding all this is the lipoprotein *cell membrane*.

The whole structure can be likened to a small factory in which a number of jobs are performed under the same roof. During normal working conditions, the whole concern is operating in harmony, with each job progressing at an appropriate rate. Some jobs are very complicated, some are simple. Disruption of certain of the jobs will bring the whole concern to a stop. Others are less important and normal working may still continue without them for a period while repairs are undertaken. Thus damage to the outer cell membrane or any of the organelles in the cytoplasm will be disruptive to some extent but the cell may still survive, just as a factory may stay in business even when the wall has been damaged and some of the minor sections disrupted.

By contrast, the nucleus of a cell is like the central computer in the office, which organizes all the work in a factory. If the computer is out of action, the whole enterprise will come to a halt. If the nucleus of a mammalian cell is damaged, the consequence may be lethal. This will be illustrated in Chapter 5, where the nucleus will be shown to be far more radiosensitive than the cytoplasm.

The cytoplasmic organelles are depicted in schematic form in Figure 2.1, which shows a few mitochondria and lysosomes together with some endoplasmic reticulum, the Golgi apparatus and the centrioles, all enclosed by the cell membrane. The problem with such a diagram is, firstly, that it has to be drawn in two dimensions, even though a cell is a three-dimensional organism; secondly, the diagram gives only a token representation of the complex relationship of these cytoplasmic organelles. While each organelle has its own function, the whole cell is more than the sum of these parts. Interaction between the organelles is essential if the cell is to remain viable.

TYPES OF MAMMALIAN CELL

The relationship depicted in Figure 2.1 will vary between the different types of mammalian cell that go to make up the various tissues of the body. While all the cells have the same basic organization of nucleus and cytoplasm, considerable differences exist. These are illustrated in Figure 2.2, which shows examples of the five groups of tissue into which mammalian cells are usually classified:

(1) *Epithelial tissues* consist of cells that grow into sheets that cover organs and line cavities. The skin is our outer covering of squamous epithelial cells. This is shown as a pavement, which becomes horny with keratin to provide a tough surface layer. The other epithelial tissue illustrated is cuboidal and this is used to line the ducts from glands, such as the

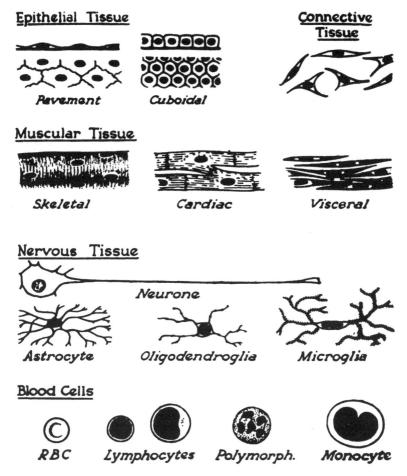

Figure 2.2. Types of mammalian cells. (Reproduced from Paul, 1975, by permission of Churchill Livingstone.)

salivary glands, or tubules, as found in the kidney. Yet another type of epithelial tissue is formed of columnar cells, which line the digestive tract and have absorptive and secretory functions.

(2) *Connective tissue* cells form the structural units of the body, such as bone, cartilage and tendon. The fibroblasts shown in Figure 2.2 are the simplest example of this type of cell, which can secrete various forms of intercellular material, such as calcium in bone or fat in adipose tissue, and also provide a loose packing of areolar tissue to support the other tissues of the body.

(3) The three types of *muscular tissue* are shown. In this tissue the cells are arranged in sheets or bundles but, as with all the cells in the diagram,

each has a nucleus as well as its specific form of cytoplasm. The cytoplasm of muscle cells gives them the property of contracting so as to produce movement or tension in the body. This is under voluntary control in the case of skeletal muscle and involuntary control in the heart and in viscera such as the intestine and bladder.

(4) *Nervous tissue* includes the brain, the spinal cord and the nerves that extend to all the tissues of the body. The diagram shows a neurone, which is an elongated cell that is specialized to conduct impulses over a distance that may be as long as that between the trunk and the toes. The three other types of nervous tissue cells are used for support and are called neuroglia.

(5) *Blood cells.* One exception to the rule that all mammalian cells have a nucleus as well as a specialized cytoplasm is the red blood cell, which is so specialized for the transport of oxygen that it ends up as a bag of haemoglobin, having lost its nucleus while it was differentiating from the progeny of stem cells in the bone marrow (see Chapter 13, Figure 13.6). The other types of blood cell produced in the bone marrow are the white blood cells, which deal with infections, and the megakaryocytes, which produce the platelets that help in blood clotting. The lymphocytes, which are also concerned with the body's defence, make up the final type of blood cell. They are responsible for immune reactions because the presence of antigens stimulates them to produce antibodies.

PROLIFERATION OF CELL POPULATIONS

The tissues of the body are formed from the above-mentioned five types of cell. Such tissues result from cell proliferation and organization, which is very active in early embryonic life but decreases as a child matures to adulthood. From then on, proliferation occurs at different rates in different cell populations, so as to maintain the functional integrity of those tissues. The cells in these tissues may undergo one of three processes: they can divide and grow in number; they can just stay alive without dividing; or they can die by apoptosis (programmed cell death) or necrosis.

Living tissues therefore can be divided roughly into three groups (Table 2.1) on the basis of their proliferation kinetics. Some adult tissues remain static with no proliferation at all. This applies to neurones, for example, in which mitosis is not possible and no cell renewal can take place. At the other extreme are the epithelial tissues, such as the epidermis and the intestinal mucosa, which continue to proliferate. The cells of these populations renew themselves throughout adult life.

There is also a middle group of organs, such as the parenchymal cells of the liver and thyroid, which, together with connective tissue and the vascular endothelial cells, have a low level of cell renewal. Endothelial cells

Table 2.1. Cell populations and their kinetic properties

| No mitosis | Low mitotic index | Frequent mitoses |
No cell renewal	Little or no cell renewal	Cell renewal
Neurones	Liver	Epidermis
Sense organs	Thyroid	Intestinal epithelium
Adrenal medulla	Vascular endothelium	Bone marrow
	Connective tissue	Gonads

Reproduced from Bertalanffy and Lau, 1962, by permission of Academic Press, Inc.

line all the blood vessels through which a flow of blood is maintained by the heart to the tissues of the body. In every tissue there is a capillary network that provides for the delivery of oxygen and other nutrients and the removal of carbon dioxide and other metabolic waste products. The combination of vascular and connective tissue provides the stroma, or framework, of all the other tissues of the body. In this middle group are cell populations where rapid renewal is possible on demand, but where cell proliferation normally occurs at a low rate in a healthy individual.

One important exception in all this is cancer, which is a disorder of cell growth. Nearly all the normal cell types may be transformed into a malignant form in which proliferation occurs without the normal self-regulatory mechanism, and these cells may then spread throughout the body. The commoner cancers are made up of epithelial cell types, and are called carcinomas. Connective tissue cells may also become malignant and result in sarcomas, while malignant bone marrow cells produce leukaemia. Cancer cells proliferate differently from normal cells and it is the prevention of such proliferation that is one of the most important properties of radiation.

Tumours are classified into two types: benign and malignant. Benign tumours have a more organized structure in that the architecture of the parent tissues is largely retained, the cells resemble those of the original tissue and the tumour remains localized without spreading throughout the body. In contrast, malignant tumours grow rapidly and invasively, with destruction of neighbouring tissue and often developing claw-like extensions. It is for this reason that such tumours are called cancers (from the Latin for crab). Unlike normal tissues, the cells of malignant tumours are an extremely heterogeneous population in terms of shape and size. The type of cell may also vary from one part of the tumour to another.

In addition to this heterogeneity, the cells in solid tumours are also variable with respect to three other functions that determine their response to ionizing radiation. This is shown in Figure 2.3 as a scheme based on three functions:

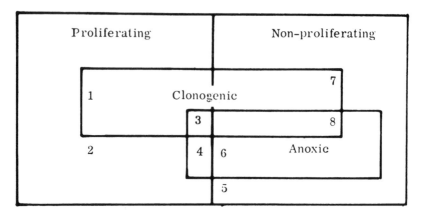

Figure 2.3. A schematic partitioning of a solid tumour based upon the proliferative, clonogenic and oxygenated status of the tumour cells. (Reproduced from Mendelsohn, 1967, by permission of the author.)

(1) Are the cells proliferating?
(2) Do the cells have clonogenic capacity?
(3) Are they oxygenated or anoxic?

It is possible to divide a tumour into eight categories on this basis. In the first category are cells that are not proliferating but have clonogenic capacity and are well oxygenated. They present the major problem in cancer treatment. Category 2 cells are oxygenated and are proliferating but they are not clonogenic, i.e. they cannot divide indefinitely. Categories 3 and 4 may not occur very often because anoxic cells are rarely able to proliferate or express any clonogenic capacity. Categories 5 and 6 contain non-proliferating, non-clonogenic cells that are either oxygenated or anoxic. The latter two categories will include the necrotic regions, which can become quite a large fraction of some solid tumours as they outgrow their blood supply (see Chapter 12, Figure 12.6). Categories 7 and 8 contain non-proliferating cells that are nonetheless clonogenic. These are sometimes called G_0 cells in the terminology used to describe the mammalian cell cycle. Category 7 would also include some cells in normal tissues such as liver and salivary gland.

THE CELL CYCLE

The growth kinetic state of a cell population depends upon how many cells are passing through their proliferative cycle and how long that cycle is. The cell cycle (Figure 2.4) is defined as the interval between the midpoint of mitosis in a cell and the midpoint of the subsequent mitosis in both

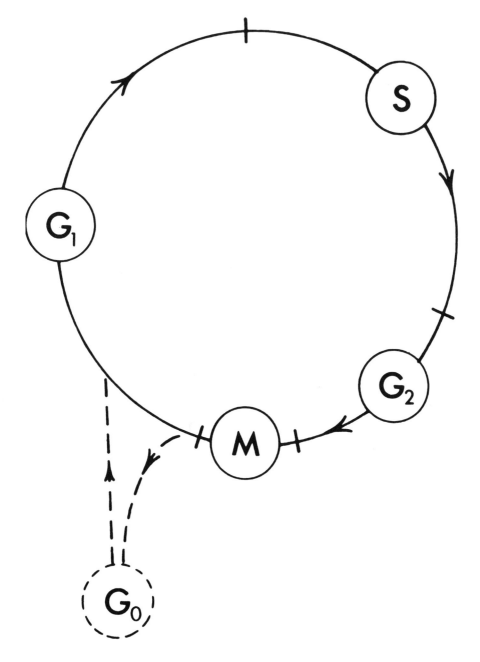

Figure 2.4. Events in the cell cycle. (Reproduced from Priestman, 1980, by permission of Farmitalia Carlo Erba.)

daughter cells. Although the words life cycle, generation cycle, mitotic cycle and nuclear cycle are sometimes used, the term cell cycle is the most commonly used. No reference will be made to the mammalian meiotic cycle.

The cell cycle follows an orderly sequence of phases between one mitosis and the next. The phase that is most easily recognized by present techniques is the DNA synthetic, or S phase. This is because DNA synthesis only occurs during that part of the cell cycle, while other cellular constituents tend to be synthesized throughout interphase (the term sometimes used to describe the intermitotic phases). Synthesis of DNA also occurs to a small extent outside the nucleus, in mitochondrial DNA. What is called unscheduled DNA synthesis (repair synthesis) may also occur following radiation damage. However, in this book the term DNA synthesis will refer to the duplication of the genome in that discrete period of the cell cycle shown in Figure 2.4 as S (the S phase). The gaps before and after the S phase are called, respectively, the G_1 and G_2 phases (where G_1 and G_2 denote gaps in the cell cycle with respect to DNA synthesis). Other molecular and biochemical processes occur during these phases. It is known that synthesis of both RNA and protein continues throughout interphase but the precise timing of all these macromolecular synthetic processes is not nearly so easy to define as the S phase. After mitosis, M, cells may spend some time in a 'resting' phase, G_0, before re-entering the G_1 phase.

Division of the cell cycle into these four phases allowed the development of a whole new subject, cell population kinetics (Chapter 3), and a totally new approach to the old problem of what controls the division of mammalian cells. It is now clear that in most cases mitosis is preceded by DNA synthesis and that the two processes are almost always correlated. This means that if we wish to study the control of cell division, we must study the initiation of DNA synthesis.

Progression through the cell cycle is based on a programme of causally connected sequential transcriptions and translations governed by a set of gene products called *cyclins*. These are a family of proteins whose concentration increases and decreases throughout the cell cycle. There are check (or transition) points before each of the two key events in the cycle (DNA synthesis and mitosis). These are then triggered by cyclin-dependent kinases (CDKs), whose activity is dependent on them combining with a cyclin. Successive combinations of activity drive cell proliferation forward (Warenius, 1997). The transition from G_1 to the S phase is initially under the control of cyclin D/CDK4 and then by cyclin E/CDK2. Progress through the S phase is initially controlled by cyclin A/CDK2 and then by cyclin A/cdc2. The transition from G_2 to mitosis is controlled by cyclin B/CDK1. The CDKs build up like water behind a 'dam' of CDK inhibitors (CKIs). Once the dam is full, surplus cyclins trigger the destruction of CKIs, the dam bursts and the cell is then committed to the S phase. There is a second 'dam' at the G_2/M transition point before the cell proceeds to mitosis.

The tumour suppressor gene p53 can play an important role in the mammalian cell cycle. If DNA is damaged (e.g. by radiation) then p53 accumulates and switches off replication in order to allow extra time for the repair of DNA damage before the S phase. If this repair fails, the p53 gene may trigger cell suicide by apoptosis. In many tumour cells the p53 gene is inactivated by mutation and cannot arrest the cycle in the G_1 phase. Such cells continue to replicate damaged DNA and accumulate more mutations. Tumour cells with p53 mutations may be more radiosensitive (see Chapter 12).

Just before mitosis, the particular form of protein synthesis necessary for this complicated process is initiated. During mitosis, the chromosomes are condensed, RNA synthesis and turnover are arrested and protein synthesis is decreased (DNA synthesis was completed sometime earlier, before the beginning of the G_2 phase, and will not recommence before the end of the coming G_1 phase).

Thus, the duration of the G_1 phase may be elongated. This brings us to the question of whether elongation of at least the initial portion of G_1 is the same as the so-called G_0 phase. There is good evidence that G_0 cells do exist in many normal tissues, including skin, bone marrow, liver, connective tissue and lymphoid tissue, but it is by no means certain that they occur in malignant cells, which may just remain in a quiescent G_1 phase. In the case of G_0 cells, activation of the genome is required before re-entry into the cell cycle, whereas cells resting in G_1 have all the genes necessary for proliferation permanently activated. Thus, quiescent G_1 cells are already committed to initiate DNA synthesis and divide, whereas G_0 cells require a specific stimulus before they are recruited into the active cell cycle. Examples of such stimulae include partial hepatectomy for liver cells, isoproterenol for salivary gland cells, thiouracil for thyroid, erythropoietin for the bone marrow stem cells and wounding for the basal cells in the epidermis. The result of such a stimulus can be that enough resting cells are triggered into proliferation to form a semi-synchronous wave of cycling cells. This might be a way of synchronizing cell populations *in vivo* but there are better ways of doing this *in vitro*.

SYNCHRONY AND SYNCHRONIZATION

Mammalian cell populations usually proliferate in asynchronous growth. Later on, in Chapters 7 and 8, it will be necessary to study the effects of radiation on cells in the various phases of the cell cycle. The way to do this is to obtain cell populations that are growing in perfect synchrony. This would require that every single cell traversed every defined point in the cell cycle (mitosis; each of the recognizable stages in G_1, S and G_2; and then the next mitosis) all together, with no deviation. This is very difficult to obtain *in vitro* and almost impossible *in vivo*. Decay in the degree of synchronization occurs when even the most highly synchronized cell population passes through successive doubling periods because of the spread in the individual cell doubling times. This decay in synchrony will be seen to occur during the one cycle of HeLa cells shown in Chapter 3, Figure 3.5.

However, some measure of the degree of synchrony is needed. It is reasonable to expect a minimum of 90% of the cells to be at the relevant point in the cell cycle (e.g. mitosis) if the population is to be considered synchronized. This is not difficult to achieve during one cell cycle by procedures such as the mitotic selection technique, and it is therefore misleading, as well as inaccurate, to use the term synchronization for procedures that produce a relatively small enrichment of a cell population and then only in one phase of a cycle, as will be shown later in Figure 2.8.

PHYSICAL METHODS OF SYNCHRONIZATION

Mitotic selection

Mammalian cells grown in monolayer cultures are less well attached to the growing surface when they are rounded up during mitosis (Figure 2.5). Gentle agitation of growth medium can shear these mitotic cells off the surface and a suspension of cells can then be obtained with a very high mitotic index. Terasima and Tolmach (1963) used this mitotic selection technique to obtain populations of HeLa cells with a mitotic index of 90%. The cells remained synchronized as they passed from the G_1 into the S phase, because the DNA labelling index also rose to 90% in a suitably short time. They also showed that the duration of the phases of the synchronized cell population was not significantly different from that in random

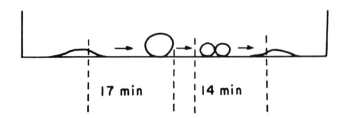

Figure 2.5. Diagram of cells growing on a plastic surface. The cells remain flattened during interphase but are rounded up for about half an hour before, during and after mitosis. (Reproduced from Sinclair, 1964, by permission of The Genetic Society of Japan.)

populations, i.e. this mechanical technique did not perturb the cells with respect to their growth parameters; furthermore, there was no loss in viability. The sort of data obtainable with such a population of HeLa cells is shown in Chapter 3, Figure 3.5, as an example of DNA labelling.

Volume selection

During the cycle, cells double in volume and an asynchronous population should include a distribution of increasing cell volumes that is relatively uniform between the smallest post-telophase cell and the largest pre-prophase cell. It should be possible to select cells from different points in such a distribution to produce a synchronized population. This can be done using a cell sorter as part of the flow cytometry technique illustrated in Figure 2.6. The cell population must be brought into a suspension of single cells and stained with a fluorescent DNA stain. A piezoelectric transducer is used to produce uniform droplets, each containing one cell. The droplets emerge as a high-velocity jet and each droplet is charged within a charging collar according to the cell volume.

In the example shown, the selection window is set to trigger drop-let charging only when cells with a mid-S DNA content are sensed. Alternatively, this droplet selection scheme allows sorting of two subpopulations in a single run. One subpopulation triggers a negative charging voltage pulse (as shown) while the other triggers a positive charging pulse. The two subpopulations are then collected on either side of the undeflected stream. With a suitable fluorescent stain, cells separated by this technique show no loss of viability and asepsis can be maintained if the flow cytometry apparatus is sterile.

An asynchronous population of Chinese hamster cells is shown in Figure 2.7a, with the usual distribution of G_1, S and G_2+M cells. Figure 2.7b shows that DNA distribution of late-G_1/early-S phase cells sorted from such a population and obviously shows good synchronization. However, this cohort of cells loses much of its synchronization later on and Figure 2.7c shows how the DNA content is spread between the G_1 and G_2 peaks, although not with the same pattern as the original asynchronous populations in Figure 2.7a. Some more applications of flow cytometry are described in Chapter 3.

CHEMICAL METHODS OF SYNCHRONIZATION

The same requirements should be applicable to chemical as to physical methods: namely, a high degree of synchronization of viable (with respect to proliferative capacity) cells at the relevant point in the cell cycle together with the absence of any perturbation of the kinetics of proliferation and macromolecular synthesis. Some chemical methods may fulfil these

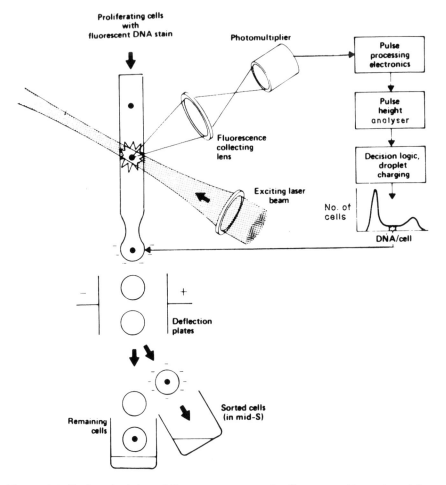

Figure 2.6. Basic principles of flow cytometry and cell sorting. (Reproduced from van Dilla and Mendelsohn, 1979, by permission of John Wiley & Sons, Inc.)

requirements, but others may produce a state of 'unbalanced growth' where the cell has a composition not shown by any cell in the course of the 'normal' cell cycle.

Chemical methods of synchronization include: (i) blocking the progress of cells at some phase in the cycle and then releasing the block so as to permit a wave of cells to resume progress through the cycle (the usual block involves the inhibition of DNA synthesis); (ii) selecting a cohort of cells in one phase by allowing them to escape through a 'window' while removing cells in the other phases. Both of these mechanisms require the use of drugs that are only active during part of the cell cycle. These are the so-called phase-

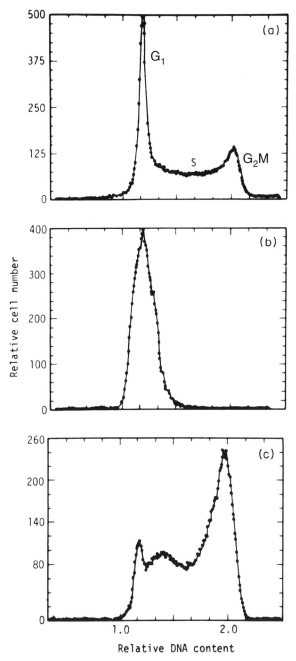

Figure 2.7. DNA distribution of CHO cell populations: (a) asynchronous; (b) synchronized at late G_1/early S; (c) later version of (b). (Reproduced from Gray et al, 1979, by permission of John Wiley & Sons, Inc.)

specific drugs that include *Vinca* alkaloids, such as vincristine, which block
the progress of cells through mitosis and kill them in the S phase, and also
antimetabolites, such as cytosine arabinoside, which kill cells specifically in
the S phase and block entry into that phase at the G_1/S boundary.

The effects of vincristine and cytosine arabinoside are shown in Figure
2.8. These drugs produce a form of synchronization in so far as there is a
peak of mitotic cells after vincristine and late G_1 cells after cytosine
arabinoside. On the left side, the diagram shows the usual distribution
between the different phases of the cell cycle of a typical growing
population. The lower distribution shows what would happen after a
treatment has depleted the cell population and cells are recruited from the
resting G_0 state. As a result, the G_1 phase contains relatively more cells than
usual, although this influx will be distributed throughout the other phases
after a short time. This phenomenon is given the term 'recruitment'. The
term 'redistribution' would be a better description of the other examples in
the diagram because only a small amount of synchronization has been

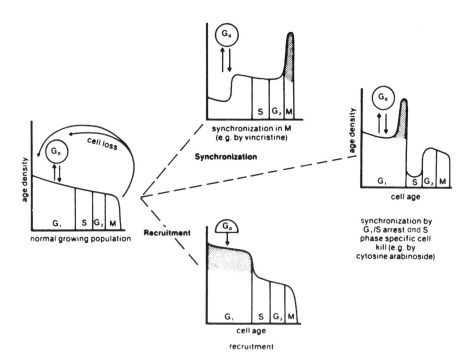

Figure 2.8. Effect of synchronization and recruitment on the distribution of the
phases of a cell population. (Reprinted from *Eur. J. Cancer* **12**, Van Putten et al,
Perspectives in cancer research, 79–85 (1976) with kind permission from Elsevier
Science, The Boulevard, Langford Lane, Kidlington, OX5 1GB, UK.)

obtained. This is the disadvantage of chemical methods of synchronization compared with the physical methods described earlier. Unfortunately, the physical methods cannot be used *in vivo*.

CIRCADIAN RHYTHM

Any study of proliferation kinetics *in vivo* must take account of the fact that most normal cell populations *in vivo* exhibit a circadian rhythm, which itself represents enough of a perturbation of the cell cycle to qualify for the description 'partial synchronization'. A significant variation in mitotic activity occurs in mouse intestinal epithelium throughout the day (Figure 2.9). By contrast, there is a negligible variation in the mitotic activity of tumour cells in the same animals during the same period. This difference might either increase or reduce the effectiveness of any deliberately induced synchronization that might be used for cancer treatment, particularly if the timing of the treatment can be chosen to take advantage of the maximum therapeutic ratio (Chapter 16). These patterns of proliferation kinetics in the different cell populations will be reflected in their response to radiation.

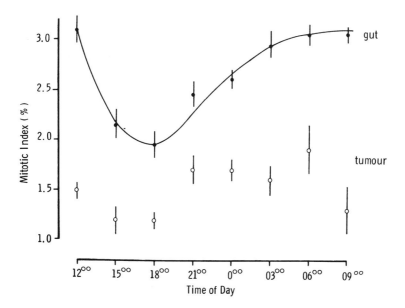

Figure 2.9. Mitotic index over a 24-h period for both intestinal epithelium and mammary tumour in C_3H mice. (Reproduced from Camplejohn and Nias, 1983, by permission of Springer-Verlag GmbH & Co. KG.)

PATTERNS OF SYNTHESIS

Radiation has specific effects upon progress through the cell cycle and this will be discussed in Chapter 7. Effects on macromolecular synthesis will be described in Chapter 5, where it will be shown that the radiation dosage required to inhibit protein and RNA synthesis is so large that it is hardly worth discussing. It is unrealistic to separate cellular macromolecules that form a functional whole, however, and the extent to which DNA synthesis is inhibited by irradiation is important. This is because of the consequence of the 'central dogma', which requires that any lasting effect on the DNA in a cell will affect its RNA and, in turn, its protein. Synthesis of DNA is used as an important marker, with mitosis, of the kinetics of cell proliferation and is the subject of the next chapter.

SUMMARY OF CONCLUSIONS

(1) The tissues of the body are built up of cells of all types to a total of nearly 10^{14} in an adult human.
(2) Each mammalian cell is a complex structure of cytoplasmic organelles and the nucleus, which is the most important element.
(3) With some exceptions, cells can proliferate and traverse the stages of the cell cycle:

$$G_1 \rightarrow S \rightarrow G_2 \rightarrow M$$

Some cells rest in G_0 but are clonogenic.
(4) A population of cells can be manipulated so that they all traverse the cell cycle in synchrony.

REFERENCES

Bertalanffy, F. D. and Lau, C., 1962. Cell renewal. *International Review of Cytology*, **13**, 359–366.

Camplejohn, R. S. and Nias, A. H. W., 1983. A study of diurnal proliferative activity in tumour and small intestine of C_3H mice bearing a transplanted mammary carcinoma. *Virchows Archiv B*, **44**, 163–171.

Gray, J. W., Dean, P. N. and Mendelsohn, M. L., 1979. Quantitative cell cycle analysis. In *Flow Cytometry and Sorting*, edited by M. R. Melamed, P. F. Mullaney and M. L. Mendelsohn. Wiley, New York, pp. 383–407.

Mendelsohnn, M. L., 1967. Radiation effects in tumors. In *Radiation Research*, edited by G. Silini. North-Holland, Amsterdam, pp. 659–675.

Paul, J., 1975. *Cell and Tissue Culture*, 5th edn. Churchill Livingstone, Edinburgh.

Priestman, T. J., 1980. *Cancer Chemotherapy – An Introduction*, Farmitalia Carlo Erba, Barnet, Herts.

Sinclair, W. K., 1964. Survival and recovery after X-irradiation of synchronized Chinese hamster cells in culture. *Japanese Journal of Genetics*, **40** (Suppl.), 141–161.

Terasima, T. and Tolmach, L. J., 1963. Variations in several responses of HeLa cells to X-irradiation during the division cycle. *Biophysical Journal*, **3**, 11–33.

van Dilla, M. A. and Mendelsohn, M. L., 1979. Introduction and Resumé. In *Flow Cytometry and Sorting*, edited by M. R. Melamed, P. F. Ullaney and M. L. Mendelsohn. Wiley, New York, pp. 11–37.

van Putten, L. M., Keizer, H. J. and Mulder, J. H., 1976. Perspectives in cancer research. Synchronization in tumour chemotherapy. *European Journal of Cancer*, **12**, 79–85.

Warenius, H. M., 1997. A cycle made for two. *British Journal of Radiology*, **70**, 125–129.

3 Proliferation Kinetics

Kinetics is the branch of physical chemistry concerned with the rates of chemical reactions; it is also used in biology, and proliferation kinetics describes the rate of growth of a cell population, which is best measured in terms of a change in total cell number. In an adult person these numbers will remain static even though a rapid turnover is occurring in individual cell populations, such as the intestinal epithelium. In contrast, the total cell number increases during childhood and in tumours.

This chapter will describe the methods used to analyse the growth of cell populations. DNA synthesis and mitosis are the most easily identifiable events in the cell cycle. Until recently, isotopic labelling of DNA and autoradiography comprised the standard method, and this is still the best way to examine the proliferative pattern of individual cells in tissues; however, flow cytometry is much less laborious and provides accurate data when the growth of a whole cell population is to be examined.

INCREASE IN TISSUE VOLUME

When there is a net increase in a total cell population, the volume of that tissue will increase. The commonest example of this is the growth of the embryonic and immature child. Direct measurements of linear parameters (length, breadth, girth) of the whole child, or its individual parts, provide quantitative data on tissue volume. The total volume of a child can also be derived from its weight, but the fact that normal growth is not exponential (except in the early embryo) and that cellular differentiation increases in relation to cellular proliferation makes the kinetics of the growing child a complicated subject for study.

The next most important example of a net increase in total cell population is found in tumours. Their cellular kinetics may be no less complicated than in some growing normal tissues but they still permit measurements of total tissue volume. The diameter of an accessible tumour must be one of the commonest of all clinical measurements in cancer work. It must be remembered that a tumour may increase in size due to proliferation of connective tissue or vascular elements, increased blood supply, haemorrhage, oedema or cyst formation, not solely because of growth in the number of tumour cells. Nevertheless, while increase in tumour diameter may provide positive evidence of tumour cell proliferation, the converse

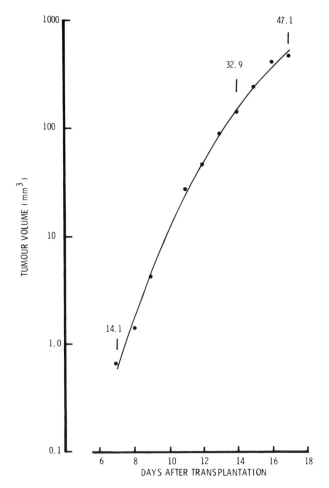

Figure 3.1. Growth curve of a C_3H mouse mammary tumour. (Camplejohn, personal communication, 1981, reproduced by permission.)

may not be true because proliferation may still continue when there is no apparent change in tumour volume.

The question arises as to whether tumours grow exponentially. The growth in volume of a transplanted mouse tumour is shown in Figure 3.1. The growth curve is not exponential but bends towards the time axis. Some tumour growth curves do remain exponential, but this may be explained on the basis of central necrosis with continued proliferation of the outer cell layers of the tumour.

Central necrosis is not the only factor confusing the evidence from serial measurements of tumour diameter. Every tumour contains a stroma of normal tissue and the relative proportions of these stromal cells to the tumour cells vary between different tumours and during the growth of each tumour. For this reason serial estimates of tumour volume, whether obtained from total weight or merely from diameter, provide only an indirect measure of the kinetics of the actual tumour cells.

INCREASE IN TOTAL CELL NUMBER

Direct estimates of total cell number allow a much more accurate measurement of the kinetics of a cell population. Where the population is homogeneous, cell counts indicate the rate of growth of such a population. Unfortunately, such homogeneous populations are rarely found except in cell cultures and ascites tumours, although clearly differentiated cell types (like peripheral blood) may be counted with almost the same degree of accuracy.

The simplest expression of an increase in the total number of a homogeneous cell population is the growth curve. This will be exponential so long as the growth conditions remain unchanged. Such a requirement is met by an established cell line in tissue culture. An example of the growth of HeLa cells over a period of 16 days, during which time the cell population doubled 13 times, which amounts to nearly four factors of ten in growth, is shown in Figure 3.2. The cell population doubling time can be calculated from such a curve and is 30 h. Such an estimate represents the *mean doubling time* of the cell population and not the mean cycle time. This is because the doubling time can only be equated to the actual cycle time in the case of a homogeneous population of cells, all of which are in exponential growth. The mean doubling time of a cell population will be longer than the mean cell cycle time whenever there is a significant proportion of the cells that are not in the *growth fraction*, and when there is a significant *cell loss* in the cell population. These terms will be explained later.

MITOTIC RATE AND MITOTIC INDEX

Cells fixed and stained at the time of mitosis are easily identified from the density of chromosomal staining. A clear definition of mitosis must be decided, ranging between the strict criterion of metaphase to a wider definition that includes all the stages from early prophase to late telophase. The wider this definition, the higher the proportion of the total cell population will be scored. A strict metaphase count often averages 2% of a mammalian cell population in logarithmic growth *in vitro*. This ratio (mitotic cells/total cells), i.e. the mitotic index of the cell population, can be used to calculate the cell cycle time if it is known what proportion of the total cycle is occupied by the stage of mitosis that is scored (i.e. cycle

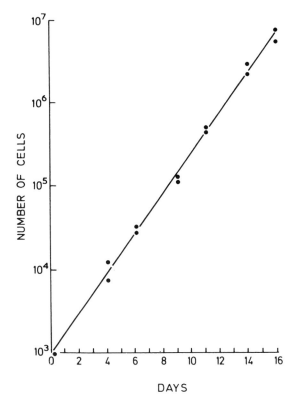

Figure 3.2. Growth curve of HeLa cells in monolayer culture. (Reproduced from Nias and Lajtha, 1968, by permission of Masson et Cie.)

time = mitotic time). Here again it must be assumed that the cell population is homogeneous with respect to growth; a correction will be needed when growth is heterogeneous.

A refinement of this method of determination from the simple mitotic index is to arrest the cells in mitosis by using the plant alkaloid vincristine (which prevents the formation of the mitotic spindle) and then measuring the rate at which cells accumulate in mitosis. (This stathmokinetic method is illustrated later in Figure 3.8.) Such a calculation must take into account the distribution of cells in the various phases of the cell cycle. The distribution of the cells will only be rectangular in the case of a population that is in a steady state, with one proliferative cell produced at each division (Figure 3.3a). The phase distribution of an expanding population will be skewed if two proliferative cells are produced at each division, because there will be almost twice as many cells in the early G_1 phase as in late G_2 phase (Figure 3.3b). This would significantly influence the results of calculations based on mitotic indices, both with and without vincristine.

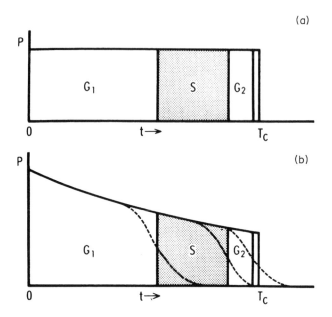

Figure 3.3. Age distribution diagrams for ideal population of cells (a) in steady state with one proliferative and one non-proliferative cell produced, and (b) expanding with two proliferative cells produced at each division and no loss of cells. Dotted lines illustrate that variation in cell cycle phase occurs under normal biological conditions. (Reproduced from Lipkin, 1971, by permission of Marcel Dekker Inc.)

TIME-LAPSE OBSERVATIONS

Direct microscopic examination for a long enough period permits the observation of cells passing from one mitosis to the next. In theory, this should be a reliable method of determining the mean cycle time of a cell population if a representative sample is observed. The only practicable way of observing a random sample of a cell population is time-lapse microcinematography, which can be used with cell populations in tissue culture. This will be illustrated in Chapter 6.

DNA LABELLING METHODS

Apart from the very brief period in the cell cycle occupied by mitosis, the only other positively measurable event in the cycle is DNA synthesis within interphase. A radioactive label can be applied to the cells using the specific DNA precursor thymidine. (BUdR can also be used; see later section on flow cytometry.) The labelled cells can then be studied by high-resolution autoradiography, which will enable the behaviour of individual cells to be

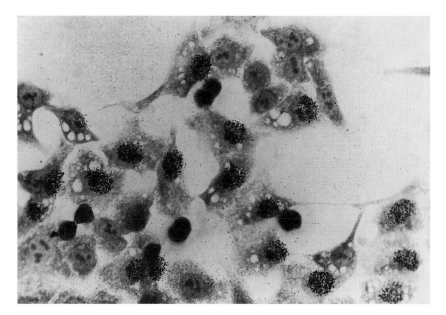

Figure 3.4. Autoradiograph of HeLa cells.

measured but will require sampling and microscopic preparations of the cell population. Alternatively, the extent of labelling can be measured by scintillation counting, which will enable a tissue to be studied *in situ* but with no positive identification of which cells are labelled, nor the extent to which they are labelled. Suitable combinations of these two techniques, repeated at intervals, will provide values for most of the kinetic parameters of a cell population.

Figure 3.4 shows an example of an autoradiograph in which black silver grains have been developed in a photographic emulsion laid over the nuclear areas of those cells in which DNA was being synthesized at the time when the radioactive isotope was applied. These cells are therefore regarded as labelled, and the others are not. A percentage labelling curve may be obtained from a series of such autoradiographs, as illustrated in Figure 3.5. A labelling period is used that is short in relation to the DNA synthetic period of the cell cycle, i.e. a 'pulse' label. Exposure of an asynchronous cell population to the radioactively labelled DNA precursor [^{3}H]thymidine for 10–30 min will label only those cells that are passing through the S period at that time. Samples of the cell population are then fixed at suitable intervals (e.g. hourly or 2-hourly) after labelling, and the relative duration of the phases of the cell cycle can be estimated to varying degrees of accuracy from such autoradiographs.

Certain cell populations in tissue culture can be synchronized to a relatively high degree with respect to the phases of the cell cycle (as

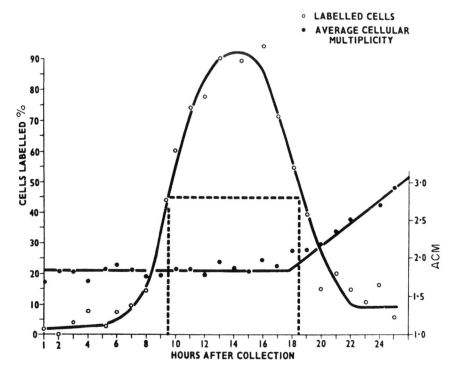

Figure 3.5. Labelling index and average cellular multiplicity (ACM) of synchronized HeLa cells. The S phase is indicated by the dotted lines. (Reprinted from *Eur. J. Cancer*, Petrovic and Nias, A comparison of the effects upon HeLa cells of isopropyl methane sulphonate and X-rays during different phases of the cell cycle, **3**, 321–328 (1967) with kind permission from Elsevier Science, The Boulevard, Langford Lane, Kidlington, Oxford OX5 1GB, UK.)

described in Chapter 2). Under these circumstances the percentage labelling curve can be used to confirm the degree of synchrony and to estimate the phases of the cycle. Figure 3.5 shows a curve obtained with HeLa cells synchronized by the mitotic selection method. Samples are taken at intervals following selection of cells that were in mitosis at zero time, and the pulse label is applied just before fixation of each sample of cells ready for autoradiography.

As the synchronized cells progress through the cell cycle, the labelling index rises from nearly zero in the G_1 phase to nearly 100% in the middle of the S phase. The index then falls as the cells progress through the G_2 phase into mitosis. It does not fall to the starting percentage because the degree of synchrony is already reduced by the time the cells reach the second half of the cycle. For this reason, although the duration of the G_1 and S periods can be estimated with some confidence, estimation of the G_2 period and the length of the total cycle time require additional data such as the curve of average cellular multiplicity (ACM), also shown in Figure 3.5.

The ACM curve remains on a plateau for the greater period and then begins to rise as cells come into mitosis. Such a curve confirms the degree of synchrony of the cell population during the first half of the cycle. This can also be estimated from the height reached by the labelling index, as well as from a determination of the mitotic index of the cells selected at zero time.

Labelled mitoses

Before flow cytometry became available, analysis of a pulse-labelled cell population provided the most reliable data on the duration of the cell cycle and its phases in a defined cell population. It had the advantage of not depending upon the labelling index (which often varies) and was not seriously affected by any partial synchrony. The method combined observations of cells at the one fixed point in the cell cycle that is easily recognizable, i.e. mitosis, with the fact that a cohort of cells was in the S phase when the population was pulse labelled.

Unfortunately fraction of labelled mitoses (FLM) are not very well demarcated, either in the sharpness of the curves or in the repetition of the second and subsequent waves. This is because cell populations are never completely homogeneous with respect to their cycle parameters. As a result, FLM curves show the pattern seen in the example in Figure 3.6 taken from the C_3H mouse mammary tumour whose growth curve was shown in Figure 3.1. Only 54% of the tumour cells were in the growth fraction (described later) and so the FLM data could only refer to this proliferating component of the cell population. A computer method (Steel and Hanes, 1971) has been used to fit the curve to the data points and derive the following values: cell cycle time $(t_C) = 11.7$ h, time in G_2 phase $(t_{G2}) = 2.8$ h, time in S phase $(t_S) = 7.5$ h and time in G_1 phase $(t_{G1}) = 1.1$ h. These values could all be calculated with some confidence because of the well-defined first wave and the reasonably well-defined second wave.

FLOW CYTOMETRY

Flow cytometry is a more convenient alternative to DNA labelling, which can also be used to measure the DNA content of cells and the growth kinetics of a cell population. The technique depends upon the use of quantitative histochemical methods, which enable the precise amount of nucleic acid and other cellular constituents to be measured by fluorescence. Thus, a suspension of single cells can be stained with a substance such as acridine orange, which fluoresces green for DNA and red for RNA. The cells then flow past sensors that can measure not only DNA and RNA content but also cell size and cell number. The technique can also be used

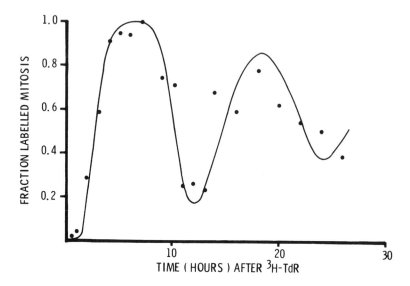

Figure 3.6. Fraction of labelled mitoses (FLM) curve for a fast-growing C_3H mouse mammary tumour. (Camplejohn, personal communication, 1981, reproduced by permission.)

for sorting cells into synchronized populations (described in Chapter 2). Figure 3.7 shows how the fractions of G_1, S and $G_2 + M$ cells in a proliferating cell population can be determined by computing the areas of the histogram.

Figure 3.8 shows an actual flow cytometry histogram obtained with the C_3H mouse mammary tumour used for Figures 3.1 and 3.6. The first peak is from normal stromal cells with a 2C (or diploid) DNA content. The second and largest peak includes tumour cells with their 2C DNA content (most tumours are aneuploid). These are the tumour cells in G_1 or G_0 phase. There is a small third peak that represents tumour cells in the G_2 phase, and the intervening cells are those in S phase. A rough estimate suggests that 62% of the tumour cells are in G_1/G_0, 26% in S and 12% in G_2 phase.

Because only 54% of such a cell population are proliferating, this means that 46% of the cells are presumably in G_0 phase. If we subtract these cells from the second peak and also the normal cells in G_2 (which will also have that DNA value), we are left with far fewer tumour cells in the 'G_1 peak'. This sort of correction might explain the apparent discrepancy with the FLM data for this tumour described in the previous section (Figure 3.6), which indicates that a smaller proportion of proliferating cells are in G_1 than in G_2.

Flow cytometry can also be used to measure cell kinetic time parameters of human tumours. Bromodeoxyuridine (BUdR) is used as a DNA synthesis label and its presence is detected immunochemically. For human tumours,

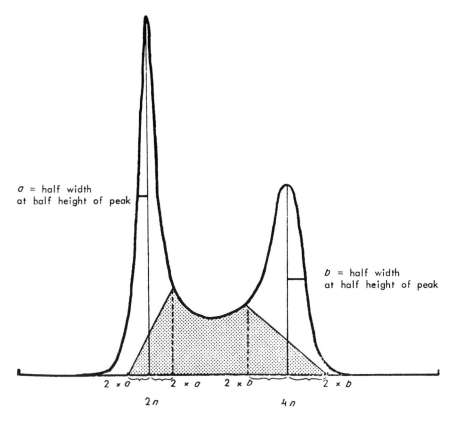

Figure 3.7. Flow cytometry. Schematic representation of a histogram obtained from an *in vitro* cell culture in the logarithmic phase of growth. Indicated are the G_1, S and $G_2 + M$ areas. (Reproduced from Kipp and Barendsen, 1978, by permission of European Press.)

the technique involves administering BUdR *in vivo* and removing a biopsy sample after a known time interval (usually 4–6 h). In this time gap, the cells that took up BUdR will have redistributed through the S and $G_2 + M$ phases because some will have divided and formed labelled daughter cells. Cells or nuclei are disaggregated from the specimen and those that have incorporated BUdR are identified using a monoclonal antibody raised against BUdR (the antibody binding site has first to be made accessible by partially denaturing DNA with HCl). To analyse on the flow cytometer, the cells are incubated with a secondary antibody (raised against the subtype of the monoclonal) labelled with FITC (green fluorescence) and the total DNA content of the cells is measured using the DNA intercalating dye propidium iodide (red fluorescence). Both the labelling index (LI) and the duration of

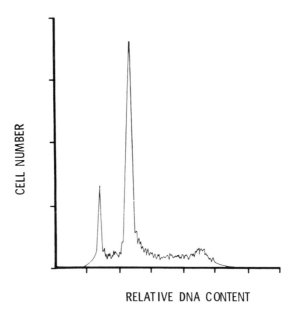

Figure 3.8. Flow cytometry of C_3H mouse mammary tumour cells. (Camplejohn, personal communication, 1981, reproduced by permission.)

the S phase (t_S) can be measured from a single sample. These parameters allow the calculation of the potential doubling time (t_{pot}).

The procedure to calculate t_S is termed the relative movement and is based on measuring the mean DNA content of the BUdR-labelled cells relative to the G_1 and G_2 populations. The basis of the technique is outlined in Figure 3.9 (Wilson, 1994). Immediately after injection there is assumed to be a uniform distribution of the BUdR cells throughout S phase such that their mean DNA content will be half-way between G_1 and G_2 (left-hand panel). To quantify this parameter, the mean DNA content of the G_1 population is subtracted from that of the BUdR-labelled cells and this is divided by the mean DNA of the G_1 subtracted from that of the G_2 cells. This will give a root mean (RM) value of 0.5.

With time, the mean DNA value of the BUdR-labelled cohort (which remains undivided) will increase as the cells progress towards G_2. A point in time will be reached when all the labelled cells will have either divided or will reside in G_2 (right-hand panel). If we make the second assumption that the progression through S phase of the labelled cells is linear, then those cells that are in G_2 represent the cells that were in early S phase at time zero. Therefore, by definition, this time will represent t_S and RM = 1. Thus, from a single biopsy (middle panel) taken at a known time greater than t_{G2} but less than $t_S + t_{G2}$, t_S can be calculated from the RM value using the assumptions that the RM value at time zero is 0.5 and that a value of unity will be reached at t_S.

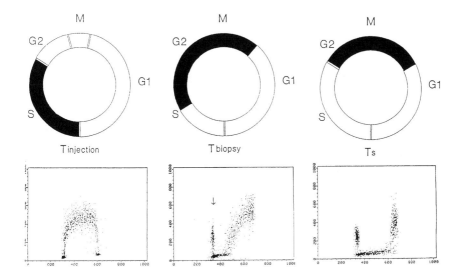

Figure 3.9. Calculation of LI, t_S and t_{pot} from a single observation. The upper panels show the movement of a BUdR-labelled cell around the cell cycle. The lower panels show the flow cytometry profiles of BUdR labelling (y-axis) against total DNA content (x-axis) that would be obtained at the times indicated. (Reproduced from Wilson, *Flow Cytometry, A Practical Approach*, 1994, by permission of Oxford University Press.)

The LI can be calculated as the proportion of BUdR-labelled cells, taking into account that some will have divided and produced two daughter cells (see arrow in middle panel) at the time of biopsy. A simple correction can be made to calculate the true LI by setting a region around the labelled, divided cells in G_1, halving this number and subtracting it from the total number of labelled cells and from the total cell number.

Another parameter, the potential doubling time t_{pot}, can be calculated from the LI and t_S by the formula:

$$t_{pot} = \frac{t_S}{LI}$$

The LI is expressed as a proportion rather than a percentage. The significance of t_{pot} is discussed later in this chapter. It is of clinical significance because it measures the maximum potential for growth in a tumour (Chapter 16).

GROWTH FRACTION AND CELL LOSS

The tissues of the normal adult 'grow', but only to the extent that 'lost' cells need to be replaced to maintain the tissues in a steady functional state. A fraction of the total cell population of any tissue will thus be 'growing' at any one time and this is called the *growth fraction*. It can be measured by flow cytometry or standard immunochemistry using the antibody Ki-67, which identifies a nuclear antigen in cycling cells as opposed to non-cycling cells. In normal adult tissue there is no net growth in the usual sense because the homeostatic mechanism maintains the tissue at a constant size so that the number of new cells exactly replaces the number of 'lost cells'. Thus the *cell loss* is unity (or 100%) in such a normal adult tissue. It is less than 100% in a tumour that continues to increase in size because it lacks a homeostatic control mechanism.

It may help to understand these proliferation kinetics if a cell population is divided into four compartments, using the word 'compartment' to describe function and not structure (Figure 3.10). The proliferating compartment represents the growth fraction from which cells may pass one way into compartments of either sterile or dead cells (cell loss). A reversible pathway also exists between the proliferating compartment and a compartment of cells in the G_0 state. These can be recruited into the growth fraction by a suitable stimulus, such as the depletion of proliferating cells by radiography. This process of 'recruitment' may apply to normal stem cell

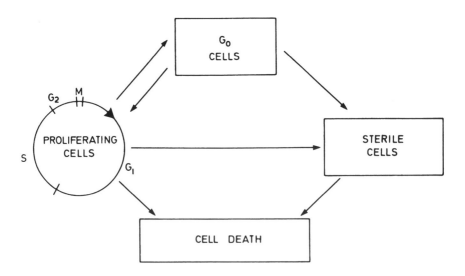

Figure 3.10. Compartments of a mixed cell population. (Reproduced from Mendelsohn and Dethlefson, 1967, by permission of Williams and Wilkins.)

populations (where the G_0 state is known to exist) as well as to resting tumour cells (where an extended G_1 state is believed to apply). Cells from the G_0 compartment may also pass irreversibly into a sterile compartment.

If the growth fraction (GF) is unity, then the doubling time of the cell population will be the same as the cycle time of its cells as long as there is no cell loss (CL). In the mixed *in vivo* cell populations found in tissues, however, this never occurs because the GF is invariably less than unity and there is always cell loss – 100% in normal adult tissues but less in tumours. The doubling time of such tissues (i.e. the time it takes for them to double in volume) will therefore be very much longer than the cycle time of their constituent cells. The scheme in Figure 3.11 shows how these various kinetic parameters are related (using the C_3H mouse mammary tumour as an example) and includes an additional parameter: potential doubling time.

POTENTIAL DOUBLING TIME t_{pot}

If some of the cells in a tissue are not proliferating (i.e. the GF is less than unity) then the rate of cell production in the population as a whole will be

KINETIC PARAMETERS

Relationships		Values for C_3H Tumour	
t_C =	CELL CYCLE TIME	11.7	hours
↑ only equal if GF is unity ↓	GROWTH FRACTION	0.54	
t_{pot}	POTENTIAL DOUBLING TIME	21.5	hours
↑ only equal if no Cell Loss ↓	CELL LOSS	0.35	
t_D =	DOUBLING TIME	32.9	hours

Figure 3.11. Relationship of kinetic parameters of a C_3H mouse mammary tumour. (Camplejohn, personal communication, 1981, reproduced by permission.)

slower than the rate that might be expected from the cell cycle time, t_C. The time taken for the number of cells to double (assuming no cell loss) will be longer than t_C and this time period is the potential doubling time, t_{pot}. If there is also some cell loss then the volume doubling time (t_D) will obviously be even longer.

The parameter t_{pot} is useful, not only as an intermediate step in the calculation of the other parameters in Figure 3.11 but also because it is not often that the GF and t_C can be directly measured in human tissues (see Chapter 15). The methods to determine those parameters require multiple samples and these are rarely available for ethical reasons. Rough estimates of t_{pot} and the GF can be made from a single sample using flow cytometry (as already described).

The relationship of the five parameters in Figure 3.11 will vary as a tumour grows. This happened with the C_3H mouse mammary tumour from which multiple samples were taken at the various time intervals shown in Figure 3.1. The volume doubling time, t_D, increased from 14.1 to 47.1 h as the tumour grew larger. It is important to remember this because the values of the parameters CL, t_{pot} and GF will all depend upon the tumour size. Only the cell cycle time, t_C, remains relatively constant, and for these tumour cells t_C is 11.7 h. (This value was obtained by the labelled mitoses technique described earlier.)

A tumour of diameter 6–7 mm is convenient for some radiation experiments and at this size the value of t_D is 32.9 h (also shown on the curve in Figure 3.1). This is the one parameter that can easily be determined in the clinic by non-invasive methods, i.e. by successive measurements either of accessible tumours directly or of pictures of those deep-seated tumours that can be delineated by X-ray techniques.

Now that we have the values for $t_D = 32.9$ h and $t_C = 11.7$ h we need to determine values for the intermediate parameters in Figure 3.11. The obvious one to go for is t_{pot}, the potential doubling time. In the laboratory, multiple samples are available and it is possible to use the stathmokinetic effect of vincristine, a plant alkaloid that prevents cells from completing mitosis. The cells accumulate in the metaphase stage because the drug interferes with the formation of the mitotic spindle. If samples of the tumour are then fixed at intervals over a few hours, the metaphase index will progressively rise. This is shown in Figure 3.12, where the metaphase collection function has been plotted on the semi-logarithmic scale that is suitable for cell populations that are growing like the C_3H mouse mammary tumour. The slope of the accumulation line can then be used to calculate the value of t_{pot} (see Aherne et al, 1977, for details of the mathematics involved). This value of t_{pot} for mouse tumours of 6–7 mm diameter was 21.5 h.

We now have values for three of the parameters in Figure 3.11. The remaining two can be calculated from the formulae:

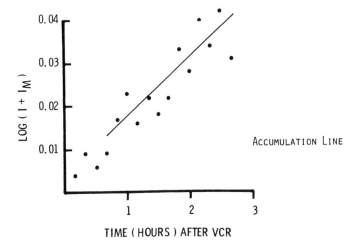

Figure 3.12. Accumulation of mitoses in a C_3H mouse mammary tumour. (Camplejohn, personal communication, 1981, reproduced by permission.)

$$GF = \frac{t_C}{t_{pot}} = \frac{11.7}{21.5} = 0.54$$

$$CL = 1 - \frac{t_{pot}}{t_D} = 1 - \frac{21.5}{32.9} = 0.35$$

The values for the five kinetic parameters have thus been derived from good evidence based upon the three independent observations (t_D, t_{pot}, t_C) that are possible with a mouse tumour.

Some old values for five different histological types of human tumour are shown in Table 3.1 for comparison. It is important to remember, however, that the only direct observations were the doubling time and the labelling index. The other parameters were calculated values. The LI was used to calculate both GF and t_{pot}. Then, this derived value of t_{pot} was used with the

Table 3.1. Mean kinetic parameters of various histological types of human tumours

Histological type	Doubling time (days)	Labelling index (%)	Growth fraction (%)	Cell loss factor (%)
Embryonal tumour	27	30	90	93
Malignant lymphoma	29	29	90	93
Sarcoma	41	4	11	68
Squamous cell carcinoma	58	8	25	89
Adenocarcinoma	83	2	6	71

Reproduced from Tublana and Malaise, 1976, by permission of the authors.

known value for t_D to calculate CL. Such a two-step calculation must obviously introduce a fair degree of uncertainty. Some applications of these methods will be described in Chapter 15 and flow cytometry estimations of t_{pot} are given in Chapter 16.

SUMMARY OF CONCLUSIONS

(1) The rate of growth of a cell population can be measured in terms of a net increase in cell number and the volume doubling time of a tissue.
(2) Time-lapse observations, DNA labelling and the mitotic index provide accurate data on individual cells.
(3) DNA flow cytometry provides the most convenient estimate of the kinetic parameters of a cell population.
(4) The kinetic parameters include cell cycle time, the phases of the cell cycle, growth fraction, cell loss and potential doubling time, all of which change when a tumour grows larger.

REFERENCES

Aherne, W. A., Camplejohn, R. S. and Wright, N. A., 1977. *An Introduction to Cell Population Kinetics*. Edward Arnold, London.

Kipp, J. B. A. and Barendsen, G. W., 1978. Comparison of DNA-histograms of cultured cells and corresponding solid tumours and their relation to data from autoradiographic analysis. In *Pulse Cytophotometry, Third International Symposium, Vienna*. European Press, Ghent.

Lipkin, M., 1971. The proliferative cycle of mammalian cells. In *The Cell Cycle and Cancer*, edited by R. Baserga. Marcel Dekker, New York, pp. 6–26.

Mendelsohn, M. L. and Dethlefson, L. A., 1967. Tumour growth and cellular kinetics. In *Proliferation and Spread of Neoplastic Cells*. Williams and Wilkins, Baltimore, pp. 197–212.

Nias, A. H. W. and Lajtha, L. G., 1968. Modification of cellular kinetics by ionizing radiation. In *Actions Chimiques et Biologiques des Radiations*, edited by M. Haissinsky. Masson et Cie, Paris, Vol. 12, pp. 95–144.

Petrovic, D. and Nias, A. H. W., 1967. A comparison of the effects upon HeLa cells of isopropyl methane sulphonate and X-rays during different phases of the cell cycle. *European Journal of Cancer*, **3**, 321–328.

Steel, G. G. and Hanes, S., 1971. The technique of labelled mitoses: analysis by automatic curve fitting. *Cell and Tissue Kinetics*, **4**, 93–105.

Terasima, T. and Tolmach, L. J., 1963. Variations in several responses of HeLa cells to X-irradiation during the division cycle. *Biophysical Journal*, **3**, 11–33.

Tubiana, M. and Malaise, E. P., 1976. Growth rate and cell kinetics in human tumours: some prognostic and therapeutic implications. In *Scientific Foundations of Oncology*, edited by T. Symington and R. L. Carter. Heinemann, London, pp. 126–136.

Wilson, G. D., 1994. Analysis of DNA – measurement of cell kinetics by the bromo-deoxyuridine/anti-bromodeoxyuridine method. In *Flow Cytometry. A Practical Approach*, 2nd edn, edited by M. G. Ormerod. IRL Press, Oxford, pp. 154.

4 Ionizing Radiations

For the majority of readers the word radiation implies X-rays and these are certainly the commonest form of ionizing radiation as far as the general public are concerned. However, there are many other forms of radiation that affect humans and are used in everyday life. The full spectrum of electromagnetic radiations was shown as Figure 1.3 in Chapter 1 and ranged from radiowaves, through microwaves and visible light, to the ionizing radiations that are the subject of this chapter and this book. All of them are forms of radiation but they vary in wavelength. For radiowaves the wavelength may be as long as 1500 m, whereas ionizing radiations have wavelengths shorter than 800 nm (8×10^{-7} m). It is only because of their very short wavelength (and very high frequency) that X-rays are damaging to biological material.

The wavelengths of various sorts of radiation are compared with the diameters of various biological objects in Figure 4.1. The objects range from

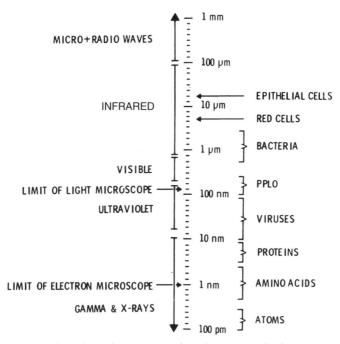

Figure 4.1. Wavelengths of sources of radiation and diameters of targets. (Reproduced from Nias, 1988, by permission of Churchill Livingstone.)

atoms to whole cells. Clearly, the wavelength of X-rays is very much shorter than the diameter of any biological structure, and the damage produced by ionizing radiations must result from disruption at the atomic or molecular level. The precise size of the biological 'target' for X-rays and the nature of this target will be discussed later. Before that, it is necessary to describe the physics of ionizing radiations, how they are produced and how they are measured. For the rest of this book the word 'radiation' will be used to mean ionizing radiation. All the other forms of electromagnetic radiation will not be mentioned again except for common properties that apply to X-rays.

Thus, radiation travels in straight lines and obeys the inverse square law: a beam of radiation has only one-quarter its intensity after it has travelled twice the distance. There are thus two ways to protect oneself from a beam of X-rays: retire to a safer distance or stand aside from the main beam. Another way is to stand behind a protective wall. Just as a beam of visible light can be shielded by a paper lamp-shade and stopped altogether by a heavy curtain, so a beam of X-rays can be collimated down to a smaller area and stopped altogether by a radio-opaque substance. The only difference is that much denser materials, such as lead or a thick layer of concrete, are needed to shield from X-rays.

X-RAYS AND γ-RAYS

Although X-rays make up only a small part of the radiation received by humans (see Figure 1.4 in Chapter 1), they are the form with which most people are familiar. X-rays are used widely in medical diagnosis and also for the treatment of cancer. Industry also uses X-rays for the testing of welds and other materials. A typical X-ray machine contains a sealed tube in which electrons are accelerated towards a metal target and X-rays are produced if the electrons hit the target with sufficient energy. The wavelength of the X-rays depends not only upon the energy of the electrons but also upon the atomic number of the metal target. The X-ray photons (or packets of energy) produced have a wavelength that is characteristic of the interaction of these two factors. Thus, an X-ray tube operating at 100 000 eV energy and using a tungsten target will produce radiation with a wavelength of 10^{-2} nm. There will inevitably be a range of energies produced by such an X-ray tube but the peak energy is the one that is usually quoted (e.g. 100 kV_p). These would be classed as soft X-rays that would not penetrate very far into biological material.

Table 4.1 shows the various energies of X-rays that are used for various purposes, including medical diagnosis and the therapy of cancer patients. As the photon energy rises, so the wavelength of the electromagnetic radiation falls and the frequency increases. Included in Table 4.1 are the

Table 4.1. Electromagnetic radiation: X-rays and γ-rays, and approximate energy ranges of interest

Photon energy		Frequency (Hz)	Wavelength (nm)	Properties
(eV)	(J)			
124 eV to	2.0×10^{-17}	3.0×10^{16}	10	Soft X-rays from excitations of inner electrons; very shallow
12.4 keV	2.0×10^{-15}	3.0×10^{18}	0.1	penetration
12.4 keV to	2.0×10^{-15}	3.0×10^{18}	0.1	Diagnostic X-rays and superficial therapy
124 keV	2.0×10^{-14}	3.0×10^{19}	0.01	
124 keV to	2.0×10^{-14}	3.0×10^{19}	0.01	Deep therapy X-rays, and rays from many radioactive iso-
1.24 MeV	2.0×10^{-13}	3.0×10^{20}	0.001	topes, e.g. ^{60}Co
12.4 MeV	2.0×10^{-12}	3.0×10^{21}	0.0001	Radiation from small betatron
124 MeV	2.0×10^{-11}	3.0×10^{22}	0.00001	Radiation from large betatron
1.24 GeV	2.0×10^{-10}	3.0×10^{23}	0.000001	Radiation produced in large synchrotrons

Reproduced from Coggle, 1983, by permission of Taylor & Francis.

γ-rays emitted by radioactive isotopes such as ^{60}Co. Because γ-rays result from discrete nuclear disintegrations, they have a single energy (e.g. 1.25 MeV for ^{60}Co). In all other respects, X-rays and γ-rays have similar properties when they interact with matter.

The tissues of the body include 'targets' of varying atomic number and the mechanism of interaction between radiation and these targets will apply to ionizing radiations of all types, including the neutrons and accelerated charged particles that will be described later. They all deposit their energy by a nuclear interaction that depends upon the structure of the target atoms. The transfer of energy occurs by one or more processes of attenuation.

With X-ray energies less than 0.5 MeV the predominant method of interaction is by the *photoelectric effect*, in which the photon is completely absorbed by the target atom, an electron is emitted and 'characteristic' radiation is produced. At higher energies between 0.5 MeV and 5 MeV *Compton scattering* is predominant. This is illustrated in Figure 4.2, which shows the neutrons and protons that form the nucleus of an atom, together with the orbital electrons in their various shells. In the Compton process the incident photon collides with an orbital electron, a recoil electron is produced and the scattered photon leaves with diminished energy. Depending upon its energy, this scattered photon may then interact with additional target atoms by further Compton scattering or by the photoelectric effect. In either case, an

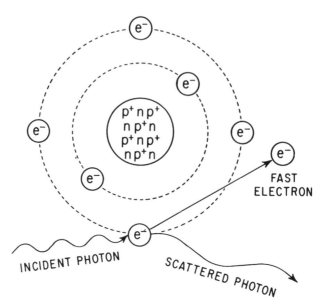

Figure 4.2. Compton scattering. (Reproduced from Hall, 1988, by permission of Lippincott-Raven.)

electron is ejected from the target atom and this leaves an unstable condition that is described by the term 'ionization'.

At still higher energies, in excess of 1.02 MeV, X-ray photons are converted into an electron and a positron by *pair production*. Positrons are positively charged electrons that are eventually annihilated by collision with ordinary negative electrons to produce two photons of energy 0.51 MeV. This is called annihilation radiation and this will then be absorbed by Compton scattering and the photoelectric effect.

ELECTRONS AND β-RAYS

In addition to the electrons produced by these three methods of absorption of X-ray photons, external electron sources are also used in certain cancer treatments. (Electrons are also called β-rays in the context of the disintegration of certain radioactive isotopes.) The attenuation of electrons is therefore an important process. Because they are negatively charged and have a very small mass, electrons will easily be deflected from their track by other electrons. A tortuous track will result so that the range of an electron (or the depth to which it can penetrate a tissue) will be much less than its track length in air. Furthermore, the greatest density of ionization occurs at the end of this track. This is because the velocity of the electron falls as its energy is degraded to a few tens of electron-volts, and then the specified ionization (measured in ion pairs/cm air) rises accordingly. This follows from the increasing probability of interaction between the atoms of the target material and the electrons when they are travelling slowly. The depth in a tissue at which this greatest density of ionization occurs will depend upon the energy of the electron source. High-energy electron beams from a betatron will ionize at an appreciable depth in tissue, whereas the 0.53 MeV β particles from a source of ^{90}Sr will deposit most of their energy within a depth of 1 or 2 mm.

RADIOACTIVE ISOTOPES

Radioactive isotopes are unstable atoms that disintegrate randomly with the emission of ionizing radiation: α, β or γ rays, or a combination of these. The same fraction of atoms disintegrates over the same time interval and so the radioactivity of the isotope decays exponentially. Figure 4.3 shows this in terms of a series of 'half-lives'. The half-life is a unique feature of each isotope, as is the type of radiation emitted and the main energy of that radiation (and therefore the depth of penetration into a tissue). The *effective half-life* is the parameter that determines the radiation dose to the tissues of

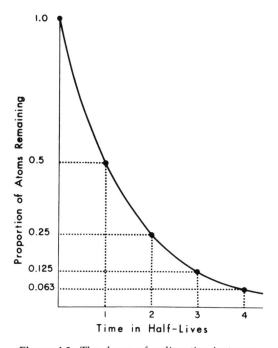

Figure 4.3. The decay of radioactive isotopes.

the body. The parameter depends upon both the basic physical half-life and the biological half-life; the latter reflects the metabolic degradation of the isotope while in the body. The relationship of the three parameters is as follows:

$$\frac{1}{\text{Effective half-life}} = \frac{1}{\text{Biological half-life}} + \frac{1}{\text{Physical half-life}}$$

Table 4.2 shows the physical half-life and type of radiation for some of the radioactive isotopes mentioned in this book. Uranium-238 has the longest half-life and the lowest energy of γ radiation. Phosphorus-32 has the shortest half-life of a β emitter and the highest energy of radiation. Strontium-90 has intermediate values. Technetium-99$_m$ is employed for nuclear medicine scanning and has only a 6-h half-life. Isotopes with even shorter half-lives are used for positron emission tomography (PET). Thus for ^{18}F it is 2 h, for ^{11}C it is 20 min, for ^{11}N it is 10 min and for ^{11}O it is 2 min. A PET facility will usually need a cyclotron on site for such isotope production.

Strontium-90 is an example of the many different artificial radioactive isotopes that can be produced by nuclear reactions involving neutrons and nuclear fission. (The radiobiology of neutrons will be discussed in Chapter 9.) The standard reaction in a nuclear power station involves the disintegration of ^{238}U, with the yield of both neutrons and radioactive isotopes such as ^{90}Sr, ^{137}Cs and ^{131}I. Strontium-90 is a beta emitter with a half-life of 28 years, while ^{137}Cs is a γ emitter with a half-life of 35 years.

These long half-lives present problems to the nuclear power industry, which has to store or reprocess these nuclear waste products without hazard to the public. Barring accidents, this can be done, but the Chernobyl

Table 4.2. Some radioactive isotopes

Radionuclide	Half-life	Radiation (MeV)
^{137}Cs	30 years	Gamma (0.66)
^{14}C	5730 years	Beta (0.155)
^{60}Co	5.3 years	Gamma (1.33)
^{3}H (Tritium)	12.3 years	Beta (0.018)
^{125}I	60 days	Gamma (0.035)
^{131}I	8 days	Beta (0.6)
^{32}P	14.3 days	Beta (1.718)
^{40}K	1.28×10^9 years	Gamma (1.46)
^{222}Rn	3.8 days	Alpha (5.5)
^{90}Sr	28 years	Beta (0.55)
^{99m}Tc	6 hours	Gamma (0.14)
^{238}U	4.5×10^9 years	Gamma (0.048)

accident showed the alternative consequences of releasing such isotopes into the environment and the food chain where the long half-life of ^{137}Cs for example, presents an enduring problem. A more acute problem arises from the release of ^{131}I. This is a volatile isotope that will quickly be taken into the thyroid gland unless non-radioactive iodine has been taken to block this uptake. It is also a γ emitter, but because the half-life is only 8 days the hazard is of short duration. (See Chapter 18 for its use in nuclear medicine.)

These nuclear waste products illustrate the fact that humans can receive ionizing radiation from both internal and external sources. Because internally deposited radioactive isotopes may accumulate selectively in critical organs, e.g. ^{131}I in the thyroid and ^{90}Sr in bone, the actual radiation dose will depend upon this factor as well as the half-life of the isotope and the energy and type of radiation emitted: β or γ rays (or α rays, discussed in Chapter 9). By contrast, the dose distribution of external sources of radiation depends on relatively simple physical principles to be discussed later.

Despite the occasional nuclear reactor accident and the residual fallout from nuclear weapons testing, the contribution of artificial radioactive isotopes to the irradiation of humans is very much smaller than that from natural sources (see Figure 1.4, Chapter 1). Thus, although uranium is naturally only slightly radioactive, it decays to radon (which contributes 32% of the sources of radiation to the public) by means of both α and γ rays. The half-life of radon is only 3.8 days but considerable quantities can accumulate in poorly ventilated buildings (Chapter 19).

RADIATION DOSIMETRY

In view of the fact that the biological effect of ionizing radiation needs to be measured on the organ or tissue of interest, the radiation dose should ideally be measured in the same site and in terms of the dose absorbed by that site. In practice, it is usually more convenient to measure the radiation absorbed by some equivalent material, or even air, and then derive the tissue dose by applying calculated or measured correction factors. National standards laboratories mainly use a very sensitive calorimeter that measures the very small increase in termperature from the absorbed radiation energy within a block of carbon as the primary standard. Such instruments are very delicate and impractical for routine use.

For accurate measurements, the air ionization chamber has been the most practical for many years, consisting of a gas-filled chamber containing two electrodes. The electric current between the two electrodes provides a measure of the amount of ionization that the radiation has produced in the defined volume of the chamber, and this may be calibrated against the primary standard to obtain the absorbed dose. The SI unit of absorbed dose is the gray (Gy), which is defined as the absorption of 1 J of radiation energy per kilogram of material. (Neutron dosimetry is described in Chapter 9.)

Geiger counters also consist of a gas between two electrodes across which a high electric potential is applied, resulting in a discharge when an ionizing event occurs. This produces an amplified electrical pulse, making the instrument very sensitive and able to count the number of photons or charged particles interacting with it. However, Geiger counters are not easily calibrated to measure absorbed dose because their response is very dependent on radiation energy.

The radiation from radioactive isotopes is often measured by scintillation counters. These convert the radiation energy into pulses of light. The size of the pulse is proportional to the energy deposited in the crystalline or liquid scintillant. The pulses of light are detected by a photomultiplier and recorded electronically. Scintillation counters can also be quite sensitive but suffer the same problems as Geiger counters in being difficult to calibrate directly to read dose and so are also used mainly to count ionizing events.

One of the most accurate liquid dosimeters uses ferrous sulphate (Fricke dosimetry). Ferrous sulphate is converted to ferric sulphate when irradiated and the yield of ferric ion can be assayed by an ultraviolet spectro-photometer (at 304 nm). The yield is directly proportional to the dose received but can only be used to measure doses greater than 1 Gy.

Because ionization chambers must be of a sufficient size (0.1 ml) to contain enough air to obtain a measurable current, the distribution of dose within smaller volumes is sometimes measured by thermoluminescent dosimetry (TLD). Small crystals of lithium fluoride or other material can be placed in an organ or tissue and irradiated at the site of interest. The absorption of radiation causes free electrons to be trapped in the crystal at higher energy levels. If such crystals are subsequently heated, the electrons release their stored energy and there is an emission of light that provides a measure of the absorbed dose. This method of thermoluminescent dosimetry can be used to measure doses of X-rays, γ-rays, electrons, protons and neutrons over a wide range from 10 μGy to 1 kGy. The crystals can be used repeatedly and some, such as lithium fluoride, are sufficiently tissue equivalent that their response does not vary greatly with energy except at very low photon energies.

Photographic film is normally very sensitive to radiation, resulting in blackening of the developed image. Its response is also strongly energy dependent but if the spectrum of the radiation is known, reasonable accuracy may be achieved in the measurement of absorbed dose down to a few tens of micrograys. Film has traditionally been used for personnel monitoring, with the holder (or 'film badge') incorporating filters to give the necessary information about radiation type and energy before the black-ening can be interpreted. Although film badges are convenient for monitoring, personnel need to decide at what site to wear the badge (e.g. near the gonads) and when to wear it. Thermoluminescent dosimetry is now becoming commonly used for this purpose because of its lower dependence on energy and the ease of automating the readout process. Small electronic pocket dosimeters based on Geiger counters may also be used to monitor personnel exposure, with the advantage of giving immediate display of the dose or dose rate received.

The history of radiation units was discussed in Chapter 1, where it was pointed out that, fortunately, there is a very close similarity between the original roentgen unit (R), which measures ionization in air, and the later unit for radiation absorbed dose (rad). The modern gray unit is exactly equivalent to 100 rad and in clinical work it has been found convenient (and perhaps safer) to use the centigray (cGy), which is then exactly the same as the old rad. This allows radiation doses to be compared in the literature, and the diagrams in this book will use cGy units to mean the same radiation dose as R and rad for general purposes when dealing with soft tissue.

The sievert unit (Sv) is the unit of dose equivalence. It has the same value as the gray unit (Gy) for ordinary X-rays but is multiplied by a weighting factor (Chapter 9, Table 9.1) when more densely ionizing radiation is involved. This will be discussed in Chapter 20, which deals with radiation protection and the problems of nuclear accidents.

The rate at which radiation is delivered to a tissue will often determine the extent of the biological effect and so the dose rate must be stated. The SI unit is Gy/s but for many purposes it is convenient to use cGy/min. When quantifying radioactive isotopes it is necessary to take into account their property of continuous disintegration, and the becquerel unit (Bq) already incorporates time in the definition of one disintegration per second. For most isotopes this unit is far too small and the megabecquerel (MBq) or gigabecquerel (GBq) is often used.

IONIZATION AND RADICAL FORMATION

There is an apparent paradox in the term 'ionizing radiation': it might be expected to mean a particular form of radiation that produces ionization in target molecules, but many molecules in aqueous solution already exist, at least partly, in an ionized state due to simple dissociation into positively and negatively charged ions that coexist in a stable equilibrium. Thus, NaCl dissociates into Na^+ and Cl^- ions, just as water itself dissociates into H^+ and OH^- ions. The consequence of X-irradiation, however, is the formation of pairs of abnormal ions (called free-radical ions) that are *not* in equilibrium. This is because of the displacement of electrons (Figure 4.2). The radiolysis of water will be described in detail later by means of a series of equations, but the first two equations illustrate the formation of free radicals:

$$H_2O \xrightarrow{\text{radiation}} H_2O^{+\cdot} + e^- \tag{1}$$

This shows the result of the ejection of electrons from the water molecule with the formation of $H_2O^{+\cdot}$ (where the dot signifies an unpaired electron). This is a free-radical ion, which is very unstable and can form neutral free radicals, which are uncharged molecules with an unpaired electron in the outer orbit:

$$H_2O^{+\cdot} \longrightarrow H^+ + OH^\cdot \tag{2}$$

Although such free radicals are more stable, they are still very reactive. Both free-radical ions and the resultant free radicals disrupt normal molecular structures and damage the biological target. This radiobiological damage is not the consequence of ionization due to simple dissociation, therefore. The important result of 'ionizing' radiation is the production of free radicals. Their formation will now be described in more detail.

When ionization occurs in air, an average of 34 eV is dissipated (probably less in liquids and solids). This does not mean that it takes that amount of energy to eject an electron from an atom, however, because that may only need about 10 eV. Two-thirds of the energy is dissipated in excitation, which is relatively unimportant in the production of X-ray damage in human tissues (although it is important with ultraviolet radiation). When an electron is knocked out of one of the outer shells of an atom, the atom becomes positively charged and is called a positive ion; the electron may then interact with another atom to form a negative ion and the two ions so produced are called an ion pair. Such an ion pair will have a very short lifetime of the order of 10^{-10} s before producing neutral free radicals, which are relatively more stable with a lifetime of up to 10^{-3} s. It is the free radicals formed from water that are responsible for about 70% of the biological effects of radiation, so they require more detailed consideration. The other half are due to direct ionization of critical biological molecules.

Radiation chemists use the technique of *pulse radiolysis* to study the nature and kinetics of radical formation. Typically, an aqueous sample is given a pulse of ionizing radiation from a linear accelerator and simultaneously the absorption spectrum of ultraviolet or visible light is measured using a spectrophotometer connected to a cathode ray oscilloscope (CRO). Because of the very short lifetime of the free radicals, an elaborate timing mechanism is used to synchronize photography of the CRO tracing with the microsecond (or shorter) pulse of electrons delivered to the sample. Analysis of the tracing provides information on the nature of the free radicals produced and their lifetime in the aqueous medium. In solid samples (and frozen aqueous samples) the free radicals have a very much longer lifetime and they may be studied futher using additional techniques such as *electron spin resonance* (Ohya-Nishiguchi and Packer, 1995). In this technique the sample is placed between the poles of a powerful magnet and determination of the perturbation of the magnetic field indicates the nature of the reactive chemical species produced by the ionizing radiation. All this involves the important scientific field of radiation chemistry, which is beyond the scope of this book (see Bensasson et al, 1993).

Following the primary absorption of radiation energy, a complicated series of events will lead to the breakage of a number of chemical bonds. Because biological material consists of 70–90% water, the radiation chemistry of water is obviously of great importance. The primary event is ionization of the water molecule to give a positive ion and a free electron:

$$H_2O \xrightarrow{\text{radiation}} H_2O^{+\cdot} + e^- \tag{1}$$

This is followed by a series of reactions leading to various forms of free radical. The initial ejection of electrons from the water molecule takes about 10^{-18} s. Around 10^{-12} s later the electrons will have become hydrated $(e^{-1} \longrightarrow e_{aq}^-)$ and the $H_2O^{+\cdot}$ free-radical ion will have produced a hydroxyl radical:

$$H_2O^{+\cdot} \longrightarrow H^+ + OH^{\cdot} \tag{2}$$

A hydrogen free radical may also be produced:

$$e_{aq}^- + H^+ \longrightarrow H^{\cdot} \tag{3}$$

together with some hydrogen peroxide:

$$OH^{\cdot} + OH^{\cdot} \longrightarrow H_2O_2 \tag{4}$$

but these latter two reactions depend upon how densely ionizing the radiation is and also on the concentration of any 'scavenger' molecules (see later section on protection and sensitization).

Thus, the radiolysis of water can be summarized in one equation:

$$H_2O \text{ radiation} \quad e_{aq}^- \quad +OH^{\cdot} \quad +H^{\cdot} \quad +H_2 \quad +H_2O_2$$
$$\xrightarrow{\hspace{3cm}} \tag{5}$$
$$(G \text{ values} = \quad 2.63 \quad 2.72 \quad 0.55 \quad 0.45 \quad 0.68)$$

The G values represent the measured yields of molecules produced by the absorption of 100 eV X-ray energy, and for ordinary radiation the highest yields are the free radicals e_{aq}^- and $OH^{\cdot}$. On the other hand the yield of e_{aq}^- may be reduced by scavenger molecules and because more densely ionizing radiation favours equation (3) the G value for e_{aq}^- may then fall to as low as 0.4. Densely ionizing radiation also favours equation (4), so the yield of

H_2O_2 will then be greatly increased. This explains the lower oxygen effect with such densely ionizing radiation (Chapter 9).

In addition to e^-_{aq}, $OH^{\cdot}$ and $H^{\cdot}$ many other free radicals are formed, but it is only proposed to discuss radiobiologically important types of reaction such as those in which aqueous free radicals react with organic biological molecules (such as DNA) and with oxygen. From a biological point of view, unless scavengers are used, it makes little difference whether a molecule is damaged directly or indirectly, although the aqueous nature of most biological targets in humans makes the indirect mechanism equally as important as direct action to produce a free-radical ion.

If the symbol RH is used to represent an organic molecule in human tissue, then the direct effect of ionizing radiation upon such a molecule may be represented by the following equations:

$$RH \xrightarrow{\text{radiation}} RH^+ + e^-$$

$$RH^+ \longrightarrow R^{\cdot} + H^+$$

Direct interaction has ionized the molecule, leading eventually to the production of the organic free radical $R^{\cdot}$. The *indirect effect* will also operate. This involves the production of the aqueous free radicals $OH^{\cdot}$ and $H^{\cdot}$, already described above, as following the ionization of the water content of most human tissues. Typical equations that may now apply to the interaction of these radicals with organic molecules in their immediate vicinity are:

$$RH + OH^{\cdot} \longrightarrow R^{\cdot} + H_2O$$

$$RH + H^{\cdot} \longrightarrow R^{\cdot} + H_2$$

The reactions of hydrated electrons will also give rise to organic free radicals. Such radicals may give rise to permanent damage, but the damage could be repaired, say, by reaction with an SH compound:

$$R^{\cdot} + -SH \longrightarrow RH + -S^{\cdot}$$

(where $-S^{\cdot}$ is relatively inert)

Figure 4.4 illustrates how the relative importance of these direct and indirect effects will vary with the ionizing density of the radiation, i.e. the distribution of ionizing events across the target and the probability of these ionizations occurring inside or outside a critical volume. It can be seen that a biological target is more likely to be damaged indirectly by radiation of low ionization density. Furthermore, the direct effect is not only more likely to operate with more densely ionizing radiation, but this will also be relatively more damaging, dose for dose. In Chapter 5 it will be shown that

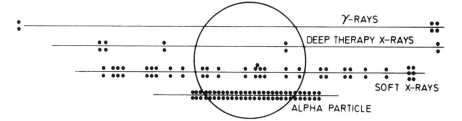

Figure 4.4. Separation of ion clusters in relation to the size of a biological target. (Reproduced from Gray, 1946, *Br. Med. Bull.* by permission of the author.)

DNA is the most important biological target and that ionizations occurring directly in the DNA and outside the DNA may result in the same reactive centres within the DNA due to the phenomenon of 'clustered damage' (see Figure 5.5).

THE OXYGEN EFFECT

In equation (5) the chemical products of the ionization of water that had the highest yield were the hydroxl radical OH$\cdot$ and the hydrated electron e^-_{aq}. The hydroxyl radical had one oxidizing equivalent, whereas the hydrated electron has one reducing equivalent, and when molecules are present in water that are oxidizable or reducible they may be attacked by the corresponding radicals. If oxygen is present in the irradiated tissue there will be an increased yield of free radicals, which are biologically damaging. The reaction of oxygen with free radicals e^-_{aq} and H$\cdot$ produces the relatively stable hydroperoxy radicals HO$_2\cdot$ and hydrogen peroxide, which are very toxic to biological structures:

$$O_2 + e^-_{aq} \longrightarrow O_2^-$$

$$O_2^- + H^+ \longrightarrow HO_2\cdot$$

$$O_2 + H\cdot \longrightarrow HO_2\cdot$$

$$2HO_2\cdot \longrightarrow H_2O_2 + O_2$$

Oxygen will also react with organic free radicals:

$$R\cdot + O_2 \longrightarrow RO_2\cdot$$

The organic peroxy radical RO$_2\cdot$ cannot easily be repaired so the radiation damage cannot be fixed. In certain parts of cells a chain reaction may even be generated, which would involve more of the original biological molecule RH:

$$RO_2\cdot + RH \longrightarrow RO_2H + R\cdot \text{ (and so on)}$$

These reactions amount to fixation of biological damage. They occur at a rate that is 30 times faster than any competing reaction, such as $R\cdot +$ cysteine, or any other hydrogen donor, which will reconstitute RH.

In summary, the oxygen effect in radiobiology involves a competition between two processes. Radiation-induced free radicals are either 'fixed' by dissolved oxygen or repaired by endogenous hydrogen donors in the particular tissue. This competition will determine the amount of radiation damage and obviously depends upon the concentration of oxygen molecules in the vicinity of the target molecule.

Because DNA is the principal target for radiation damage, the most important example of the oxygen effect involves DNA free radicals. These may be repaired by reduction, involving a hydrogen donation from a sulphydryl compound such as glutathione. Alternatively they may be fixed by oxidation, involving the addition of molecular oxygen or other electron-affinic compound. This will lead to altered DNA structure, such as breaks in the phosphodiester backbone. The effect of dissolved oxygen is reduced as the ionization density increases, because more densely ionizing radiation favours equations (3) and (4) (on p. 57) and oxygen is produced in the tracks of dense ionization.

PROTECTION AND SENSITIZATION

By far the best clinical radiation sensitizer is oxygen dissolved in the tissues at a phyiological concentration. Under normal conditions, of course, oxygen is usually present in the cellular environment so that sensitization can only be demonstrated by comparison with the situation when tissues are (presumably abnormally) hypoxic. If the concentration of oxygen molecules in the vicinity of the irradiated tissue is reduced, this will swing the radiation chemical competition in favour of the endogenous hydrogen donors in that tissue.

The balance may be affected in the opposite direction by the addition of protective compounds, such as those containing the sulphydryl group —SH (e.g. cysteamine and cysteine). In terms of reactions, then, as a result of this competition, while oxygen is more damaging because of the effect already discussed:

$$R\cdot + O_2 \longrightarrow RO_2\cdot$$

a compound containing an —SH group will have the following effect:

$$R^{\cdot} + {-}SH \longrightarrow RH + {-}S$$

The sulphydryl group has enabled the ionized molecule to be restored to its normal state. In practice, most —SH compounds investigated so far have proved toxic in the concentrations necessary to be effective in clinical use. A new class – the thiophosphates – are not toxic, however, but are not protective until they are transformed by enzymes inside living cells. A good example is WR-2721 (Ethiofos; see Chapter 11). Most cells contain measurable amounts of —SH groups, but the concentrations are not high enough to compete successfully with atmospheric O_2 for the $R^{\cdot}$ radical. As well as protection by the mechanisms discussed, there are also several other ways by which protective compounds may operate (see Chapter 11).

Alternative sensitizers to oxygen must not only act by intracellular binding of naturally occurring radioprotectors (such as the —SH compounds) but may also act by swinging the radiation chemical competition in favour of the oxidative pathway and against the reductive. The main products of the irradiation of water are the $OH^{\cdot}$ radicals, which are oxidative, and the hydrated electrons (e_{aq}^{-}), which are powerful reducing agents. Any compound that is *electron-affinic* will tend to be radiosensitizing. This is the mechanism of action of the nitroimidazole class of compounds, which have been used clinically on the assumption that they mimic the oxygen effect in those hypoxic tissues to which they can diffuse. They are also one of the class of *bioreductive drugs*, i.e. they are activated by metabolic reduction in tumour cells to form highly effective cytotoxins. These are discussed in Chapter 11.

Compounds that interfere with DNA synthesis may also be sensitizers, and so may the other cytotoxic chemotherapeutic agents used in conjunction with radiotherapy. Strictly speaking, such compounds should be used at a non-toxic level if true radio-sensitization is to be shown (cf. oxygen). Most therapeutic regimes of combination chemotherapy and radiotherapy show only an additive effect from the two cytotoxic modalities (see Chapter 11).

In summary, the biophysical effects of radiation involve the attenuation of either an incident X-ray photon (producing a fast electron) or an incident fast neutron (producing a recoil proton) in tissues, leading to the production of ion pairs and then free radicals. These interactions lead to the breakage of chemical bonds and biological effects, which are the subject of the next chapter.

SUMMARY OF CONCLUSIONS

(1) X-rays are electromagnetic radiations of such short wavelength and such high frequency that they cause ionization.

(2) Interaction with matter occurs by the photoelectric effect, by Compton scattering or by pair production, depending upon the energy of the radiation.
(3) The higher the photon energy, the shorter the wavelength and the greater the penetration of irradiated tissue.
(4) Radiation also occurs as α, β and γ rays. Radioactive isotopes are unstable atoms that emit such radiation as they decay.
(5) Radiation doses can be measured chemically, and by ionization chambers, film badges, thermoluminescent material and scintillation.
(6) The SI units of radiation are the gray (Gy), the sievert (Sv) and the becquerel (Bq).
(7) Ionization of molecules leads to the formation of free-radical ions. The radiolysis of water produces OH·, H· and e^-_{aq} radicals.
(8) Radiation sensitization and protection depends upon the competition between oxygen fixation and hydrogen donation.

REFERENCES

Bensasson, R. V., Land, E. J. and Truscott, T. G., 1993. *Excited States and Free Radicals in Biology and Medicine*. Oxford University Press, Oxford.
Coggle, J. W., 1983. *Biological Effects of Radiation*, 2nd edn. Taylor & Francis, London.
Gray, L. H., 1946. Comparative studies of the biological effects of X-rays, neutrons and other ionizing radiations. *British Medical Bulletin*, **4**, 11–18.
Hall, E. J., 1988. *Radiobiology for the Radiologist*. Lippincott, Philadelphia.
Nias, A. H. W., 1988. *Clinical Radiobiology*, 2nd edn. Churchill Livingstone, Edinburgh.
Ohya-Nishiguchi, H. and Packer, L., 1995. *Bioradicals Detected by ESR Spectroscopy*. Birkauser Verlag, Basle.

5 Subcellular Radiobiology

The tissues of the body are built up of mammalian cells, which form the basic biological units. For most of the purposes of this book it will be convenient to regard cells as the biological target of ionizing radiation. The primary biophysical effects of radiation were described in Chapter 4 in terms of the radiolysis of water, which, after all, constitutes the majority of the body substances. Most biological targets are a good deal more complex than water, however, and this chapter will consider the consequences to a mammalian cell of radiation damage at the biochemical level, where organic molecules are interacting in a complex manner. This is usually in the context of the various organelles, or subcellular structures, that were described in Chapter 2.

Those organelles were compared to the various departments of a factory, whose smooth running would be more or less disrupted depending upon where any damage was inflicted. Damage to the central computer would bring the whole factory to a standstill. Damage to one or more of the outlying departments might still permit a considerable amount of production to continue as long as the central computer was able to function. In that analogy the central computer was able to function. In that analogy the central computer is the nucleus of the cell and this will be the subject of greatest emphasis in this chapter.

Before that, some attempt must be made to find out just how important is the response of the cytoplasmic organelles to radiation. The problem is how to recognize radiation damage in such discrete structures that are of considerable functional importance to the cell. Damage to mitochondria might be recognized by changes in electron microscopic appearance or by changes in their contribution to energy production in the cell, detected by biochemical assays of the enzymes needed for both anabolic and catabolic activity. Damage to the lysosomes might have untold effects in biochemical terms. Then, thirdly, the endoplasmic reticulum is the site of enzymatic and other protein synthesis using the RNA template.

RADIATION BIOCHEMISTRY

How is it possible to separate damage to one organelle from that to another? Functional tests have to be used because the clearest of electron microscopic changes can only represent a static view of what is, in reality, a dynamic organization in the cell as a whole. This dynamic organization consists of a complex of macromolecules, with the same type of molecule often distributed in such different cellular compartments as the nucleus, mitochondria and elsewhere in the cytoplasm, where the biochemical environmental conditions are different. Because of this, the same macromolecule may have different radiosensitivities in different compartments.

Following irradiation, macromolecules may undergo degradation, cross-linking and breakage of internal structures. The major specific effects of biochemical importance can be summarized as follows for the different classes of molecules: carbohydrates suffer degradation; lipids undergo oxidation (chain reaction); and proteins suffer breakage of secondary and tertiary bonds. Nucleic acids show a range of effects following irradiation, including change or loss of base, hydrogen bond breakage between chains, single-strand breaks, double-strand breaks (both chains simultaneously) and cross-linking within the helix to another DNA molecule or to protein.

EFFECT OF RADIATION ON MACROMOLECULAR SYNTHESIS

The roles of cyclins, cyclin-dependent kinases (CDKs) and CDK inhibitors in the control of progress through the cell cycle, and the role of p53 in apoptosis, was described in Chapter 2. Figure 5.1 repeats the diagram of the cycle to show the first gap G_1 (and G_0) before DNA synthesis (S) begins, and the second gap G_2 after it is completed and before mitosis (M). During the S phase, mammalian cells contain greater quantities of DNA polymerase than during G_1 and G_2. Those enzymes responsible for the formation of the substrates for DNA synthesis, i.e. deoxyribonucleoside triphosphates, will also increase in activity during the S phase and then diminish again. The two checkpoints in the cell cycle were described in Chapter 2: the first near the beginning of G_1 where a cell may be arrested in G_0 before progressing to S, and the second in the G_2 phase when the cell cycle may either be arrested again or progress into mitosis without further interruption.

All these temporal positions will prove important in later chapters of this book, where radiation and/or chemical agents will be shown to have specific effects upon progress through the cell cycle and on the proliferation of cell populations. As far as macromolecular synthesis is concerned, the radiation dosage required to inhibit RNA and protein synthesis is too large to merit further separate mention. It is unrealistic to separate cellular macromolecules that form a functional whole, however, and the extent to which DNA synthesis is inhibited by irradiation is important because, from the central dogma, any lasting effect on DNA must affect RNA and protein.

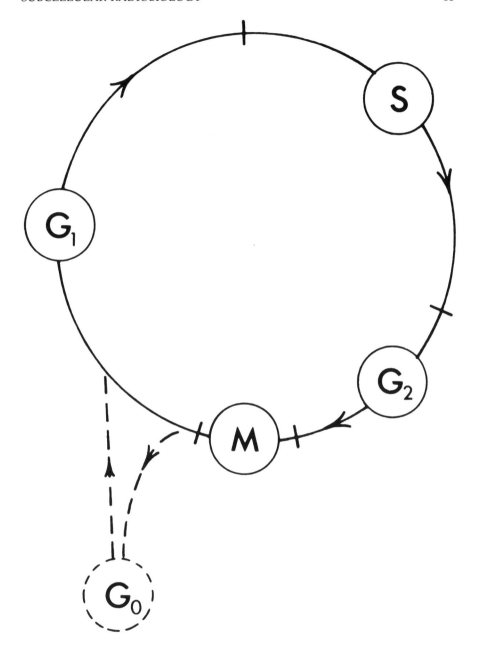

Figure 5.1. The cell cycle. (Reproduced from Priestman, 1980, by permission of Farmitalia Carlo Erba.)

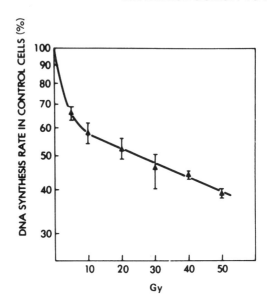

Figure 5.2. Dose–response curve for the effect of X-rays on the rate of DNA synthesis in normal human fibroblasts. (Reproduced from Painter, 1986, by permission of *Int. J. Radiat. Biol.*, Taylor & Francis)

Figure 5.2 shows an X-ray dose–response curve for DNA synthesis in human cells *in vitro*. DNA synthesis is clearly inhibited by a biphasic pattern, but the dosage scale (in Gy) shows how relatively insensitive the synthesis of this macromolecule is to radiation in the lower dose level of a few gray, which will be shown in later chapters to have a marked effect upon the survival or proliferative capacity of such cells. This example only serves to illustrate the consequences of irradiation upon macromolecular synthesis in mammalian cells.

We must remember, however, that most of the metabolism in cells is linked by common substrates, enzymes or co-factors. The whole cell can be considered as a collection of multi-enzyme systems. Nevertheless, irradiation of such systems with doses of biological interest (less than 50 Gy) produces insignificant damage to most of the components. This remains true even for radiation damage to rate-limiting factors of these multi-enzyme systems, which might affect the rates of many steps of the system. However, as the reaction proceeds from one step to the next, this 'insignificant' damage may either multiply or accumulate to become larger, so that the rate of the final step may be altered significantly. There may be significant damage to the cell by this mechanism of 'amplification'. Such damage can rarely be identified as cytoplasmic in origin, however.

Rather than consider the radiation effects on these cytoplasmic organelles, it might be more useful to think of a cell as just a bag of enzymes. This is far too simple, of course, because the enzymes are enclosed not only in the outer cell membrane but also in a complex arrangement of internal membranes (which some cell biologists consider to be in continuity). It has been thought that radiation damage to these membranes is responsible for the killing of cells. Such damage to the cell membrane and/or intracellular membranes (e.g. nuclear, mitochondrial and lysosomal membranes) would be expressed as altered permeability, resulting in transfer of unwanted molecules from one cellular compartment to another. This would produce unbalanced metabolism and would finally lead to cell death.

At the dose levels used in this book, however, there is no evidence for the direct involvement of membrane damage in the killing of cells except for apoptosis (see Chapter 6). After a mean lethal dose of several grays, cells divide at least once before they die and it is clear that the radiosensitive target is unlikely to be membrane. Most of the evidence points to the nucleus, rather than the cytoplasm.

RADIOSENSITIVITY OF THE NUCLEUS

Radiosensitivity of the nucleus has been shown by two types of experiment. Firstly, α-irradiation was used from polonium (a decay product of radon, Chapter 19). Because of its short range it could be delivered either to the cytoplasm or to the nucleus of cells in tissue culture by the exact positioning of the tip of a fine needle upon which the polonium had been deposited (Figure 5.3). When a dose in excess of 250 Gy was delivered to the *cytoplasm* it had no effect upon the proliferation of these cells. By contrast, the mean lethal dose to the *nucleus* was less than 1.5 Gy. This experiment shows that the nuclear region of the cells is at least 100 times more radiosensitive than the cytoplasm.

The other type of experiment compared the radiation effect of tritiated (^{3}H-labelled) water with that of tritiated thymidine. Thymidine is a specific requirement for DNA synthesis and so tritiated thymidine will be localized in the chromosomes in the cell nucleus, whereas tritiated water will be evenly distributed throughout the whole cell (the nucleus and the cytoplasm). The result showed an even greater difference in radiosensitivity, in that more than 1000 times the radioactivity from tritiated water was required to equal the amount of cell damage produced by tritiated thymidine. This sort of experiment ignores the detailed molecular structure of the cell, however, because the sensitivity of its DNA should more properly be compared with that of its RNA and protein molecules (next section).

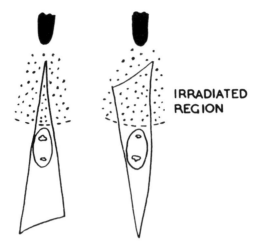

Figure 5.3. Alpha irradiation of most of the cytoplasm of a fibroblastic cell, one end at a time, using a polonium-tipped microneedle (the black object). (Reproduced from Munro, 1961, by permission of *Annals of the New York Academy of Sciences*)

MOLECULAR RADIOBIOLOGY

Radiation effects at the molecular level can best be understood in the setting of what is now a classical part of the central dogma of molecular biology, which states that RNA is transcribed from DNA (Figure 5.4). The genetic information of the cell is transferred from the nucleus by *messenger RNA* (MRNA) to ribosomes in the cytoplasm. Protein synthesis then occurs at the site of the ribosomes, where the necessary amino acids are assembled by *transfer RNA* (tRNA) along the MRNA template. Because cells are continuously synthesizing new proteins, there is also a requirement for RNA synthesis throughout the cell cycle, whereas DNA synthesis is confined to only a part of the cycle.

If the tritium-labelling experiment described earlier is extended using tritiated amino acids such as glycine or serine (for protein) in comparison with tritiated uridine (for RNA) and tritiated thymidine (for DNA), then the sensitivity of cells to tritium can be compared for the whole sequence of the

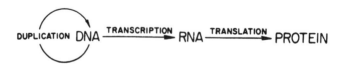

Figure 5.4. The central dogma of molecular biology.

central dogma, and the following order of sensitivity to tritiated cell components is found:

$$DNA > mRNA > rRNA \text{ and } tRNA > \text{amino acids}$$

with damage to DNA being eight times as effective as damage to these particular amino acids. This is a much more sophisticated approach to molecular radiobiology and enables the relative sensitivity of the various cellular targets to be compared. If the pathway is extended, then it can be stated that radiation damage to the cell is followed by expression of molcular damage in the following sequence:

$$DNA \longrightarrow RNA \longrightarrow \text{proteins} \longrightarrow \text{lipids and other macromolecules}$$

The relationship between intracellular damage to DNA and the response of the cell (lethal or otherwise) to radiation is one of the fundamental problems of molecular radiobiology. Absolute sensitivities of living cells to the lethal effects of radiation vary widely but, in general, mammalian cells are particularly sensitive. In well-oxygenated suspensions, radiation doses of the order of a few grays suffice to prevent division of the large majority of the cells. From purely chemical radiation considerations, the amount of molecular damage that can arise from the absorption of such small amounts of radiation is extremely small. Most of the large macromolecules, such as proteins and enzymes, that are essential to the functioning of the cell are represented many times in its structure. It would not be expected that damage to a few of these molecules would bring about such a drastic response to radiation. However, there are not many nucleic acids in that structure. The DNA molecule and its sequences of bases is unique. It is not surprising, therefore, that damage to DNA is presumed to be the main cause of lethality in cells after moderate doses of radiation.

Table 5.1 shows some of the damage produced in a mammalian cell nucleus by 1 Gy of low, linear energy transfer (LET) radiation. Such a dose will produce a large number of ionizations in the nucleus but far fewer DNA lesions, such as sugar or base damage, DNA–DNA and DNA–protein cross-links, DNA single- or double-strand breaks and chromosome

Table 5.1. Damage in a cell nucleus from 1 Gy

Ionizations in cell nucleus	100 000
Ionizations directly in DNA	2 000
DNA single-strand breaks	1 000
DNA double-strand breaks	40

Reproduced from Goodhead, 1994, by permission of *Int. J. Radiat. Biol.*, Taylor & Francis.

aberrations. Only 40 double-strand breaks (dsb) are produced per Gy per cell (i.e. only 1 dsb per chromosome per Gy), but these are the critical lesions causing cell death. Track structure analysis shows that 50% of dsb are not simple but will have other types of DNA damage nearby. This is called *clustered* damage. Figure 5.5. shows a cluster of ionization events impinging on the DNA double helix. These clusters are a few nanometres in size and formed by single tracks. They will be more difficult to repair because their complexity increases with increasing LET. By contrast, single-strand breaks are relatively easily repaired. DNA repair enzymes have now been identified and the molecular biology of the repair of radiation damage will be discussed in Chapter 7.

The double helical structure of DNA is a complex molecule. One way of getting information on the effects of radiation is to simplify the problem by the study of single strands of DNA. These can be obtained by lysis of cells under alkaline conditions. High-speed centrifugation of such DNA in a sucrose gradient can then be used to determine the molecular weight of the single strands. Molecular weight is found to decrease with increasing radiation dose: it falls to a minimum within 30 s of irradiation and then begins to rise back towards the starting level within 20 min. A more sensitive alternative takes advantage of the different rates of elution of damaged and undamaged DNA from membrane filters. The degree of retention on the filter is a measure of the number of single-strand breaks (ssb) and the subsequent repair of such breaks.

In the living situation, of course, DNA is double-stranded. The *'Comet' assay* (Fairbairn et al, 1995) is a sensitive and rapid method for detecting DNA double-strand breaks in individual cells. The original assay has now been adapted to involve a more rigorous lysis of the nucleus of single cells embedded in agar, leaving naked DNA. This is then exposed to an electric field, which stretches the DNA into a tail (or comet). (Many readers will remember seeing comet Hale–Bopp in 1997, with its characteristic blunt head and misty tail). The length of the tail is proportional to the number of strand breaks, which will be dominated by dsb at neutral pH.

Another technique is pulsed-field gel electrophoresis, which uses the fact that fragments of DNA carry a negative charge. When incorporated into an agarose gel, they migrate under an electric field at a speed that is inversely proportional to their size. The movement of the DNA is detected by staining with a DNA-specific fluorescent dye after electrophoresis. DNA of known molecular weight is used to calibrate the movement of irradiated DNA in the gels. The technique gave similar values for the rate of dsb rejoining as were found by the neutral elution technique (Iliakis et al, 1991). Similar values were found for the rate of rejoining of chromatin breaks measured by the premature chromosome condensation (PCC) technique (see later).

It seems reasonble to correlate these laboratory phenomena of the repair, or rejoining, of dsb in DNA with the biological phenomenon of recovery

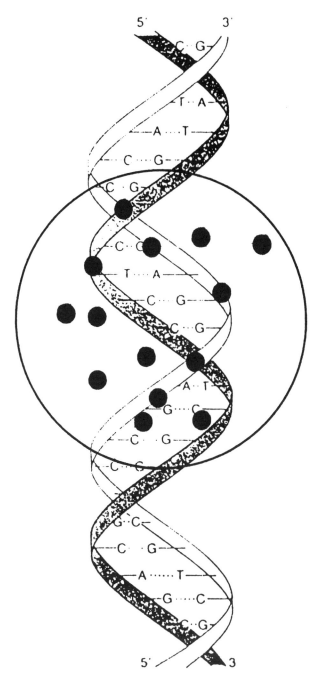

Figure 5.5. A cluster of ionizations impinging on DNA. (Reproduced from McMillan and Steel, 1997, by permission of Edward Arnold.)

from sublethal or potentially lethal damage because the time scale for the repair of such breaks approximates to that for recovery from radiation damage. However, there are many intermediate steps that must be shown to occur before the biochemical 'repair' of DNA can be equated to 'recovery' from sublethal radiation damage. This will be discussed in Chapter 7. The only intermediate step in the argument that will be discussed in this chapter concerns damage to DNA at the chromosomal level.

Chromosome aberrations cannot be studied until the cell has progressed through the cycle to the next mitosis after irradiation. Before that, the *premature chromosome condensation* (PCC) technique can be used. Interphase cells in which damage is to be assessed (e.g. human cells) are fused with a mitotic hamster cell, which forces the human chromosomes to condense prematurely, making chromosome breaks visible. Using this technique, the yield of PCC initial breaks per cell is only 6 per cell per Gy (Iliakis et al, 1991) compared with 40 dsb per cell per Gy; so about 6 dsb are produced for every PCC, but 90% of PCCs are repaired and only four remain as permanent breaks. The technique can be used to analyse damage to cell populations that may no longer be able to divide.

CHROMOSOME DAMAGE

Except for cells in the lymphocyte series and the oocyte, which may show death during interphase (apoptosis), mammlian cells respond to moderate doses of radiation by mitotic death, i.e. the cells do not die immediately after irradiation but begin to die when they come into mitosis (Chapter 6). At this stage abnormal mitotic figures may be evident, containing chromosomal aberrations, anaphase bridges and fragments, leading to mechanical failure of the genetic process and genetic loss. Metabolic activities may continue, however, and such cells may remain 'alive' in that they may show no loss of functional integrity. Nevertheless, the cells are doomed to die because they have lost their capacity for unlimited proliferation, i.e. their reproductive integrity: they are 'sterilized'.

Some cells sterilized by radiation may enlarge to 'giant' proportions and become polyploid, i.e. have an increased number of chromosomes, but others may not show immediate overt chromosomal damage even by the most sophisticated cytogenetic techniques. The damage to the most sensitive target, the DNA, may only need to be at the genetic level, whereas very large losses of genetic information will not be visible under the light microscope. Even a small chromosomal fragment (e.g. an interstitial deletion) may involve the loss of several megabases of DNA. The usual sterilizing effect of irradiation is explicable by a mechanism of damage to the DNA template, amounting to a change in the code.

Even severe damage to function may well not be demonstrable by cytogenetic methods, only by the techniques of molecular biology. DNA miscoding would be shown by a change in the base ratios. Such damaged cells may be capable of several life cycles before their proliferative capacity fails, because although new RNA synthesis will be affected, existing RNA will code for protein synthesis for some time before miscoding begins to be noticeable. Genomic instability may then become manifest. This accounts for the known phenomenon of radiation-damaged cells proliferating into colonies of 10 cells (or more) before cell division ceases (Chapter 6). Genetic change of a greater extent will lead to reproductive death, which may be manifest as overt chromosomal damage.

Chromosome staining techniques using Giemsa have revealed considerable detail in the form of banding patterns along the length of each individual chromosome. This adds another dimension to the study of chromosomal aberrations because it allows the detection of balanced, transmissible changes not visible with conventional solid staining. The various banding methods have had a great impact on clinical and cancer cytogenetics, allowing recurrent types of aberration to be related to various malformations and neoplasms. Standardized patterns are used universally for the accurate mapping of genes.

More recently, the technique of fluorescence *in situ* hybridization of chromosome-specific molecular probes – '*FISH painting*' – has been used to reveal aberrations. Figure 5.6 shows how chromatin from one pair of homologues is specifically and distinctively coloured (here, black). The break-up and redistribution of material from this chromosome can then be traced with considerable accuracy, and frequently reveals that aberrations are more complicated than might be inferred from conventional staining. Several chromosomes can be painted using different colours (here, black and hatched) to study exchange interactions in detail. (The letters refer to the S & S system of nomenclature for designating chromosome aberrations; Savage and Tucker, 1996.)

Paints are available for every human chromosome, so the dissemination of material from one chromosome to another can be charted with considerable accuracy. The method is much simpler than the banding techniques and is particularly valuable for long-term follow-up studies in radiation accident situations (see Chapter 20) because it detects the transmissible changes. In the study of primary radiation-induced exchanges the FISH technique has indicated that many of the aberrations that were assumed, from conventional staining, to be simple two-break types are in fact multi-break 'complex' exchanges. This means that there has previously been an underestimate of the damage produced in chromosomes by radiation.

If the irradiation is delivered early in the cell cycle before DNA synthesis has begun then the chromosomes will not yet have duplicated and damage

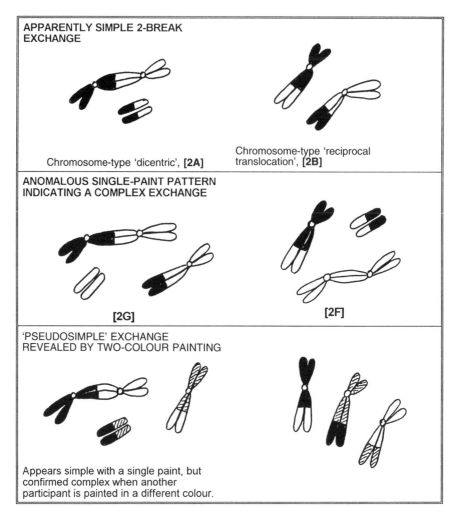

APPARENTLY SIMPLE 2-BREAK EXCHANGE

Chromosome-type 'dicentric', **[2A]**

Chromosome-type 'reciprocal translocation', **[2B]**

ANOMALOUS SINGLE-PAINT PATTERN INDICATING A COMPLEX EXCHANGE

[2G]

[2F]

'PSEUDOSIMPLE' EXCHANGE REVEALED BY TWO-COLOUR PAINTING

Appears simple with a single paint, but confirmed complex when another participant is painted in a different colour.

Figure 5.6. Diagram of FISH-painted chromosomes. (Savage, personal communication, 1997, reproduced by permission.)

will occur to whole chromosomes. This may be visible at the next mitosis as *chromosome-type aberrations*. By contrast, *chromatid-type aberrations* may follow irradiation later on in the cell cycle when each chromosome will have divided into two chromatids held together only at the centromere, so that the damage may only be evident in one of the two chromatids of a pair. A large number of permutations and combinations may then be evident in the mitotic figure of an irradiated cell population. This has been the subject

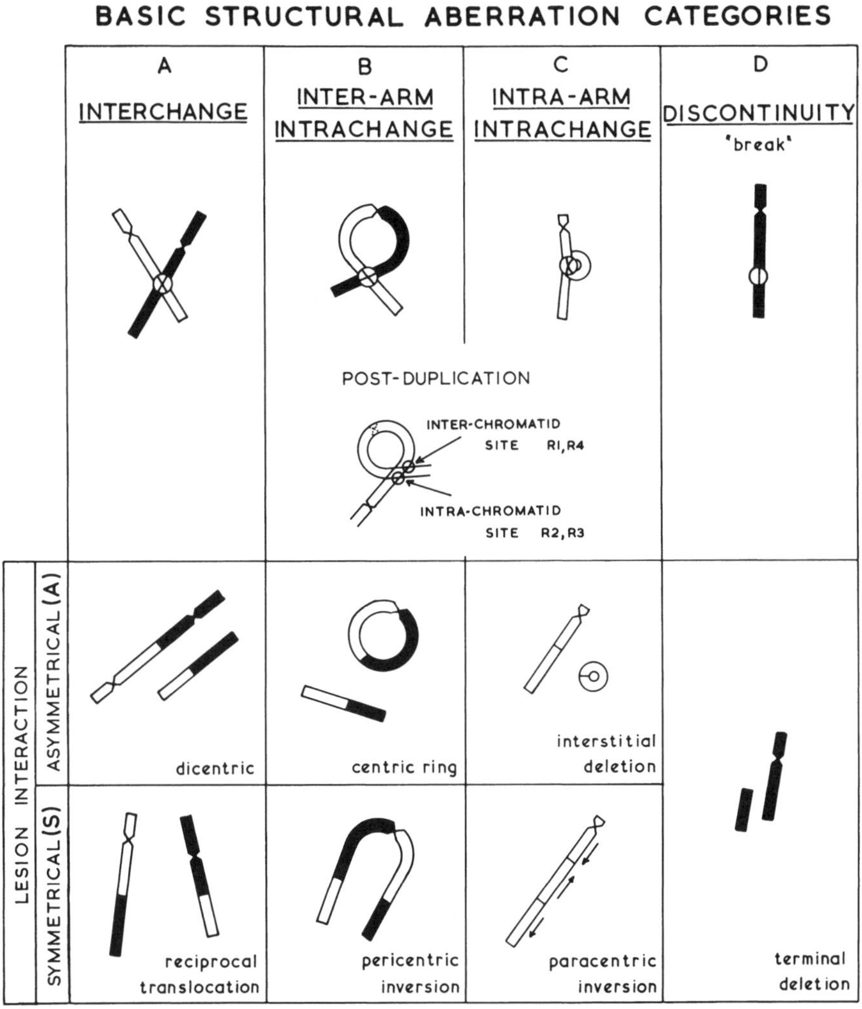

BASIC STRUCTURAL ABERRATION CATEGORIES

Figure 5.7. Basic structural aberration categories. (Reproduced from Savage, 1983, by permission of *Clin. Cytogen. Bull.*)

of extensive studies by geneticists who have devised a nomenclature to describe the aberrations (Savage, 1983).

There are four basic categories of aberration (Figure 5.7). One of them (D), the 'discontinuity' or 'terminal deletion', can be thought of as being derived from a single break. The others (A–C) all require the interaction of a minimum of two breaks. Of these the interchange (A) is the commonest form for *chromosome-type* aberrations, and the two rejoining modes, which yield either a dicentric or a reciprocal translocation, are thought to be equally likely, although, as pointed out above, the latter are only visible if specialized staining techniques are employed. Because the dicentrics are much easier to score, this is the basis of a technique of biological dosimetry (see later) that can be used in radiological protection to supplement physical dosimetry in the event of a suspected accidental exposure to radiation (Lloyd and Purrott, 1981). With *chromatid-type* aberrations, the added possibility of interaction between breaks in the sister chromatids makes the various forms of intra-arm intrachanges (C) the commonest aberration.

The asymmetrical forms, which are always accompanied by acentric fragments (and therefore lead to severe genetic loss), are termed 'unstable' because cells containing them are rapidly lost from the cycling cell population, leaving only the 'stable' symmetrical forms to be transmitted. In the long term, therefore, little obvious chromosome damage is detected unless specialized staining techniques are employed.

The unstable dicentric aberration (Figure 5.7) appears to be the most consistent index of radiation damage and represents about 60% of all observed unstable aberrations following acute irradiation. It has a low background frequency (about 1 in 1000 cells) in lymphocytes obtained from normal persons exposed only to background radiation. The presence of two centromeres in the aberration usually gives it a very distinctive appearance. The acentric fragments can also be recognized as *micronuclei*, which correlate with loss of cell survival.

Chromosome aberrations used to be classified into one- or two-hit lesions, depending on whether one or two ionizing events would be required for their production. But, although the majority of chromosome aberrations involve the interaction of two lesions, track segment analysis has now shown that both of these lesions may be produced by the passage of one ionizing track. Alternatively, the two lesions may be produced by independent tracks. Thus an exchange, like a dicentric, can be either a 'one-track' or a 'two-track' aberration (one cannot tell which, by inspection). It is this that determines the theoretical shapes of dose–response curves.

With low-LET radiations, the majority of exchanges are two-track at higher doses, their predominance tending to decrease as the dose, or dose rate, is lowered. This explain the curvilinearity of low-LET dose–response curves (Chapter 8). In the case of high-LET radiations (Chapter 9), ionization density in the tracks ensures that, in all cases (at least at the doses that can be used) both lesions are always produced by the same track, hence their dose–response curves are always linear and there is no dose rate effect.

It is clear that the principal lesion for the production of chromosome aberrations by radiation is the DNA double-strand break. Experimental work with restriction endonucleases (which produce defined sequence dsb) leads to the production of all types of aberrations: *chromosome type* if given in G_1; *chromatid type* if given in S or G_2. Efficiency of production is extremely high. There is also evidence that single-strand breaks, which are produced by radiation at a very much higher rate than dsb (Table 5.1), hardly ever lead to aberration formation in the normal course of events. This is because a dsb is more difficult to repair than an ssb (Chapter 7).

Experiments with animals and data from studies on irradiated patients have shown that the aberration yield in lymphocytes following a uniform whole-body irradiation is similar to that obtained when blood samples are given the same dose *in vitro*. Therefore, it is possible to construct *in vitro* calibration curves relating radiation dose to aberration yield, and these form the basis of the biological dosimetry technique. In practice, most overexposures are to X- and γ-radiation and a number of laboratories have established *in vitro* curves for that.

The National Radiological Protection Board (NRPB) laboratory has produced calibration curves for all types of external radiation likely to be encountered in an accident. Figure 5.8 shows a selection of the curves for different types of radiation. The dose–response is curvilinear with X- and γ-

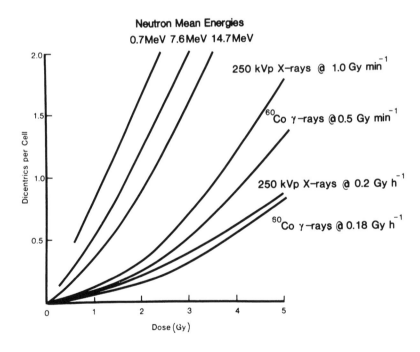

Figure 5.8. Dose–response curves of dicentric aberration yields for several qualities of radiation. (Reproduced from Lloyd and Purrott, 1981, by permission of Nuclear Technology Publishing.)

rays and lower dose rates are less effective. For neutrons, the more densely ionizing the radiation (i.e. the lower the neutron energy), the more linear the dose–response (Chapter 9).

SIZE OF RADIATION TARGET

Even with the most sophisticated chromosomal staining techniques, the evidence from these aberrations represents a very crude picture of the damage following doses of X-irradiation in the mean lethal dose range of 1–2 Gy. We must bear in mind that the average DNA content of a mammalian cell corresponds to a gross molecular weight of about 6×10^{12} Da. Even if this weight is divided among 20–50 mammalian chromosomes, molecules in excess of 1×10^{11} Da could conceivably be involved. Such large molecules might be about 10 cm long if they exist as continuous DNA duplexes, yet a complete radiation lesion can be produced by a cluster of ionizations (Figure 5.5) within a 'target size' of a few nanometres, which is comparable to the diameter of DNA.

It used to be assumed that some ionizing events may only be sublethal and that two or more sublethal events must be necessary before the damage would be lethal. Radiobiologists then had to choose between two 'target theories' with a requirement either for one sensitive site to be hit twice or more or for one hit to occur in two or more sensitive sites within the cell. Track structure analysis (Goodhead, 1994) shows that neither of these target theories is valid because lethal damage occurs with very soft X-rays (less than 1 keV). These produce single electron tracks, which are so short that it is difficult to assume interaction between separate sublethal events. The shapes of the cell survival curves for X-radiation can just as well be explained on the basis of single hits, many of which are repaired by processes that become saturated at higher doses. (The various target theories will be discussed in Chapter 8.)

It follows that the size of the critical target in a mammalian cell can be estimated from the effects of this low-LET radiation, which is reparable. Lethal damage can occur with an energy deposition of about 100 eV (about four ionizations) within a moderate cluster of about 2 nm. This is roughly the diameter of a DNA double helix. Such very soft (< 1 keV) X-rays are relatively much more damaging than the hard (> 200 keV) X-rays used in radiotherapy, although they are of limited clinical importance because of their very short range in tissue. The lethal damage from high-LET radiation (Chapter 9) involves a higher energy deposition of about 400 eV (15 ionizations) within a large cluster of 5–10 nm, but such lesions are not repairable.

All this evidence serves to show the very small size of the radiation target in mammalian cells. It is clear that the DNA double helix is the site of that target, although associated membrane structures may also be involved.

SUMMARY OF CONCLUSIONS

(1) The nucleus of a mammalian cell is very much more radiosensitive than the cytoplasm and other organelles.

(2) DNA is more sensitive than RNA, and RNA is more sensitive than protein, in terms of cell death.

(3) In terms of macromolecular synthesis, however, DNA is relatively resistant to radiation.

(4) In terms of DNA structure, radiation damage can be detected by assaying single- and double-strand breaks.

(5) When cells are irradiated early in the cycle, chromosome aberrations will be detectable at the next mitosis. Chromatid aberrations follow irradiation later in the cell cycle. 'FISH painting' is used to identify aberrations.

(6) Unstable dicentric aberrations and micronuclei provide an index of radiation damage that is dose dependent.

(7) Calibration curves enable accidental radiation exposures to be estimated in terms of such chromosome aberrations.

(8) The size of the critical cellular target of radiation is about 2 nm, similar to the diameter of a DNA double helix.

REFERENCES

Fairbairn, D. W., Olive, P. L. and O'Neill K. L., 1995. The comet assay: a comprehensive review. *Mutation Research*, **339**, 37–59.

Goodhead, D. T., 1994. Initial events in the cellular effects of ionizing radiations: clustered damage in DNA. *International Journal of Radiation Biology*, **65**, 7–17.

Iliakis, G., Blocher, D., Metzger, L. and Patelias, G., 1991. Comparison of DNA double-strand break rejoining as measured by pulsed field gel electrophoresis, neutral sucrose gradient centrifugation and non-winding filter elution in irradiated plateau-phase CHO cells. *International Journal of Radiation Biology*, **59**, 927–939.

Lloyd, D. C. and Purrott, R. J., 1981. Chromosome aberration analysis in radiological protection dosimetry. *Radiation Protection Dosimetry*, **1**, 19–27.

McMillan, T. J. and Steel, G. G., 1997. DNA damage and cell killing. In *Basic Clinical Radiobiology*, 2nd edn, edited by G. G. Steel. Edward Arnold, London.

Munro, T. R., 1961. Irradiation of selected parts of single cells. *Annals of the New York Academy of Sciences*, **95**, 920–931.

Painter, R. B., 1986. Inhibition of mammalian cell DNA synthesis by ionizing radiation. *International Journal of Radiation Biology*, **49**, 771–781.

Priestman, T. J. 1980. *Cancer Chemotherapy – An Introduction*. Farmitalia Carlo Erba, Barnet, Herts.

Savage, J. R. K., 1983. Some practical notes on chromosomal aberrations. *Clinical Cytogenetics Bulletin*, **1**, 64–76.

Savage, J. R. K. and Tucker, J. D., 1996. Nomenclature systems for FISH-painted chromosome aberrations. *Mutations Research*, **366**, 153–161.

6 Radiation Cell Damage

The first task in this chapter is to clarify what is meant by the term cell death. The death of a person is clearly understood to mean the cessation of life. Bodily functions come to a halt and degeneration follows. The same applies to cell death; the cell ceases all its functions and degenerates. However, a problem arises when the effects of radiation are considered in terms of the proliferative capacity of a cell. This is a particular parameter that is used quite commonly to express *cell survival*, particularly in the context of tumour tissues where the capacity of cells to continue proliferating presents the clinical problem in the cancer field. It is therefore necessary to understand what is meant by loss of cell survival because that measure of 'cell death' will be used frequently in this book and in other radiobiological literature. In contrast to dead cells, these have lost proliferative capacity but may remain very much alive with respect to all the other metabolic activities and secretory powers of cells that are otherwise undamaged.

The study of cell death, in its true sense, presents the obvious problem that a dead cell rapidly disintegrates and cannot be studied because it is no longer visible. In an organized tissue the debris of such a dead cell will be rapidly removed by phagocytosis and there will only be negative evidence of its death. The cell culture technique enables this phenomenon of true cell death to be studied. Figure 6.1 shows photographs of Chinese hamster fibroblasts that were first shown in Chapter 5 (Figure 5.3) being irradiated by alpha particles from a polonium source. An apparently undamaged cell is illustrated in Figure 6.1a; Figures 6.1b–d show a cell degenerating during the 4 days after irradiation. The cell is degenerating because the nucleus was exposed to a very large dose of alpha irradiation. The remnant of the cell is still visible but is clearly disorganized. It would be difficult to study such a cell *in vivo* because it would long since have been removed by phagocytosis. Quite clearly the whole architecture of the cell is disrupted and there is no question that the cell is dead in every respect.

In those days, the word pyknosis was used to describe what happened to such a dying cell. Nowadays the term *apoptosis* would probably be used, to distinguish from simple necrosis. (Apoptosis is discussed later.) One of the first changes occurs in the nucleus where the chromatin strands (i.e. the DNA) condense to form a compact mass. At this stage the dying cells are easily distinguishable from the surrounding live cells, which will not be so heavily stained in a histological preparation. Figure 6.2 shows what

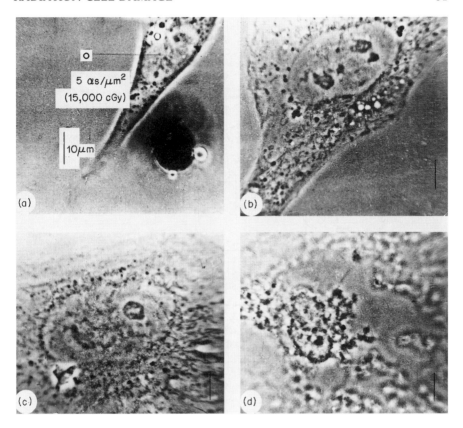

Figure 6.1. Effect of alpha particles on Chinese hamster cells. (a) Normal cell being irradiated by polonium source (back disc). (b) Cell enlarged 2 days later. (c) Further enlargement after 3 days. (d) Degeneration after 4 days. All scale lines are 10 μm. (Reproduced from Munro, 1970, by permission of Academic Press, Inc.)

happens to a tumour during the days after it has been irradiated. The proportion of tumour cells that show 'pyknosis' rises to a maximum 2–3 days after irradiation and then falls away as the dead cells are removed by phagocytosis. However, before irradiated cells die in this way they may grow into giant cells.

GIANT CELLS

Figures 6.3b and 6.3c show the nuclei of two more fibroblasts, before and after irradiation. The only differences between these two photographs is that the cell nucleus in Figure 6.3c is very much larger than that in Figure

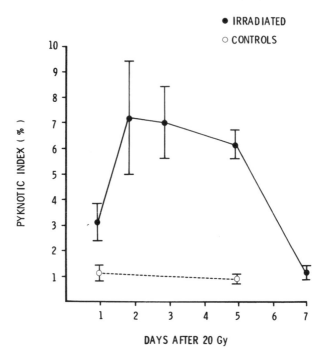

Figure 6.2. Changes in pyknotic index of C_3H mouse mammary tumours after 20 Gy irradiation. (Reproduced from Jones and Camplejohn, 1982, by permission of Springer-Verlag GmbH & Co. KG.)

6.3b despite the fact that they were photographed at the same magnification. (Figure 6.3a shows a lymphocyte for comparison.) The cell nucleus in Figure 6.3c is quite reasonably described as that of a giant cell. If it were not for the difference in magnification, it would not be possible to distinguish the one cell from the other because all the normal architectural features are present. Here, again, the second cell of the pair has received a large dose of irradiation but there is no sign of death. Metabolic functions have continued and when the DNA content of this cell was measured by an integrating microdensitometer it was found to be more than 20 times that of the cell in Figure 6.3b. (The DNA content of irradiated cells was discussed in Chapter 5.)

Giant cells like these are characteristic of the effects of radiation upon cell populations. What has happened is that while the process of mitotic division has been inhibited, all other metabolic functions have continued normally, especially macromolecular synthesis. The rate of cell enlargement is shown in Figure 6.4, which shows how cells grew exponentially in volume for at least 6 days, after an X-ray dose of 12 Gy, until the mean volume was 10–20 times that of normal cells. Thereafter, the rate of

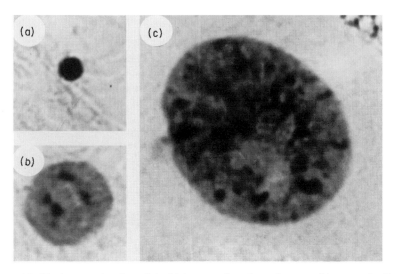

Figure 6.3. Feulgen-stained nuclei of (a) normal rat lymphocyte, (b) normal cell and (c) giant cell 8 days after irradiation. (Reproduced from Nias and Paul, 1961, by permission of *Int. J. Radiat. Biol.*, Taylor & Francis)

enlargement decreased until a plateau was reached about 12 days after irradiation. During the period of exponential growth the cell volume doubled in 34 h. This rate of growth in *volume* can be compared with that of unirradiated HeLa cells, which double in number every 20 h under the same conditions when proliferation would be the normal rule.

By contrast, an irradiated cell cannot grow in number, only in volume. In terms of proliferative capacity such a cell is 'dead' but it is not dead in any other capacity. Quite clearly the mitotic apparatus has proved to be the most radiosensitive of the cell constituents. As far as the control of cancer growth is concerned, this is a most satisfactory conclusion. The phenomenon will apply equally to normal cell populations, however.

Giant cell formation will only be evident in those cell populations that normally undergo mitotic division and will therefore be synthesizing the extra complement of DNA, RNA and protein preparatory to such mitotic division. There are many types of mammalian cell that remain stationary in terms of such a proliferative process and the effect of irradiation would not be manifest in terms of giant cell formation in such cells. As far as mitotic activity is concerned a classification into three types of normal cell population was given in Table 2.1 in Chapter 2 and this will indicate which cell populations might be expected to show giant cell formation after irradiation. Added to that classification must be the wide variety of tumours that, although growing relatively slowly, continue proliferation without any physiological restraint.

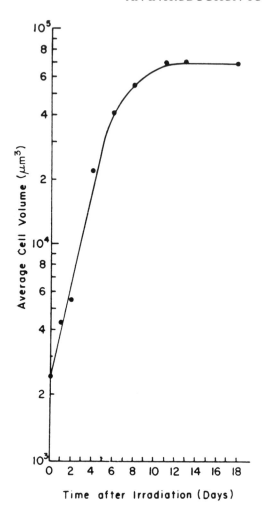

Figure 6.4. Enlargement of HeLa cells after irradiation. (Reproduced from Tolmach and Marcus, 1960, by permission of Academic Press, Inc.)

INTERPHASE DEATH AND APOPTOSIS

The term interphase death has been used to describe what happens to irradiated cells that die before they reach the next mitosis; in contrast to mitotic death, which obviously means the death of a cell at the time of mitosis. The word necrosis might be used but biologists use the term 'apoptosis' to distinguish from ordinary necrosis because it is involved in many normal biological processes like embryonic and T-cell development,

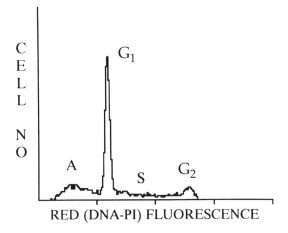

Figure 6.5. A DNA histogram of L1210 lymphoma cells incubated from 18 h in arginine-deficient medium. Label A indicates the sub-G_1 peak from apoptotic cells. (Reproduced from Ormerod, *Flow Cytometry: A Practical Approach* 2nd edn, 1994, by permission of Oxford University Press.)

metamorphosis and hormone-dependent atrophy. It can also be induced by cytotoxic processes, such as irradiation (Blank et al, 1997). The word actually means 'falling leaves' (as in the autumn fall) and can be regarded as a form of cell suicide, or programmed cell death. There is condensation of nuclear chromatin, compaction of cytoplasmic organelles and cell shrinkage. In contrast to necrotic cells, apoptotic cells maintain cell membrane integrity following nuclear fragmentation. The fragmentation of DNA can be measured by flow cytometry. Figure 6.5 shows such a DNA histogram where there is a sub-G_1 peak (labelled A) from apoptotic cells.

Apoptosis involves several tumour suppressor genes, including p53, in normal cells. Normal p53 acts as a 'molecular policeman', monitoring the integrity of the genome (Lane, 1992). If DNA is damaged by irradiation, p53 accumulates and switches off replication (Chapter 2) to allow extra time for it to repair. If the repair fails, however, p53 may trigger cell suicide by apoptosis. In tumour cells, p53 is inactivated by mutation and cannot carry out this p53-dependent process.

The mean lethal dose (D_0) for loss of reproductive capacity (and, remember, this is not death in the absolute sense) is about 1.5 Gy. At that comparatively low dose level, mitotic death is the more common form of death for the majority of mammalian cell types. If, however, an enormous dose of several hundred grays is delivered in one dose to a cell population, then this is such a large physical insult to the biology of the cell that disruption and death occur rapidly by necrosis. Immediate death of this nature is still described as interphase death. It is the sort of death that might occur with a very high temperature or any other physical damage that does not have the discrete effect of ionizing radiation due to the very short wavelength of an X-ray beam. Interphase death is therefore an uncommon phenomenon as far as the main subject matter of this chapter is concerned and will not be discussed any further.

It is because the small lymphocyte does not normally go through a reproductive cycle in the peripheral blood, and dies by apoptosis after irradiation, that alternative assays had to be developed to indicate radiation response. One technique has been used to transform 'T' cells (in the jargon of cell-mediated immunity) so that they go through at least one mitotic cycle, including the period of DNA synthesis. Phytohaemagglutinin (PHA) is used to stimulate the lymphocytes from their resting, or G_0 state. Thymidine labelling of the transformed cells can then provide an index of the degree of transformation, and this index has been found to be depressed if the G_0 cells are irradiated. With this technique a radiation dose–response curve has been obtained for small lymphocytes. (The dose–response curve was biphasic with a mean lethal dose (D_0) of 235 cGy for the sensitive component but 40% of the lymphocytes were very radioresistant; Chamberlain et al, 1980.)

The slope (or D_0 value) of that dose–response curve seems to suggest that lymphocytes are much less radiosensitive than other types of mammalian cell (which have D_0 values around 150 cGy), but this is a misleading comparison because these curves are not *survival* curves in terms of reproductive integrity (one of these will be shown in Figure 6.7 in this chapter). They can only be used as a functional test for comparing the effects of different types of radiation on the DNA synthesis that occurs in lymphocytes during the limited number of cell divisions stimulated by PHA.

There is no equivalent test of the radiation response of cells like the neurones, which cease mitosis from the time of birth and appear to be very resistant to radiation. Damage can be manifest by their behaviour in physiological terms, i.e. changes in action potential all along the nervous fibre, but in terms of loss of function and death they are quite resistant. Quite clearly it is not possible to put the neurone to any test of proliferative capacity.

RADIATION CELL DEATH AND REPRODUCTIVE CAPACITY

For the remainder of this chapter the simple words 'cell death' will be qualified to give the more technical meaning that is applicable to the remaining material of this book. This is concerned with the proliferation of mammalian cells and how this may be impaired by ionizing radiation. Enough has been said in the earlier paragraphs of this chapter to warn the reader that *survival* and *reproductive death* will be commonly used and no

Table 6.1. Classification of damage

No damage	Survival of normal reproductive capacity
Sublethal damage	Survival of normal reproductive capacity after time for recovery
Potentially lethal damage	Survival of normal reproductive capacity after time for recovery in stationary phase
Non-lethal damage	Survival of reproductive capacity, but slow growth
Lethal damage	Loss of reproductive capacity

further apology will be offered when this is no longer emphasized. Instead of using the word 'death' the word 'damage' will be used, as in Table 6.1 where five types of damage are listed, together with the heading 'No damage' for completion's sake.

No damage

It is important to include such a heading of 'No damage' in order to be absolutely clear what is to be regarded as a normal cell in these terms of reference. Every student of biology should be aware of the variations that occur in all biological species and in all cell populations. Operational definitions have to be made and this book is no exception to that. For the purposes of Table 6.1 the definition 'No damage' means that the cell has an indefinite capacity for proliferation and satisfies all the functional tests that are available. It is a convenient assumption to make that if the cell has reproductive integrity then it is normal in all these respects. This is not to say that cells that have no reproductive capacity are not normal in their particular function in the body, as has already been discussed above with the neurones, but reproductive capacity is the present topic of this section.

Sublethal damage

The second category of damage is headed 'Sublethal damage'. This will be discussed in greater detail in Chapter 7. It is a form of damage that is chiefly evident at low dose levels and is shed after the passage of a relatively short period of time; a half-time of 1 h has been found for many cell populations. (But a biphasic pattern is found for some tissues.) After this relatively short period of time, cells that have suffered such sublethal damage and have had the opportunity to repair this damage then have all the characteristics of undamaged cells. This phenomenon is demonstrated by a two-dose experiment.

Potentially lethal damage

This third category of damage will also be described in Chapter 7. Potentially lethal damage is perhaps an unfortunate term because the damage is manifest in those cell populations that are proliferating and well nourished. It is repaired, however, in cells that remain stationary because of some nutritional defect or a lowering of temperature if the cells are in culture. This happens during a relatively short period of time: about the same length of time as applied to the repair of sublethal damage. When such potentially lethal damage has been repaired, more cells will survive. The damage is only lethal if the cells are stimulated to divide during the time interval. The way to test for this potentially lethal damage is to stimulate proliferation and compare cells so stimulated with those that have been allowed to rest for a few hours. The importance of this phenomenon is that tumour cell populations include some cells that are resting (or quiescent) due to some nutritional deficiency, so that the radiation used for treatment may be less effective due to this recovery process.

Non-lethal damage

This fourth category of damage is also a slightly misleading term because damage without lethality is somewhat of a contradiction. The term describes the situation where although some of the cells of an irradiated population have in fact died, some of the others that remain alive have suffered heritable lesions (sometimes called lethal mutations). Although these lesions do not prevent proliferation, they do affect the rate of such proliferation. Such non-lethally damaged cells are also more sensitive to a second treatment with radiation. Non-lethal damage can be observed by clone size analysis (described later in this chapter). More recently, the term *genomic instability* has been used to describe a transmissable chromosomal instability that has been demonstrated in haemopoietic stem cells. This results in a diversity of aberrations in the clonal progeny many cell divisions later, with delayed apoptotic cell death (Kadhim et al, 1995). The phenomenon may be a key feature of the evolution of radiation-induced malignancy (Chapter 19), although the genetic background that produces an apoptotic response may well eliminate potentially leukaemic cells and actually reduce the probability of leukaemogenesis. While genomic instability may lead to increased cancer risk, induced hyper-radiosensitivity (Chapter 8) may have the opposite effect.

Lethal damage

This final heading in Table 6.1 refers again to cell death, but with respect to mitotic death (rather than the interphase death that affects salivary glands, spermatogonial stem cells and lymphocytes), because the radiation doses under consideration here are at more modest levels. Lethal damage is manifest by loss of reproductive integrity, and this will now be described.

LOSS OF REPRODUCTIVE INTEGRITY

In 1955 Puck and Marcus used a culture technique for mammalian cells that had long been used by bacteriologists for assaying the viability of bacterial cells. This involves 'plating' diluted suspensions of bacteria on a surface of nutrient agar in a Petri dish and examining the colonies of bacterial growth that subsequently appear. Puck and Marcus used an equivalent technique with a nutrient medium that would support the growth of mammalian cells. They plated single cells in Petri dishes; these cells attached to the glass surface and those that were viable proliferated to form colonies. The following year they published their classical paper (Puck and Marcus, 1956), which showed that radiation reduced the viability of such mammalian cells in terms of a loss in colony-forming ability (see Chapter 1, Figure 1.1).

Figures 6.6a and 6.6b show examples of this technique in practice. The Petri dish on the left shows a number of black circles. At this low magnification this is the appearance of the colonies that are the progeny of single mammalian cells that have been allowed to grow over a period of 10 days. Each colony may consist of 1000 or more cells but the minimum

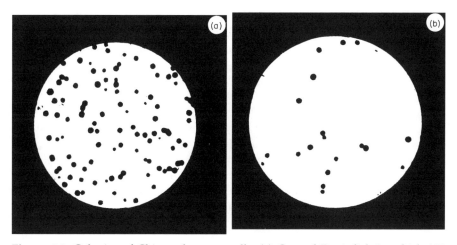

Figure 6.6. Colonies of Chinese hamster cells. (a) Control Petri dish in which 100 single cells were seeded and allowed to proliferate for 5 days before staining. There are 95 colonies, hence 95% plating efficiency. (b) 100 cells were also seeded into this dish, which was then treated with 600 rad of X-rays. There are 19 colonies corresponding to a surviving fraction of $19/95 = 0.2$

requirement for 'survival of colony-forming ability' is usually taken as a 50-cell colony. This will be the result of 5–6 cell divisions; most genetic injury would have been expressed by then.

The Petri dish on the right was seeded with the same number of mammalian cells but these cells had been given a dose of X-rays at the single-cell stage. It is clear that only a small proportion of these single cells were able to grow into colonies that are visible to the naked eye. The consequence of the radiation dose is a loss in the colony-forming ability of the single cells and this is the measure of survival that is used as the index of cell viability or, conversely, cell death.

If a number of Petri dishes are seeded with aliquots of these single cells that have been treated with a range of X-ray doses then a variable number of colonies will result. Taking the Petri dish with the unirradiated cells as the 'control', then the number of colonies there represents 100%, or a surviving fraction of unity. The colony counts from the dishes containing irradiated cells are then compared with this control number and the dose–response is derived in terms of the surviving fractions. Figure 6.7 shows a dose–response curve obtained in this way, with radiation dose plotted on a linear horizontal scale. Because the surviving fraction is plotted on a logarithmic vertical scale, the resultant shape of the radiation dose–response curve is mainly a straight line. Increasing the radiation dose to 2100 cGy results in nearly four decades of exponential decrease in cell survival, down to 10^{-4}. One is accustomed to the precision of physical parameters but it is pleasing to note that biological parameters can also obey precise rules. A detailed discussion of these parameters will be found in Chapter 8.

Radiation dose–response curves like these are used throughout radio-biology nowadays. They provide a basis for comparison of a number of environmental conditions: namely, the irradiation of different cell types and the response of the same cell type to different forms of ionizing radiation. The usual experimental design involves a large number of Petri dishes or screw-capped plastic bottles seeded with aliquots of cells that are irradiated with suitable doses under suitable environmental conditions. The one disadvantage of a technique like this is that the precise fate of each single cell cannot be analysed. Statistical analysis is employed and a reasonable degree of precision is therefore obtainable. If the detailed fate of single cells does need to be followed, then the technique must be much more time consuming and painstaking, namely pedigree analysis.

PEDIGREE ANALYSIS

In this technique a small number of cells is studied by time-lapse cinephotography and the pedigrees obtained are illustrated in Figure 6.8. The number of cells that can be followed in this way is severely limited, of

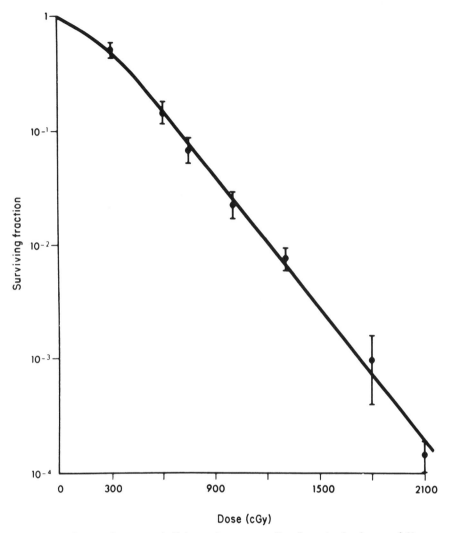

Figure 6.7. Survival curve of Chinese hamster cells after single doses of X-rays. (Reproduced from Nias, 1974, by permission of Simon Fraser University, BC, Canada.)

course, but quite important information can be obtained. Nowadays, an image analysis technique might be used, such as the dynamic microscopic image processing scanner (DMIPS) that was used for the low dose–response data to be shown in Chapter 8 (Figure 8.4).

For the upper pedigree in Figure 6.8 an unirradiated cell has been photographed and six cell divisions have occurred during the 150-h period

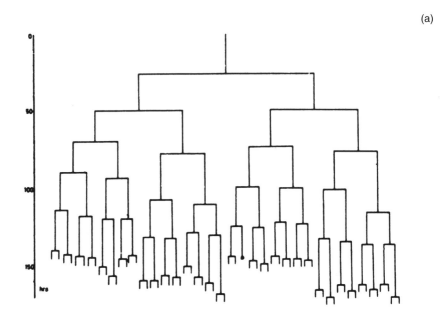

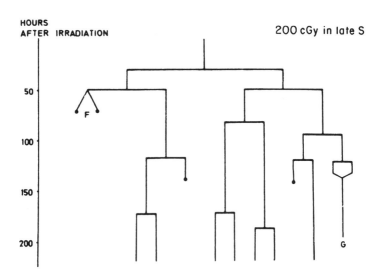

Figure 6.8. Pedigrees of L cells: (a) control cell; (b) cell treated with 200 cGy. F=fragmentation; G=giant cell; and dots indicate cell death. (Reproduced from Trott, 1969, by permission of WILEY–VCH Verlag GmbH, Postfach 10 11 61, DH 69451, Weinheim.)

of observation, with a remarkably uniform division pattern. The mean generation time was 25 h and only one of the progeny has died, so the unirradiated cell has proliferated into a colony of 62 cells (i.e. the cell has 'survived'). By contrast, the lower pedigree shows what happens to a cell after irradiation. Only four divisions have occurred, four cells have died and two have fused to form a giant cell, so there are only seven cells after 200 h (i.e. the irradiated cell has failed the test of 'survival').

Pedigrees like these underline the random nature of radiation effects upon cell populations, including the fact that an irradiated cell may undergo as many as four divisions before mitotic division ceases and also that the variation in the intermitotic time is random. The size of colony from one of these pedigrees is obviously variable and the problem here is that so few of these pedigrees can be obtained in any one period of time. As an alternative, clone size analysis can provide almost the same amount of information.

CLONE SIZE ANALYSIS

In this technique the clones that have been grown in the sort of Petri dishes depicted in Figures 6.6a and 6.6b are examined under a dissecting microscope and the number of cells per clone enumerated. Figure 6.9 shows the clone size distributions after a series of doses given to Chinese hamster cells, as used for Figure 6.7. It shows how the mean clone size decreases with increasing radiation dose. The horizontal scale is expressed in terms of the number of cell divisions. In effect this is the total cell number on a log scale to the base 2. With this technique a clone that has undergone zero cell divisions is of course a giant cell, and there are clearly more giant cells with the larger radiation doses. What is clear from Figure 6.9 is that there is no simple criterion of radiation damage, rather there is a spectrum of damage. Although this is dose dependent, there is no 'all or nothing' effect, which is hardly surprising with a random form of physical damage such as a beam of ionizing radiation.

At the right-hand end of the clone size distribution are the large clones that have grown up from irradiated cells but are indistinguishable from those of unirradiated control cells. The majority of the control cells have completed 6–10 divisions and there are clones of this size after each of the three radiation doses; however, the higher the dose, the fewer the large clones. At the extreme left-hand end of the distribution are the small clones of cells that have divided once or twice and the giant cells that have not divided at all. The higher the radiation dose, the more there are of these very small clones of cells that have not been able to reproduce.

The central part of the distribution consists of clones of intermediate size that have the ability to reproduce but grow very much more slowly than

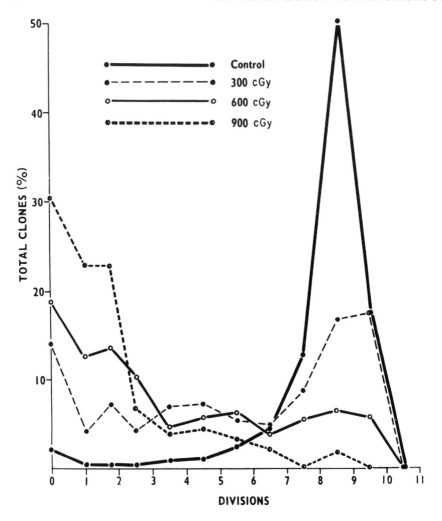

Figure 6.9. Clone size distributions of Chinese hamster cells 5 days after irradiation. (Reproduced from Nias, 1968, by permission of *Cell Tissue Kinet.*)

they would have done before irradiation; these are the progeny of cells that have suffered non-lethal damage. Earlier in this chapter, the term *genomic instability* was used to describe the phenomenon that may be shown to persist *in vivo* for many cell generations.

In vitro, this heritable form of damage is characterized not only by slower growth but by a lowered plating efficiency and an increased sensitivity to repeated treatment. In cell cultures this form of damage is only of importance after a form of treatment that leaves *no* full-size clones in the surviving cell population. (This is shown in Figure 6.11 after drug

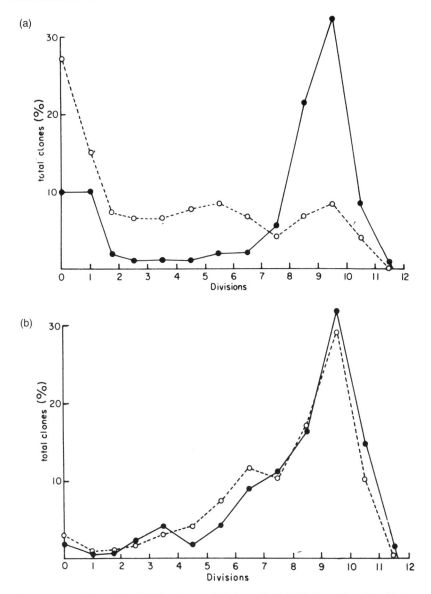

Figure 6.10. Clone size distributions of HeLa cells: (a) 10 days after irradiation with 300 cGy X-rays, (b) same cell populations 10 days after (a). (○) Irradiated; (●) control. (Reproduced from Nias, 1968, by permission of *Cell Tissue Kinet.*)

treatment.) However, the random nature of radiation damage nearly always leaves a few large clones of apparently undamaged cells. Because the large clones (9–10 divisions) each contain about 1000 cells and the small clones (4–5 divisions) only contain about 25 cells, it only needs a few large clones

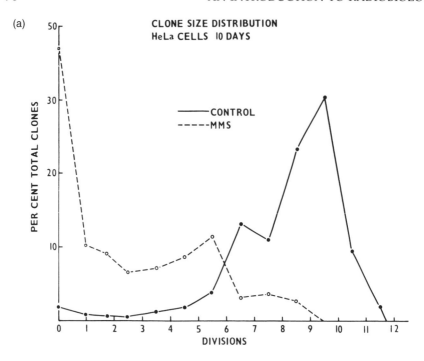

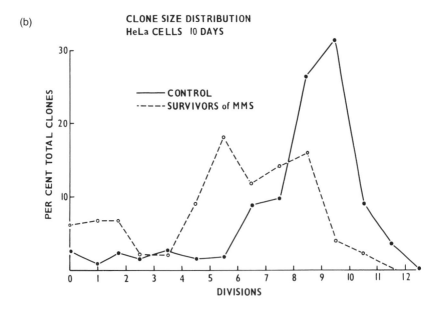

Figure 6.11. Clone size distributions of HeLa cells: (a) 10 days after treatment with MMS (100 µg/ml for 15 min); (b) same cell populations 10 days after (a).

to provide enough undamaged cells to outnumber the more slowly growing non-lethally damaged cells in the small clones.

This is shown by comparing the clone size distributions in Figure 6.10. In the first distribution, HeLa cells were studied 10 days after a dose of 300 cGy and the clone size distribution of these irradiated cells is obviously different from that of the control cells, with a fair number of small clones but also some large clones. The second distribution shows the result after just another 10 days' growth of those two cell populations. By this time there is no longer any difference between the clone size distributions. The progeny of the large clones in Figure 6.10a now predominate in Figure 6.10b and both cell populations are now growing at exactly the same rate. Thus, the non-lethally damaged cells have been diluted out and the end result is only that the total number of cells will be lower in the population that was irradiated 20 days earlier. These cell numbers will be shown as a pair of growth curves in Chapter 7 (Figure 7.3).

By contrast, the clone size distributions in Figure 6.11 show what happens to HeLa cells 10 days after a dose of the monofunctional alkylating agent methyl methane sulphonate (MMS), which has a similar effect on cell survival as 300 cGy. Figure 6.11a shows *no* large clones after MMS treatment. Perhaps not surprisingly, after a further 10 days the survivors of the MMS treatment still do not show the same clone size distribution as the control cells (cf. Figure 6.10b). The cells were probably suffering from 'genomic instability' (described earlier under 'non-lethal damage').

SUMMARY OF CONCLUSIONS

(1) The strict definition of cell death means the loss of all functions and viability.

(2) After modest doses of radiation, however, mammalian cells may lose the capacity to proliferate but remain viable with respect to metabolic functions.

(3) Such cells may become giant in size – up to 20 times the normal volume.

(4) After irradiation some particular cell types may die by apoptosis during interphase, but mitotic death is much more common overall.

(5) Some irradiated cells suffer a non-lethal form of damage, which is the consequence of genomic instability.

(6) Radiobiologists assay the biological effect of a dose of radiation in terms of cell survival, which is defined as the clonogenic capacity of the individual cells.

(7) Pedigree analysis shows that a few divisions of damaged cells may follow a radiation dose, but that a surviving cell can proliferate into a clone containing at least 50 cells.

(8) Clone size analysis shows that the larger the dose, the smaller the average clone. After irradiation, however, some undamaged cells grow into large clones and these cells soon outnumber the damaged cells from small clones.

REFERENCES

Blank, K. R., Rudoltz, M. S., Kao, G. D., Muschel, R. J. and McKenna, W. G., 1997. The molecular regulation of apoptosis and implications for radiation oncology. *International Journal of Radiation Biology*, **71**, 455–466.

Chamberlain, S. M., Kirk, J. and Nias, A. H. W., 1980. Variation in neutron RBE values for human lymphocytes. *International Journal of Radiation Oncology, Biology, Physics*, **6**, 341–344.

Jones, B. and Camplejohn, R. S., 1982. Cell kinetic response of an experimental tumour to irradiation. *Virchows Archiv B*, **40**, 405–410.

Kadhim, M. A., Lorimore, S. A., Townsend, K. M. S., Goodhead, D. T., Buckle, V. J. and Wright, E. G., 1995. Radiation-induced genomic instability: delayed cytogenetic aberrations and apoptosis in primary human bone marrow cells. *International Journal of Radiation Biology*, **67**, 287–293.

Lane, D. P., 1992. p53, guardian of the genome. *Nature*, **358**, 15–16.

Munro, T. R., 1970. The relative radiosensitivity of the nucleus and cytoplasm of Chinese hamster fibroblasts. *Radiation Research*, **42**, 451–470.

Nias, A. H. W., 1968. Clone size analysis: a parameter in the study of cell population kinetics. *Cell and Tissue Kinetics*, **1**, 153–165.

Nias, A. H. W., 1974. The oxygen enhancement ratio of mammalian cells under different irradiation conditions. In *Proceedings of the 5th International Hyperbaric Conference*, Simon Fraser University, BC, Canada, pp. 650–659.

Nias, A. H. W. and Paul, J. 1961. DNA content of giant cells produced by irradiation. *International Journal of Radiation Biology*, **3**, 431–438.

Ormerod, M. G., 1994. *Flow Cytometry. A Practical Approach*, 2nd edn. IRL Press, Oxford.

Puck, T. T. and Marcus, P. I., 1956. Action of X-rays on mammalian cells. *Journal of Experimental Medicine*, **103**, 653–684.

Tolmach, L. J. and Marcus, P. I., 1960. Development of X-ray induced giant HeLa cells. *Experimental Cell Research*, **20**, 350–360.

Trott, K. R., 1969. Mortality rate and recovery in pedigrees of irradiated mammalian cells *in vitro*. *Studia Biophysica*, **18**, 127–135.

7 Reparable Damage

This chapter deals with three types of radiation damage that may have only a temporary effect on cells. They may then recover from these effects and be restored to normal viability. Although the radiation doses involved in these phenomena may also produce lethal damage in some cells, this will be discussed in the next chapter. At this stage it is convenient to make an artificial distinction and only consider what happens to those cells that do *not* lose their viability after undergoing division delay, sublethal damage or potentially lethal damage.

DIVISION DELAY

It was seen in Chapter 2 how cells may be delayed in their progress through the cycle by a chemical such as cytosine arabinoside, which can be used for synchronization (Figure 2.8). The cells are held up at the G_1–S transition point because DNA synthesis is inhibited by the chemical. This chapter deals with a form of division delay that is produced by radiation and is expressed as a delay in progressing through the cell cycle towards mitosis. The period of this division delay is not only radiation dose dependent but also varies with the point in the cell cycle at which the dose is delivered.

Figure 7.1 shows this for synchronized HeLa cells irradiated at different points during their 20-h cycle. The average amount of delay for a full cycle is about 1 min/cGy but the amount varies at different points in the cycle. It is only 0.4 min/cGy when the cells are in the middle of the G_1 phase. At later times there is progressively more delay as cells progress through the S phase until a maximum of 1.4 min/cGy is reached, when cells are irradiated near the end of the cycle in the G_2 phase; G_2 delay is thus the most important.

It is assumed that this division delay process is designed to allow cells time to survey DNA damage before an irreversible commitment to mitosis. This allows either repair of the damage and then resumption of the cell cycle, or removal of irreparable cells by cell death.

The pattern can be explained on the basis of a dose-dependent inhibition of the synthesis of those macromolecules necessary for progress through the cell cycle up to and including mitosis (Warenius, 1997). The particular macromolecules involved are the cyclins and p53 (see Chapter 2). Cyclin B and cdc2 levels are reduced after irradiation in the S phase and this will

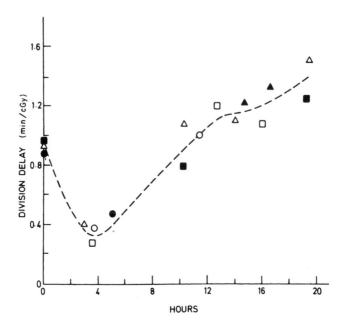

Figure 7.1. Division delay of HeLa cells irradiated at different times after synchronization by mitotic selection. (Reproduced from Terasima and Tolmach, 1963, by permission of Biophysical Society)

lead to G_2 delay. If DNA is damaged in the G_1 phase, p53 accumulates and switches off the cycle to allow time for the cell to repair radiation damage before it enters the S phase. If this repair fails, p53 may trigger cell death by apoptosis. On balance, the result of delaying irradiated cells prior to the G_1 and G_2 check-points will be an increase in survival. Such an increase in survival is also found with cells that are not proliferating when they are irradiated and undergo the process of recovery from potentially lethal damage, PLDR (described later).

Because the G_2 phase is relatively short, there is very little time for such cells to repair this damage and overcome the inhibition of protein synthesis. This is the reason why the duration of division delay is maximal for cells irradiated in the G_2 phase and is less and less evident in cells irradiated during earlier phases of the cell cycle. Damage to cellular targets at these earlier points in the cell cycle can often be repaired in a matter of an hour or so and cells are then more likely to be restored to an apparently normal state before they reach that critical point preceding mitosis. Thus, irradiation has little effect upon the progress of cells from the G_1 phase into the S phase. On the other hand, depression of DNA synthesis may lead to a prolongation of the S phase and this will be more evident in cells irradiated later in the S phase. However, cells irradiated earlier in the S phase will have more time for the damage to be repaired before the end of the cycle, so division delay from that cause remains minimal. Damage to cells irradiated in mitosis is less easily repaired but this will not be manifest until the end of the *subsequent* cell cycle as a prolongation of that G_2 phase.

POSITION OF G_2 BLOCK

Drug studies have been used to determine the position of the X-ray-induced 'G_2 block'. These are shown in Figure 7.2 for three cell lines. Arrows for X-ray, actinomycin D, puromycin and cycloheximide show the positions of the blocks produced by these agents in the cell cycle. All three examples use the same time scale. Example (a) shows HeLa cells blocked by a dose of

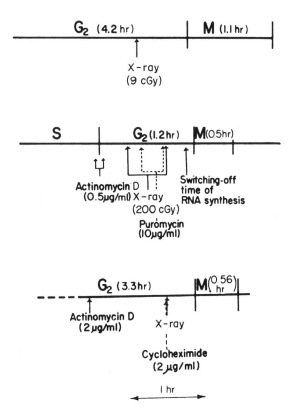

Figure 7.2. The position of the G_2 block: (a) HeLa cells; (b) L5178y mouse leukaemia cells; (c) CHO cells. (Reproduced from Okada, 1970, by permission of Academic Press, Inc.)

only 9 cGy. Example (b) shows L5178Y mouse leukaemic cells to be blocked in the same position either by X-rays or by the protein synthesis inhibitor puromycin, which also inhibits recovery of X-ray-induced block. Example (c) shows a similar finding for Chinese hamster ovarian (CHO) cells where, again, the X-ray block is at the same position as that produced by cycloheximide, another inhibitor of protein synthesis. In both (b) and (c) the drug actinomycin D, which inhibits DNA-dependent RNA synthesis, produces a block at an earlier point in the cycle when the last necessary messenger RNA synthesis occurs. The evidence is very conclusive for a precise point in G_2 where synthesis of a protein is inhibited by radiation.

Recovery from the G_2 block is characterized by the reappearance of mitotic cells; the time required for this to occur provides the measure of radiation-induced division delay. There is a further complication in that the first cells entering mitosis are probably cells recovering from a G_2 block produced by low doses of irradiation. After high doses, the first cells entering mitosis will be those that were in the earlier G_1 and S phases of the cycle at the time of irradiation. These cells, being less sensitive to delay than the later cells, overtake the G_2-blocked cells and enter mitosis before them. This leads to the so-called 'inverse dose rate effect' when irradiation is administered at a lower dose rate (Chapter 17).

In summary, the delay of G_2 cells is mainly due to G_2 block. The delay of S-phase cells is partly due to depression of DNA synthesis and partly due to a prolongation of the G_2 period. The delay of cells irradiated in G_1 does not actually occur in the G_1 phase; it can be expressed as a very slight prolongation of the S phase and a prolongation of G_2. The whole phenomenon of division delay is worthy of study but the total period of delay is short in relation to the length of the cell cycle following doses of a few grays. After higher doses an increasing proportion of cells will suffer lethal damage and then division delay will be almost irrelevant.

The end result of the several mechanisms is illustrated by the growth curves of HeLa cells in Figure 7.3. After 3 Gy, the irradiated cell population continues to increase at the same rate as that of the control cells for the first 2 days. Then there is a slowing in the rate of increase but by the eighth day the growth curve of the irradiated cell population resumes at the same rate as that of the control cells. The inflection in the irradiated cell curve is the result of division delay, together with lethal and non-lethal damage (the latter was shown by clone size analysis in Chapter 6, Figure 6.10). Division delay from 3 Gy will be about 5 h (Figure 7.1); lethal damage will reduce the surviving fraction by 65% and non-lethal damage will result in 50% of slowly growing clones of cells. The dashed line in Figure 7.3 shows the net effect of all these processes in terms of the proportion of the irradiated cell population (19%) that both survives and regrows at the same rate as the control cells. Division delay soon becomes negligible and the slowly growing non-lethally damaged cells eventually become outnumbered by

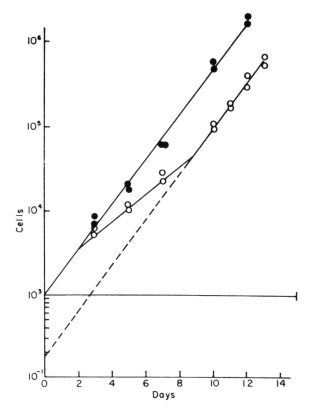

Figure 7.3. Growth curves of HeLa cells after 3 Gy (○); control (●). (Reproduced from Nias, 1968, by permission of *Cell Tissue Kinet.*)

the faster growing cells that have survived normally. These then predominate so that the surviving cell population grows at a normal rate. Only the total number is reduced as a consequence of the radiation.

These surviving cells will not only have recovered from a short period of division delay but they will also have recovered from sublethal and potentially lethal radiation damage. The rest of this chapter will be devoted to this phenomenon and also to potentially lethal damage.

RECOVERY FROM SUBLETHAL DAMAGE

The shape of single-dose radiation cell survival curves will be discussed in greater detail in the next chapter. The 'shoulder' portion of such curves needs to be considered at this stage, however. A shoulder on a survival

curve means that damage must be accumulated for an effect to be
produced. The curve with the closed circles in Figure 7.4 illustrates this
shoulder and the fact that cells that survive doses in the straight-line region
must first have accumulated damage that is sublethal. If the sublethal
damage (SLD) were to become fixed, one would expect the survival curve of
cells irradiated for a second time to lie along the line of that original curve.
In practice, however, the results of irradiating again the survivors of a first
dose of 505 cGy are shown in curves that are displaced upwards from that
original curve: by a smaller amount after a 2.5-h interval and by a larger
amount after 23 h.

Because the width of the shoulder of a survival curve provides a measure
of the capacity of the cells for SLD, changes in the width can be used to
measure changes in this capacity. Upward extrapolation from the straight
part of the survival curve to the vertical axis provides an 'extrapolation
number' (N) that is 6.8 for the main curve in Figure 7.4. The curve for cells

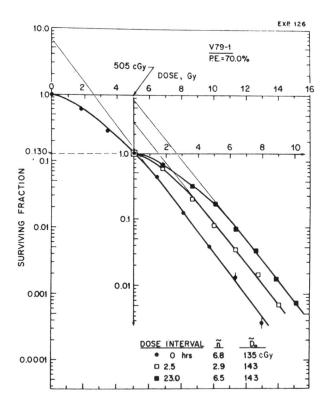

Figure 7.4. Single and fractionated dose–response curves of V79 cells. (Reproduced
from Elkind and Sutton, 1960, by permission of Academic Press, Inc.)

given second doses of irradiation after a 2.5-h interval extrapolates to 3, while the extrapolation number for the curve after 23 h has risen back to the initial value of 6.8. The slope of the straight part of all these curves (defined as D_0 in the next chapter) has a very similar value. One can therefore conclude from this example that after 2.5 h the cells that survive the first dose have resumed half their capacity for SLD and by 23 h the cells have survived as though they had never been irradiated, and have a full capacity for SLD. The shoulder has been reconstructed!

The extra dose required amounts to the size of the reconstructed shoulder. For a given biological effect (such as reduction to a surviving fraction of 0.01) the single dose required will be D_1, while the total dosage required from two doses will be D_2. The dose increment is then $D_2 - D_1$. This value is the same as D_q, the quasi-threshold dose (defined in Chapter 8), which is one parameter for describing the size of the shoulder. This D_q might loosely be called the 'wasted' radiation before the more effective exponential dose–response becomes operative. Some values of D_q for mouse cell populations are shown in Table 7.1.

Some mammalian cells have a broad shoulder on their survival curves and split-dose experiments then show a considerable amount of repair of SLD. Other types of cell show only a small shoulder on their survival curves and much less repair of SLD. If the shape of the curves is described by the linear quadratic equation $-\alpha/\beta$ (see Chapter 8), then it is the quadratic component that causes the curve to bend and results in the sparing effect of a split dose. If a survival curve has a large shoulder, there will be a small α/β ratio because β is more important than α, and vice versa. Some d/β ratios are shown at the end of this chapter, in Table 7.2.

An example of the time course of such recovery from sublethal damage (SLDR) is shown in Figure 7.5 for cells held at either 37 °C or 24 °C during various time intervals between fixed first and second doses of X-rays. The curve for 37 °C shows a prompt increase in survival at 0.5 h and this rises to a maximum by 2 h, when there is an increase in survival similar to that shown after 2.5 h in Figure 7.4. After this maximum the 37 °C curve then

Table 7.1. Recovery capacity of mouse cells

Cell type	D_q (cGy)
Normal bone marrow	100
Leukaemic bone marrow	115
Mammary carcinoma	230
Osteosarcoma	280
Skin	350
Intestine	450
Stomach	550

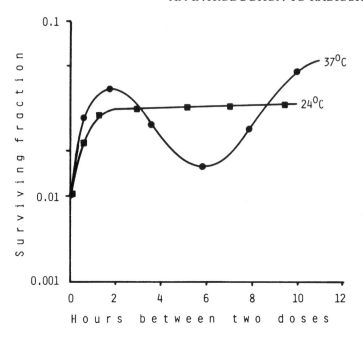

Figure 7.5. Time course of survival of V79 cells irradiated with a first dose at zero time and a second dose at increasing time intervals at 37 °C and at 24 °C. (Reproduced from Elkind et al, 1965, by permission of Academic Press, Inc.)

drops to a minimum value at about 6 h and this might be thought to mean some loss of the ability of cells to recover from SLD.

The 24 °C curve shows the true situation. At this reduced temperature there is still an immediate increase in survival during the first hour between two doses of X-rays, although the rise appears slower and the increase is less. There is no subsequent fall to a minimum value, however.

The pattern of survival at 37 °C is the result of the combined effect of SLDR and progression of cells through the phases of the cell cycle. An unirradiated population of cells will normally be asynchronous and be distributed through all the phases of the cycle. Radiosensitivity and radioresistance vary throughout the cycle, however (Chapter 8), and so the first dose of radiation will preferentially kill cells that are in the more sensitive phases. Those that survive will be in the more radioresistant phases and so will become partially synchronized. They will also have suffered SLD, from which they will recover during the next few hours. Recovery leads to increased survival but as time goes on such previously radioresistant cells will progress into the more radiosensitive phases of the cell cycle by the time of the second dose of radiation.

These opposing effects will thus lead first to the maximum and then to the minimum survival level. The surviving cells will also suffer division delay due to the first dose of irradiation. Finally, they will undergo division and the surviving fraction will rise again after 6 h as shown in Figure 7.5. The curve for cells maintained at 24 °C shows what happens when there is no progression through the sensitive and resistant phases of the cell cycle, so that the minimum and subsequent rise in survival is not seen. The initial rise represents SLDR, uncomplicated by progression.

Figures 7.4 and 7.5 apply to asynchronous populations of cells. The question arises: what happens to cells given first doses of irradiation at different stages in the cell cycle and do they also recover from SLD? The answer is provided in Figure 7.6, which shows the two-dose response in synchronized cells given a first dose at four points in the cycle: at 2.5 h (G_1), 7 h (early S), 10.6 h (late S) and 13 h (G_2). In all four cases there is an immediate rise in survival. The effect appears to be greatest in S-phase cells but it also occurs in G_1 and G_2 cells. In summary, cells show SLDR throughout their cycle, but more in the S phase.

REPAIR MECHANISM

The action of radiation on living cells used to be explained by various *target theories* (Lea, 1955). These included mathematical models such as the single-hit multi-target equation, which happens to fit the majority of mammalian cell survival curves, and the linear-quadratic equation, which can be used for the shoulder portion of curves (Chapter 8). They assumed that the shoulder is primarily due to the interaction of sublethal lesions or the accumulation of SLD. By contrast, the *repair model* (Alper, 1984) assumes that the shoulder is the result of the repair of single lesions produced by small amounts of radiation energy over small distances (i.e. single tracks) in proportion to the dose. The model presumes that lesions produced by X-radiation can be repaired by a process that becomes saturated with increasing dose. This saturable repair mechanism was sometimes called Q repair (of SLD) in contrast to P repair (of potentially lethal damage, PLD).

The most important lesions in cellular radiobiology take the form of point mutations (i.e. changes in the molecular structure of the DNA genetic material) and these occur at a rate that is directly proportional to the dose of radiation. The lesions will include changes in the bases of the nucleic acid, breakage in the continuity of the strands of the double helix and abnormal cross-links formed in the DNA or between it and cellular proteins. The most important lesion for lethality is the double-strand break (Chapter 5), in which the structure of the DNA is interrupted at about the same position in both strands. This will be lethal if it is not repaired.

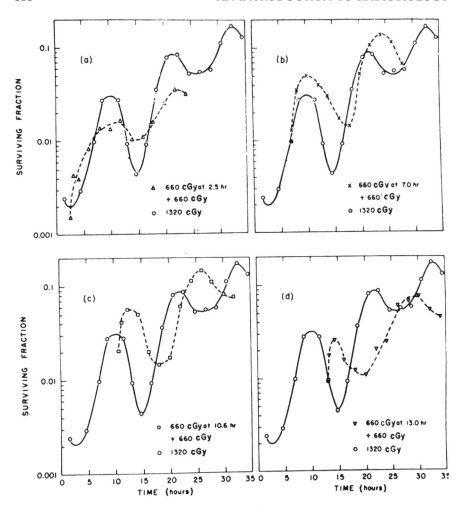

Figure 7.6. Two-dose response of synchronized V79 cells. The solid line shows the response to a single dose of 1320 cGy. The dotted lines show the response to a first dose of 660 cGy given at the four times and then followed by second doses of 660 cGy given at increasing time intervals thereafter. (a) 2.5 h, (b) 7 h, (c) 10.6 h, (d) 13 h. (Reproduced from Sinclair, 1964, by permission of The Genetics Society of Japan.)

Single-strand breaks are much less of a problem because a gap with clean ends can be filled by the action of DNA polymerase and then one of the DNA ligases joins the ends. The defective region in the damaged strand is returned to its original form by relying on the complementary information stored in the unaffected strand.

Things are not so simple in the case of a double-strand break (dsb). Even if the ends are clean, a simple ligation must lead to a change in sequence because damaged bases will have been removed. Even a very efficient repair system may lead to the accumulation of mutations. There are certain genetic diseases where the cells are defective in enzyme repair functions (e.g. ataxia telangiectasia) and such cells can be three times more radiosensitive than normal repair-proficient cells. Some lesions may be misrepaired and the resultant non-lethal damage may lead to the induction of cancer (Chapter 19).

Molecular biologists have cloned genes related to DNA repair that are mutated in some radiosensitive cell lines. This work has led to the discovery of a number of repair genes: XRCCl was the first to be cloned in 1990 and this gene produces a protein that is important in the repair of single-strand breaks; XRCC5 produces the Chinese hamster version of the human Ku86 protein and the human A–T (ataxia telangiectasia) protein, which are involved in damage recognition and repair of double-strand breaks. This work has provided a putative mechanism for dsb repair that involves a protein complex (PK) consisting of three components: Ku86, DNA–PK catalytic subunit (DNA–PKcs) and Ku70. Under normal circumstances these three proteins do not join together into the DNA–PK complex, but when they encounter a radiation double-strand break, Ku70 and Ku86 form a heterodimer that binds to the DNA end, recruiting DNA–PKcs and activating the complex. The activated DNA–PK complex then phosphorylates down-stream proteins and the dsb ends are rejoined by ligation (Gordon and McMillan, 1997).

In the past, the use of inhibitors of DNA, RNA and protein synthesis showed that only the RNA inhibitor actinomcyin D had any effect on recovery. This is shown in Figure 7.7 by the considerable reduction in the shoulder of the survival curve for cells irradiated after treatment with a dose of actinomycin D. The cells were synchronized at the G_1–S border by the chemical method (using hydroxyurea) and then irradiated 4 h later when they would have progressed towards the end of the S phase. The next chapter will show that cells are most radioresistant at this point in the cell cycle and that this radioresistance takes the form of a large shoulder on the survival curve. The size of the shoulders of the curves in Figure 7.7 is shown by the D_q dose, which is 595 cGy for the right-hand curve. The left-hand curve has a much smaller shoulder, with a D_q of 170 cGy. (In terms of the linear-quadratic model, the curves would have smaller and larger α/β ratios, respectively.) Clearly the treatment with actinomycin D has reduced the capacity of the cells for sublethal damage.

The biophysical relationship between the density of ionization and radiobiology will be discussed in Chapter 9 but in this present chapter it is only necessary to remember that the lethal lesions of low-LET radiation are produced by an energy deposition of about 100 eV within a moderate

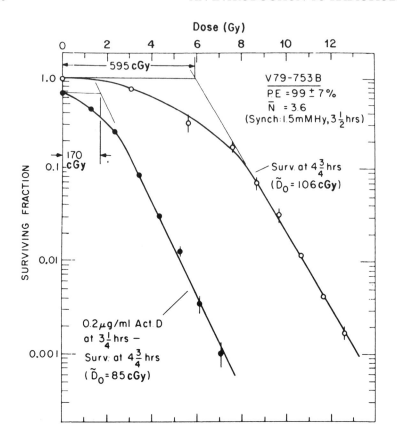

Figure 7.7. Effect of actinomycin D on the dose–response curve of synchronized V79 cells in the S phase. (Reproduced from Elkind and Redpath, 1977, by permission of Plenum Press.)

cluster of about 2 nm diameter (Chapter 5), and that these lesions can be repaired. By contrast, the dominant lesions produced by high-LET radiation involve energies of about 400 eV within a large cluster of 5–10 nm, and these lesions are *not* repairable (see Chapter 9). It is for this reason that the more densely ionizing the radiation, the smaller the shoulder on the survival curve and the less the recovery from SLD.

It has already been shown that recovery proceeds quite well at a reduced temperature and it will be shown in Chapter 10 that oxygen must be reduced to a minimal level before recovery is inhibited. Further light will be shed upon this question by considering the other mechanism of recovery, from potentially lethal damage. The two phenomena will be seen to be related in part.

RECOVERY FROM POTENTIALLY LETHAL DAMAGE

This other form of recovery, from potentially lethal damage (PLD), occurs in cell populations that are not actively proliferating. These would be tissues with a negligible growth fraction (Chapter 3), which will include many tumours but also some normal tissues. Recovery from PLD (PLDR) has been demonstrated in cell cultures that have been allowed to grow into a densely crowded 'plateau phase' when they stop proliferating. A series of radiation doses is delivered and if the cells are then diluted and plated out in fresh growth medium straight away, for the usual assay of proliferative capacity, then a typical response curve for single doses is found. If, however, the cells are left in plateau phase for 6–12 h without medium change before being plated out, the survival curve is flatter (Figure 7.8), i.e. survival is increased. (With medium change, the cells resume proliferation and there is no PLDR.) With PLDR, the amount of recovery is dose dependent: the higher the dose, the more the recovery (in contrast to SLDR).

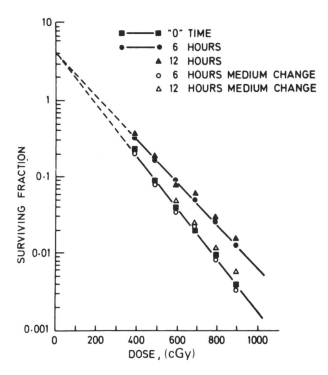

Figure 7.8. Survival curves for plateau-phase cells with varying delays after irradiation. (Reproduced from Hahn and Little, 1973, by permission of Elsevier Science-NL, Sara Burgerhartstraat 25, 1055 KV Amsterdam, The Netherlands.)

The D_0 values of these two curves are 1.25 Gy without recovery and 1.55 Gy with recovery, and the two curves extrapolate back to the same number.

The phenomenon can easily be demonstrated in tissue cultures, which can be manipulated to mimic non-growth fractions found *in vivo*. Thus, cells growing exponentially at 37 °C do not recover from PLD, which is 'fixed' within a few minutes at that temperature. By contrast, if the same cells are cooled down to 20 °C and held at that temperature, the damage is not fixed and recovery occurs. Thus the damage is only potentially lethal, although it can be expected to be lethal in a proliferating tissue at 37 °C. Recovery also occurs if the normal progression of cells through the cycle is inhibited in any other way, such as by incubating them in balanced salt solution instead of complete culture medium, or if certain metabolic inhibitors are used, such as the protein synthesis inhibitor cycloheximide.

Clearly PLDR is dose dependent, unlike SLDR, which is dose independent over a wide range of doses. But although the two forms of recovery are different, they may be additive under appropriate conditions. A special technique is needed to enable the study of the two different recovery phenomena. Figure 7.9 shows the result of comparing the survival of cells kept for a 20-min period in hypertonic saline (0.5 M) with that of cells kept for 20 min in isotonic saline (0.14 M). The two survival curves with open symbols show the result of this comparison after single doses of irradiation. Cells placed in hypertonic saline cannot repair potentially lethal damage but cells in isotonic saline can do so during the 20-min period.

The two survival curves with closed symbols show cell survival after second doses of irradiation have been delivered 2 h after the first dose. In each case the shoulder is 'reconstructed' and the exponential curve shows a displacement typical of complete SLDR. Figure 7.9 thus shows that SDLR and PLDR can be independent phenomena under these particular conditions, but can also be combined. The final amount of radiation damage may vary between the two extremes shown by the survival curves.

In the case of stationary cell populations the uppermost curve will apply after two doses of irradiation and the next curve after only one. In the case of growing cell populations the lower two curves apply: the lowest after single doses of irradiation and the other one after two doses separated by a time interval of 2 h.

HALF-TIME OF RECOVERY

Such time intervals are best considered in terms of 'half-time', i.e. a time interval after which half the damage has been repaired. In terms of DNA damage, the various biochemical techniques described in Chapter 5 showed the initial rate of dsb rejoining to have a half-time of 10–12 min after a dose of 25 Gy and 15–20 min after 50 Gy (Iliakis et al, 1991). The premature

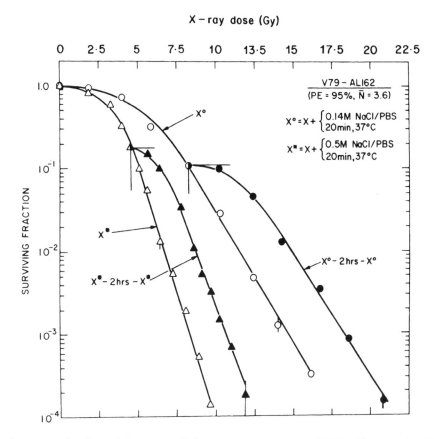

Figure 7.9. Single and fractionated dose–response curves of V79 cells treated with isotonic or hypertonic saline. (Reproduced from Utsumi and Elkind, 1979, by permission of Academic Press, Inc.)

chromosome condensation (PCC) technique for measuring the rate of rejoining of chromatin breaks showed the much longer half-time of 87 min. These were measured using plateau-phase Chinese hamster ovarian (CHO) cells.

At the cellular level, the time course of recovery from radiation damage follows the sort of exponential curve shown in Figure 7.5, where the precise time of completion of the process is uncertain but the half-time can be measured with more confidence. In that example the half-time for repair of SLD was about 1 h. A similar half-time applies to the *repair* of PLD. The half-time for *fixation* of PLD is only 2 min, however, when proliferating cells are maintained at 37 °C immediately after irradiation. If they are cooled to 20 °C the fixation of potentially lethal lesions is inhibited and the damage can be repaired.

These half-times apply to the examples shown in this chapter where cells were examined *in vitro*. In the case of tissues *in vivo*, however, recovery can be a slower process with a biphasic pattern of short and long half-lives. Table 7.2 shows such half-lives reported for various animal tissues (together with the α/β ratios that apply to such tissues). (In the tumour example to be shown in Chapter 10, Figure 10.13, the first maximum was not reached until 6 h after the first dose.) Table 7.2 also shows examples of smaller and larger values of α/β ratio, implying a larger or smaller capacity for repair of SLD.

Cells irradiated in the G_1 phase can repair both forms of damage but the amount of PLD repair is only half that of SLD repair in the case of S-phase cells. Mitotic cells can neither repair PLD nor accumulate SLD. The consequence of this difference between the radiosensitivity of cells irradiated in the different phases of the cell cycle will be demonstrated in the next chapter in terms of their cell survival curves.

SUMMARY OF CONCLUSIONS

(1) Even modest doses of radiation may reduce cell survival but in certain cases radiation may have only a temporary effect from which cells may recover.
(2) Cells will be delayed by radiation in their progress through the division cycle. On average, division delay amounts to 1 min per cGy but cells irradiated in the G_2 phase suffer more delay and G_1 cells suffer less delay.
(3) Sublethal damage (SLD) can be shown to explain the shoulder on a cell survival curve. All cells can recover from SLD with a half-time of about 1 h *in vitro*, but longer *in vivo* with a biphasic pattern. Repair inhibitors may delay this.

Table 7.2. Parameters for biphasic repair of sublethal damage

Tissue	α/β Ratio	Repair half-life	
		Short (min)	Long (h)
Mouse kidney	2.1	9	5
Pig skin	5.19	10.2	5.38
Mouse lung	4.01	19.2	1.92
Rat spinal cord	2.0	42	3.8

Adapted from Canney and Millar, 1997, by permission of BIR.

(4) The amount of repair of SLD is correlated with the size of the shoulder of a cell survival curve, expressed either as the D_q or the α/β ratio.

(5) Molecular mechanisms have been described for the repair of DNA double-strand breaks.

(6) Cells that are not proliferating at the time they are irradiated will recover from damage that is potentially lethal. Potentially lethal damage (PLD) is rapidly fixed by proliferating cells, however, with a half-time of only 2 min.

(7) Both SLD and PLD can be shown to be independent phenomena.

REFERENCES

Alper, T., 1984. Implications of repair models for LET effects and other radio-biological phenomena. *British Journal of Cancer*, **49** (Suppl. VI), 137–143.

Canney, P. A. and Millar, W. T., 1997. Biphasic cellular repair and implications for multiple field radiotherapy treatments. *British Journal of Radiology*, **70**, 817–822.

Elkind, M. M. and Redpath, J. L., 1977. Molecular and cellular biology of radiation lethality. In *Cancer: A Comprehensive Treatise*, Vol. 6, edited by F. F. Becker. Plenum Press, New York, pp. 51–99.

Elkind, M. M. and Sutton, H., 1960. Radiation response of mammalian cells grown in culture. 1. Repair of X-ray damage in surviving Chinese hamster cells. *Radiation Research*, **13**, 556–593.

Elkind, M. M., Sutton-Gilbert, H., Moses, W. B., Alescio, T. and Swain, W., 1965. Radiation response of mammalian cells grown in culture. V. Temperature dependence of the repair of X-ray damage in surviving cells (aerobic and hypoxic). *Radiation Research*, **25**, 359–376.

Gordon, A. T, and McMillan, T. J., 1997. A role for molecular radiobiology in radiotherapy? *Clinical Oncology*, **9**, 70–78.

Hahn, G. M. and Little, J. B., 1973. Plateau-phase cultures of mammalian cells: an *in vitro* model for human cancer. *Current Topics in Radiation Research*, **8**, 39–83.

Iliakis, G., Blocher, D., Metzger, L. and Pantelias, G., 1991. Comparison of DNA double-strand break rejoining as measured by pulsed field gel electrophoresis, neutral sucrose gradient centrifugation and non-unwinding filter elution in irradiated plateau-phase CHO cells. *International Journal of Radiation Biology*, **59**, 927–939.

Lea, D. E., 1955. *Actions of Radiations on Living Cells*, 2nd edn. Cambridge University Press, Cambridge.

Nias, A. H. W., 1968. Clone size analysis: a parameter in the study of cell population kinetics. *Cell and Tissue Kinetics*, **1**, 153–165.

Okada, S., 1970. *Radiation Biochemistry*, vol. 1, Academic Press, London, p. 227.

Sinclair, W., 1964. Survival and recovery after x-irradiation of synchronized Chinese hamster cells in culture. *Japanese Journal of Genetics*, **40**, supplement 141–161.

Terasima, T. and Tolmach, L. J., 1963. Variations in several responses of HeLa cells to x-irradiation during the division cycle. *Biophysical Journal*, **3**, 11–33.

Utsumi, H. and Elkind, M. M., 1979. Potentially lethal damage versus sublethal damage: Independant repair processes in actively growing Chinese hamster cells. *Radiation Research*, **77**, 346–360.

Warenius, H. M., 1997. A cycle made for two. *British Journal of Radiology*, **70**, 125–129.

8 Intrinsic Radiosensitivity

This chapter will describe the way in which the radiosensitivity of *individual cells* is determined. The radiosensitivity of tissues and individuals will be discussed in later chapters.

When Puck and Marcus plotted their values for surviving fraction against radiation dose, they found the dose–response curve shown in Figure 8.1. The shape of this curve is characteristic for X-radiation, i.e. it is the sort of dose response that would apply to conventional radiotherapy. After an initial shoulder region, the larger the dose on a linear scale, the smaller the surviving fraction on a logarithmic scale. This exponential relationship has been found for all mammalian tissues in which it has been possible to test the radiation response of the constituent cells by some quantitative method. This means that larger tumours require larger doses of radiotherapy to cure them, assuming that every single tumour cell must be 'sterilized'. The fact that the normal-tissue tolerance dose is smaller for larger volumes is an unfortunate limitation in radiotherapy in view of this theoretical requirement for a larger tumour dose. Be that as it may, the essential feature of survival curves for mammalian cells is their exponential shape following the initial shoulder region when X-rays are used.

The curve in Figure 8.1 illustrates the response of cells to *single* doses of radiation. The response of cells in a tissue to a dose fractionated over several weeks will depend upon a number of factors (Chapter 16), including the size of the individual fraction doses. The biological effect of these doses can be predicted from the cell survival curves obtained with those cell populations that are relevant to the clinical problem.

The usual method of comparison between such curves is by describing their shape using the two parameters D_0 and N (Figure 8.2). Parameter D_0 describes the slope of the exponential portion of the curve after the initial shoulder, and it is the dose (in cGy) required to reduce the surviving fraction to a value of $1/e$ (where e is the exponential function), which equals 0.37. Thus, D_0 is the mean lethal dose for that cell population and the value can be read off the graph as the extra dose required to reduce survival from 10% to 3.7% or from 1% to 0.37%. The dose required to reduce survival from 100% to 37% might be called D_{37} but this is a misleading parameter because it includes the shoulder portion of the curve.

The size of the shoulder of a cell survival curve is described by extrapolating the exponential portion upwards to the vertical axis of the graph (Figure 8.2). This point on that logarithmic scale is then called, quite

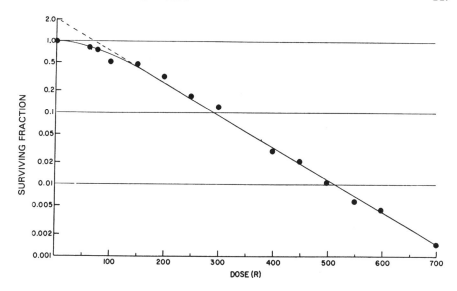

Figure 8.1. Radiation dose–response of human cancer cells *in vitro*. (Reproduced from Puck and Marcus, 1956, by copyright permission of The Rockefeller University Press.)

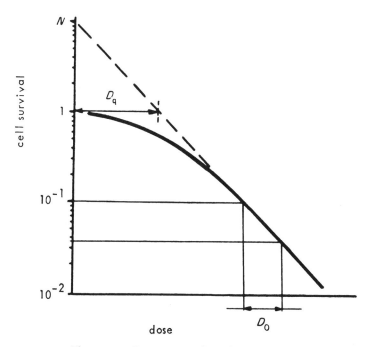

Figure 8.2. Parameters of a cell survival curve.

Table 8.1. Parameters of cell survival curves (aerated cells after 300 kV irradiation)

Cell	N	D_0 (cGy)	Coefficient of initial slope
CHO	3.24 ± 0.36	193 ± 7.4	0.106 ± 0.04
HeLa	3.22 ± 0.23	150 ± 3.5	0.48 ± 0.24

Reproduced from Nias and Gilbert, 1975, by permission of John Wiley & Sons, Inc.

simply, the extrapolation number, N. The point where this extrapolated line crossed the horizontal axis (at 100% survival) may be described as the quasi-threshold dose D_q (in cGy). This may loosely be considered as an amount of 'wasted' radiation attributable to sublethal damage (Chapter 7), for that cell population, after a large dose has been given.

The shapes of cell survival curves can thus be compared using the parameter D_0 to describe the exponential slope and either of the parameters N or D_q to describe the extent of the shoulder. Most mammalian-cell X-ray survival curves have D_0 values between 100 and 200 cGy, extrapolation numbers between 1 and 5 and D_q values between 50 and 250 cGy (see Table 8.1). The curve shown in Figure 8.1 has typical values, with $D_0 = 100$ cGy, $N = 2$ and $D_q = 65$ cGy.

Later in this chapter it will be seen that the shoulders of survival curves for tissues tend to be larger than those for single cells but that the final slope, D_0, remains the same for a particular cell type. The D_0 value can be regarded as a measure of the *intrinsic* radiosensitivity of that cell population, whereas the clinical radiosensitivity depends also upon the size of the shoulder and the cellular environment.

Because it is not always possible to obtain the full extent (particularly a final slope) of a survival curve for cells taken from human tissues, an alternative parameter is sometimes used: the *mean inactivation dose*, $\bar{D}$ (Fertil et al, 1984). This is derived from the area under the whole survival curve and is 'the average dose to kill a cell' (averaged over all doses). By contrast, D_0 is derived from the exponential slope of a survival curve and is 'the dose to kill an average cell' over that range of doses. The D parameter is useful for comparing the radiosensitivity of human cell lines (see Chapter 12).

TARGET THEORY

Except for the shoulder portion, the mammalian survival curve is exponential in shape. A survival curve for virus particles is entirely exponential, with no shoulder at all. This implies a random process of cell killing, which is to be expected from the random distribution of ionization. The original target theory proposed that there are critical sites in cells that must be hit if the cell is to be killed. Exponential survival curves would then be expected if a single hit in a single target is sufficient to cause cell death (as with viruses). Most survival curves for mammalian cells do not fit such a simple exponential shape, however, and some form of multi-event model had to be proposed. The old nomenclature of 'hits' and 'targets' can now be changed to the nomenclature used to explain chromosome aberrations (Chapter 5) in terms of lesions in the DNA produced by one or more ionizing tracks. Nevertheless, it may be of interest to describe the three classical models:

(1) The simple multi-target model suggests that there are two or more targets in a cell that must each receive a single hit before the cell is killed. The model is described by the algebraic equation:

$$f = 1 - (1 - e^{D/D_0})^N$$

where f is the surviving fraction after a dose D, D_0 is the mean lethal dose and N is the extrapolation number. The model can also make an assumption that N is the number of targets that must be hit. This seemed appropriate for Figure 8.1, where the curve extrapolates to the whole-number 2 and it is reasonable to think in terms of two strands of DNA as targets. Unfortunately, most curves do not extrapolate to whole numbers nor to multiples of two. Furthermore, the simple multi-target model implies a zero slope to the curve at zero dose, and most survival curves have a detectable initial slope as in Figure 8.1.

(2) The best fit for most curves is obtained by an equation that combines the simple multi-target model with a single-event component. This gives the initial slope at low doses and then the final exponential slope. The equation for this is:

$$f = e^{-D/D_1} [1 - (1 - e^{-D/D_2})]^N$$

where D_1 and D_2 refer to the initial and final slopes.

Figure 8.3 compares the curves that fit these first two models, where the important difference lies in the presence or absence of an initial slope. It has to be said that the radiobiological data are not always accurate enough to make the distinction. However, the data nearly always give the best fit to an exponential final slope and this is not in accord with the third model, which is represented by the linear quadratic equation:

$$f = e^{-(\alpha D + \beta D^2)}$$

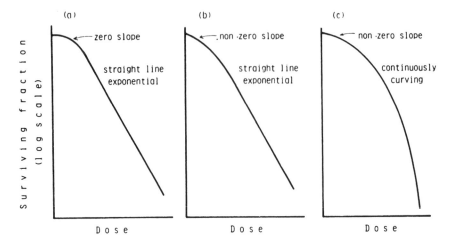

Figure 8.3. Three of the models used to fit the survival data when mammalian cells are treated with single doses of X-rays: (a) multi-target; (b) multi-target plus single hit component; (c) linear-quadratic. (Reproduced from Coggle, 1983, by permission of Taylor & Francis.)

where α and β determine the relative importance of single-hit and two-hit events. There is a continuously bending survival curve that has the expected initial slope but it never becomes exponential, even at high doses.

(3) The linear-quadratic α/β model has been applied to iso-effect data, which have an important bearing on the tolerance of normal tissues to the fractionation regimes of dose and time used in radiotherapy (discussed in Chapter 16, Figure 16.12). Nevertheless, cell survival data do not really support application of the α/β model because most survival curves do not fit the linear-quadratic equation. The first ever survival curve for mammalian cells in 1956 (Figure 8.1) shows nearly two logarithmic decades of exponential data, and my own data have extended over four decades (see Chapter 6, Figure 6.6). The evidence did not fit the continuous curve required by the linear-quadratic model. On the other hand, individual doses of fractionated radiotherapy lie more frequently over the low-dose range (i.e. the shoulder portion) of survival curves, so it may be reasonable to apply the model in so far as it fits that *initial* range of survival data. (See Chapter 16 for a discussion of the use of the model in radiotherapy.)

Because one of the most important radiobiological mechanisms that applies to fractionated radiotherapy is recovery from radiation damage (Chapter 7), which is related to the shoulder of the survival curve, it is important to establish an alternative to the target models that can be applied to the biological data. The three models assumed that the shoulder arises primarily from physical considerations, such as the accumulation of 'sublethal' damage or the interaction of sublethal lesions, so either one sensitive site had to be 'hit' twice or more, or one 'hit' had to occur in two or more sensitive sites within the cell.

However, there is increasing evidence that neither of these target theories is valid because lethal damage occurs with very soft X-rays (< 1 keV). These produce single-electron tracks, which are so short that it is difficult to assume interaction between separate sublethal events (see 'Target size' in Chapter 5). Although the majority of chromosome aberrations involve two lesions in the DNA, both of these lesions can be produced by one ionizing track or, alternatively, the two lesions can be produced by independent tracks. An exchange, like a dicentric, can be either a 'one-track' or a 'two-track' aberration and this determines the shape of the survival curve.

With the low-LET radiations considered in this chapter, the majority of exchanges are two-track at higher doses. Their predominance tends to decrease as the dose, or the dose rate, is lowered. This explains the shoulder on the curves. With high-LET radiations (Chapter 9), ionization density in the tracks ensures that in all cases both lesions are always produced by the same track. Hence, their survival curves are linear and there is no dose rate effect (see Chapter 17 for dose rate effects).

Another explanation for the shape of the cell survival curves for X-radiation was the *repair model* (discussed in Chapter 7), which assumed that all survival curves were one-hit exponentials but that the shoulder was the result of some dose-dependent repair process (e.g. a pool of repair enzymes or radical-scavenging molecules) that may have a limited capacity. As the radiation dose increased, the process became saturated and its efficiency decreased. Perhaps the DNA–PK complex of proteins involved in the repair of DNA strand breaks (Gordon and McMillan, 1997), also described in Chapter 7, is a candidate for the so-called 'repair substance' required by the repair model.

THE INITIAL SLOPE OF SURVIVAL CURVES

The precise shape of the shoulder portion of mammalian cell survival curves is not always known for certain. This is because, unlike the curve shown in Figure 8.1, the majority of the mammalian cell survival curves published in the radiobiological literature are derived from biological data where survival has been measured over the higher range of dosage, where an exponential dose–response is to be expected. There are fewer data for lower dose levels where the 'shoulder' portion of a survival curve is found. In the absence of 'shoulder' data the existence of an initial slope can only be inferred from the shape of the exponential portion of the survival curve, and there is obvious uncertainty. When cell survival has been measured after low doses, however, there may still be some uncertainty due to the fact that the biological assay system contains small errors. At the lowest dosage where survival is highest, it may not be possible to demonstrate a surviving fraction that is significantly lower than unity.

There is evidence, however, that very low radiation doses (or dose rates) are more effective per unit dose than larger doses. This *low-dose hypersensitivity* (HRS) occurs with doses up to 30 cGy. With higher doses, by contrast, the opposite mechanism occurs and there is *induced radioresistance* (IRR). Figure 8.4 shows data obtained by a DMIPS (dynamic microscopic image processing scanner) with Chinese hamster cells irradiated with X-rays or neutrons. The inset in the figure shows this HRS/IRR phenomenon very clearly with X-rays and also shows that it does not occur with neuron irradiation. The HRS/IRR phenomenon has also been shown to apply *in vivo* with skin, kidney and lung in fractionated radiotherapy (Chapter 16) when very small doses per fraction are used (Joiner et al, 1996). If a small conditioning dose (below 30 cGy) is first given, cells are protected from the HRS phenomenon so there is an adaptive mechanism, possibly associated with the amount and rate of DNA repair.

Most earlier studies used doses of 50 cGy and above, so that the HRS/IRR phenomenon could not be seen. Two examples will be illustrated where cells were exposed to 'shoulder' doses and the initial slope of the survival curves was derived directly. A computer program was used to calculate the shape of the survival curve that best fits the biological data. The initial slope of the survival curves was calculated for those examples where 'shoulder' data were available.

Figure 8.5 shows the response of Chinese hamster ovarian (CHO) cells irradiated with X-rays or Co γ-rays. There are data points at 50 cGy intervals over the shoulder region of the acute X-ray curve. This shows a small initial slope with a coefficient that is only just significantly different from zero (Table 8.1). This direct estimate of the initial slope of the CHO cell survival curve after X-irradiation is obviously more reliable than the estimate derived from the exponential slope of the curve shown for protracted γ-irradiation. However, inspection of the data leads one to doubt whether the apparent difference between the curves is significant and whether they actually do cross over.

By contrast, Figure 8.6 shows that the initial slope of the acute X-ray survival curve for HeLa cells has a much larger coefficient (Table 8.1). The curve also has data points at 50 cGy intervals over the shoulder region and there is a well-defined initial slope that has a D_0 value of 312 cGy, which is only about twice the value of the final D_0 of 150 cGy.

The curves in Figures 8.5 and 8.6 both had similar extrapolation numbers and the cells have the same capacity to recover from sublethal damage. By contrast, Figure 8.7 shows a diagram of the curves for bone-marrow

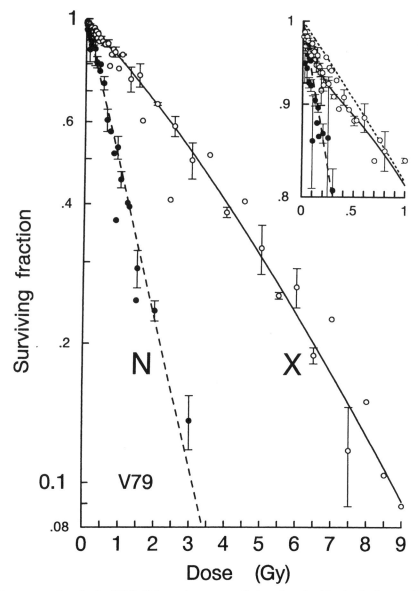

Figure 8.4. Survival of V79 Chinese hamster cells irradiated with single doses of X-rays or neutrons. (Reproduced from Joiner et al, 1996, by permission of Elsevier Science-NL, Sara Burgerhartstraat 25, 1055 KV Amsterdam, The Netherlands.)

damage (A) and lung damage (B). Curve A has both a steeper initial slope and a smaller extrapolation number than curve B. This difference has been utilized in the treatment of patients with acute leukaemia who are given doses of total body irradiation (Chapter 14) before bone marrow

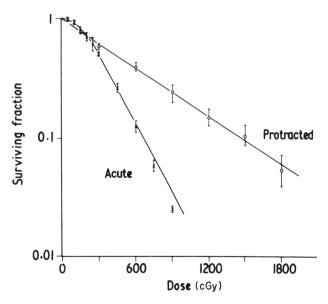

Figure 8.5. Survival curves for CHO cells irradiated in air with 300 kV X-rays and protracted ^{60}Co γ-rays. (Reproduced from Nias and Gilbert, 1975, by permission of John Wiley & Sons, Inc.)

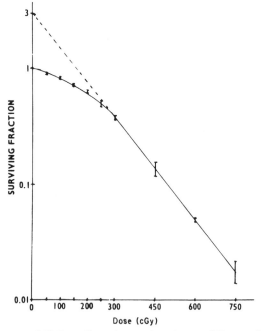

Figure 8.6. Response of HeLa cells to increasing doses of X-rays. (Reproduced from Nias and Gilbert, 1975, by permission of John Wiley & Sons, Inc.)

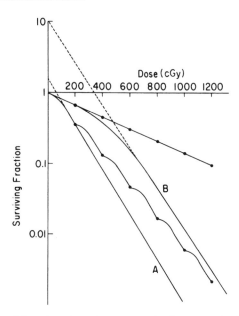

Figure 8.7. Effect of dose fractionation on survival curves of cells with limited (A) or large (B) capacities to accumulate and repair sublethal injury. Curve A represents bone marrow stem cells and curve B represents the cells responsible for radiation pneumonitis. (Reproduced from Peters et al, 1979, **131**, 243–247, by permission of Radiological Society of North America.)

transplantation. The diagram shows how repeated treatments with 200 cGy doses will lead to more leukaemic bone-marrow damage than lung damage, due to differences in the shoulder size and repair capacity of the two cell populations.

SPHEROID CULTURES

One example of variability in the size of the shoulder of a cell survival curve is shown in Figure 8.8. These curves are derived from an assay technique that is intermediate between the *in vitro* single-cell monolayer culture used for Figure 8.1 and the *in vivo* tissue assays that will be described later on. With this technique, cells are cultured *in vitro* but kept in suspension, where they grow into multicellular 'spheroids' that are morphologically similar to nodules of cancer.

As the spheroids grow in size, the radiation response changes and this is shown by the four survival curves in Figure 8.8. From single V79 cells (a), to 30 μm spheroids (b), the change in response amounts to an increase in extrapolation number from 10 to 200 for the same value of D_0 of 170 cGy.

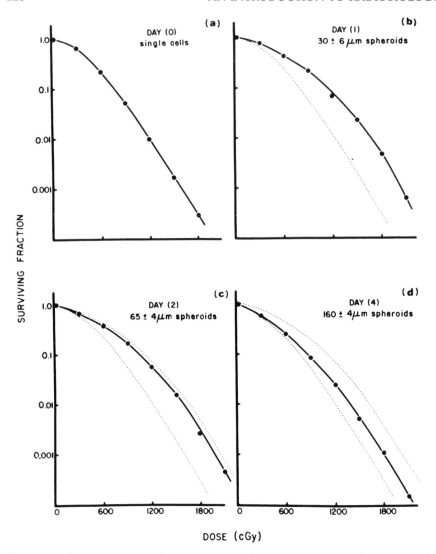

Figure 8.8. Survival curves of cells grown as spheroids. The broken line in (b) is the curve from (a); the broken curves in (c) and (d) are the same as the two curves of (b). (Reproduced from Sutherland and Durand, 1976, by permission of Elsevier Science-NL, Sara Burgerhartstraat 25, 1055 KV Amsterdam, The Netherlands.)

This change is entirely attributable to the increasing intercellular contact resulting from the three-dimensional form of the spheroid. However, as these grow larger, to 65 μm (c) and 160 μm (d) in diameter, the extrapolation number falls to 104 and then to 41, owing to the increasing proportion of non-cycling cells, which are more radiosensitive.

In even larger spheroids there are hypoxic cells in the centre and so this technique is particularly useful for the study of radiosensitizing drugs such as the nitroimidazoles (Chapter 11), where a quantitative assay is needed not only of the degree to which hypoxic cells can be made more radio-sensitive but also of the extent to which the drug can diffuse into the necrotic centre of a tumour. The multi-cellular structure of these spheroids presents the same sort of diffusion problem for oxygen and other nutrients as is found in tumour tissues *in vivo*. The oxygen effect will be discussed in Chapter 10 but these multicellular spheroid data for aerated cells are consistent with one of the conclusions that may be drawn from Table 8.1: namely, that values for N and D_q tend to be higher for survival curves derived from tissue than from single-cell assays, perhaps because of the cell-to-cell interaction of repair enzymes.

At the end of this chapter Table 8.4 provides a list of the parameters of the X-ray survival curves for the various cell populations shown in this chapter and in Chapters 12 and 13. The table provides some basis for comparison between the radiosensitivity of different types of cell assayed either in cultures *in vitro* or in tissue *in vivo*. Not all the assay systems are strictly comparable, however, and the appropriate chapters in the book should be consulted for details.

PHASE SENSITIVITY TO RADIATION

Under the special conditions of a cell culture laboratory, it is possible to manipulate a cell population so that all the cells are passing through the phases of the cycle synchronously (see Chapter 2). It is found that, with the exception of mitosis, cells are most radiosensitive towards the end of the G_1 phase and the beginning of the S phase. They then become progressively more resistant as they progress through the S phase but become more sensitive when they pass into the G_2 phase before the next mitosis. When this experiment is done under ideal conditions, the ratio of surviving fractions can amount to a factor of 200 (see Figure 8.10).

It would be more realistic to look at the sort of survival curves shown in Figure 8.9, where the difference in radiosensitivity is only fourfold. Under clinical conditions this fourfold ratio might still be useful, and it is one possible explanation for the synergistic effect of radiation combined with certain chemotherapeutic agents. Chemical synchronization was discussed in Chapter 2 with agents such as cytosine arabinoside as an example. With cytosine arabinoside, cells are delayed in their progress through the cell cycle at the sensitive point at the end of G_1 and the beginning of S (see Figure 8.11).

The two survival curves shown in Figure 8.10 have a difference in shape that is qualitatively similar to that of the spheroid culture curves shown in

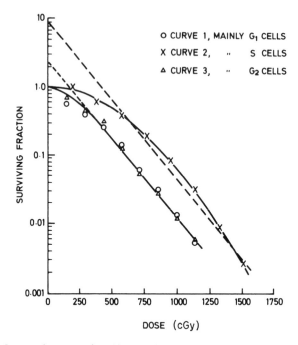

Figure 8.9. Survival curves for Chinese hamster (lung) fibroblasts irradiated with 250 kV X-rays in air during the three phases of the cell cycle. (Reproduced from Sinclair, 1967, by permission of the author.)

Figure 8.8. The final slopes have a similarity that is emphasized by the dotted lines. The main difference is the size of the shoulders: larger for cells irradiated in the S phase, smaller for cells irradiated in the G_1 and G_2 phases. Unlike the spheroid culture curves, both of the curves in Figure 8.9 were obtained from the survival of single cells. The differences are due only to the position in the cycle when they were irradiated.

Looking at the parameters of these survival curves, it is seen that the curves for synchronized cells have a D_0 value of about 2 Gy, which is not very different from the value of 1.7 Gy found when similar cells were being grown into spheroids. If the size of the shoulders of the curves in Figure 8.9 is measured in terms of extrapolation number, N, then the values are $N = 2$ for single cells in G_1 and G_2 and $N = 8$ for single cells irradiated in the S phase. (The extrapolation numbers are listed in Table 8.2.) The value for the asynchronous single cells (Figure 8.8) was $N = 10$, and thus the survival curve of an asynchronous population of single cells is very similar in shape to that of a synchronized cell population irradiated in the S phase.

In general, it can be stated that the radiosensitivity of a heterogeneous population of cells is dominated by the most resistant component, and the survival curve has an extrapolation number that is approximately the same

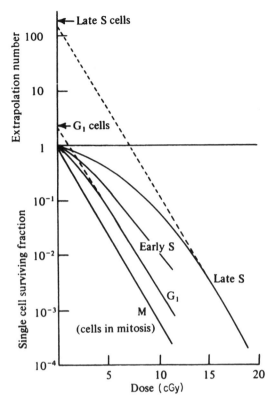

Figure 8.10. Survival curves for Chinese hamster cells at different stages of the cell cycle after synchronization by both mitotic selection and tritiated thymidine treatment. (Reproduced from Sinclair and Morton, 1966, by permission of Academic Press, Inc.)

Table 8.2. Shoulder size of V79 cell survival curves

Culture condition	Extrapolation no.	Fig. no.
Fully synchronized in mitotic phase	1	8.10
Partially synchronized in G_1 and G_2 phases	2	8.9
Partially synchronized in S phase	8	8.9
Asynchronous single cells	10	8.8
Asynchronous spheroid	200	8.8
Fully synchronized in late S phase	200	8.10

as that of this component. This means that although cells in the G_1 and G_2 phases of the cycle are more sensitive, cells in the S phase are no more resistant than average, certainly when synchronized by the mitotic selection technique used for the curves in Figure 8.9.

One problem with even the mitotic selection technique, however, is that there is still some degree of heterogeneity of the cell population, and the presence of even a few of the resistant S-phase cells can obscure the true sensitivity of cells in the more sensitive phases. This has been dealt with by adding a further step to the mitotic selection technique. Cells that are only supposed to be in the G_1 phase are treated with tritiated thymidine of high specific activity; this has the effect of killing any S-phase cells that happen to be present. Figure 8.10 shows the survival curves that are then obtained. The final slopes are still similar but there is a much greater difference in the size of the extrapolation numbers. The value for mitotic cells is the lowest possible at unity, while the late-S cells show an even higher value than before (approaching 200), which was what was found for the cells irradiated in the 30 μm spheroids discussed earlier (Table 8.2).

All these observations support the hypothesis of Sinclair (1972) that there is some factor 'varying during the S period, which also plays a part in controlling lethal radiation damage'. This may have something to do with the repair complex discussed earlier with the *repair model* to explain the shoulder of X-ray cell survival curves. Concentration of repair enzymes would influence the extrapolation number of cell survival curves. This could result in changes of N for survival curves taken at different stages in the mitotic cycle. Furthermore, repair enzymes would be more likely to remain in equilibrium, in higher concentration, in cells in contact with each other. This happens in spheroids and organized tissues, which are shown to have larger extrapolation numbers to their survival curves (see Table 8.3).

TIME COURSE OF PHASE SENSITIVITY

Another way of looking at the survival pattern of synchronized cells cultured *in vitro* is depicted in Figure 8.11. The upper panel (a) refers to V79 Chinese hamster cells (as used in Figure 8.10) and shows how their survival varies throughout the 12 h of the cycle that follow synchronization. The phases of the cycle are shown from labelling data. Clearly, the S phase occupies a considerable proportion of the cycle, from about 2 to 8 h. A higher survival level occurs for much of this period (which is, of course, why the curve for S-phase cells typifies the response of the whole population). There is one peak of survival in the later portion of the S phase.

The lower panel (b) refers to data obtained with HeLa cells (used for Figures 8.1 and 8.6). These cells have a very much longer G_1 phase than Chinese hamster cells and it is evident that there is another peak of survival towards the beginning of this G_1 phase. From the end of the G_1 phase onwards the patterns shown in Figure 8.11 are very similar and it can be

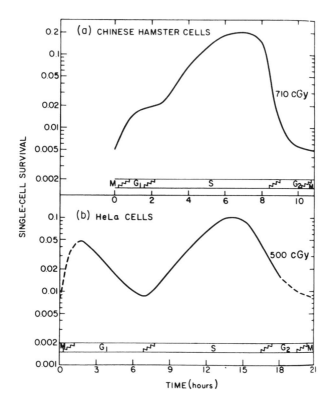

Figure 8.11. Age response of (a) Chinese hamster cells and (b) HeLa cells to X-rays. (Reproduced from Sinclair, 1972, by permission of Elsevier Science-NL, Sara Burgerhartstraat 25, 1055 KV Amsterdam, The Netherlands.)

concluded that both cell lines show the most *sensitive* responses at mitosis and at the G_1 to S transition point, whereas they are *resistant* towards the end of the S phase and then fairly sensitive in the G_2 phase.

For this reason, it is misleading to state that cells are radioresistant during the whole of the S phase, because this is not so. Nor are they necessarily sensitive throughout the G_1 phase. It is tempting to speculate that the extra peak of resistance in G_1 occurs whenever a cell population has a long G_1 phase, and this is likely to be found in tumours because they often include cells in an elongated G_1 phase (see Chapter 2).

Cells in a G_0 phase are known to be relatively radioresistant too, but this is due to recovery from potentially lethal damage in such resting cells, expressed as an increase in the value of D_0 rather than N (see Chapter 7). The true radiation response of some of these cells is likely to be complicated by the fact that they exist in an extended G_1 or G_0 phase because of

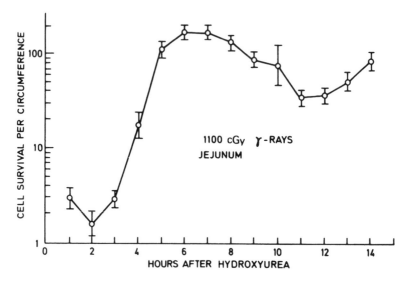

Figure 8.12. Variation in the survival of mouse intestinal crypt cells following exposure to 1100 cGy of γ-rays at various times after treatment with hydroxyurea. (Reproduced from Withers, 1975, **114**, 199–202, by permission of Radiological Society of North America.)

nutritional deprivation. This will also tend to reduce survival of clonogenic capacity, but such an artefact is difficult to exclude when cell populations are being assayed *in vivo*.

It is not easy to obtain effective synchronization of cell populations *in vivo* so as to study these patterns of radiosensitivity and radioresistance in the tissues of the body. Chemical methods of synchronization have to be used (see Chapter 2). Figure 8.12 shows how intestinal stem cells vary in radiosensitivity as they proceed through the remainder of the cycle, after being blocked at the beginning of the S phase by the antimetabolite hydroxyurea. (The assay is described in the next section; see Figure 8.13.) At 2 h the stem cells are still in early S, where they are most radiosensitive; by 6–8 h they have progressed to late S, where they are much more resistant. If survival at this point in time is compared with that from the same radiation dose delivered to an asynchronous cell population (Figure 8.13), the result is almost identical. As is shown for cultured cells (Figure 8.11), it is the early-S cells that are more radiosensitive. The late-S cells are no more radioresistant than the population taken as a whole. However, there is a very large difference in cell survival – 100 times. This is the consequence of combining a drug treatment with X-radiation at different time intervals (see Chapter 11).

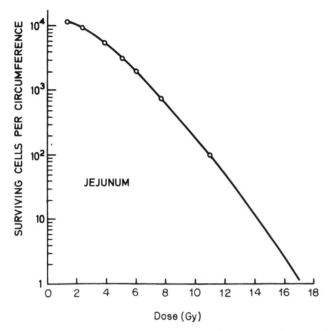

Figure 8.13. Composite single-dose survival curve for intestinal stem cells irradiated in C₃H mice. (Reproduced from Withers et al, 1975, by permission of Elsevier Science Inc., 655 Ave. of the Americas, New York NY 10010-5107.)

DOSE–RESPONSE CURVES *IN VIVO*

Intestinal crypt assay

The intestinal crypt assay is one of the techniques for measuring the radiosensitivity of cells in their normal environment, and was used to obtain the data shown in Figure 8.12 for the phase sensitivity of intestinal epithelial cells. The cell population originates in the crypts of Lieberkuhn and if a large enough dose of radiation is absorbed then many of the crypts are left with only one viable cell. In mouse experiments such cells repopulate the crypts very quickly (the cell cycle time is less than 12 h), so that after 3 or 4 days a histological section across the lumen of the irradiated intestine will show a number of regenerating crypts around the circumference. This number is dose dependent and a survival curve can be drawn, as in Figure 8.13.

The D_0 of this curve is 130 cGy over the dose range above 1150 cGy but it is difficult to derive values for the shoulder region of the curve at lower doses. This is because it is estimated that the total number of stem cells may amount to more than 10 000 per circumference, but it is not possible to count much more than 100 regenerating crypts. Over the dose range below 1100 cGy the shape of the cell survival curve can only be determined from multi-fraction experiments (Withers et al, 1975). The very large shoulder region on the curve might suggest a large value for N and D_q, i.e. a large capacity for the cells to recover from sublethal damage (see Chapter 7). The fractionation experiments show that this depends upon the size of the fraction dose, however. With a typical clinical fraction dose of 200 cGy, for example, the D_q is 120 cGy, but this value rises to 430 cGy over the high-dose range above 1150 cGy, where the survival curve adopts its final exponential slope. (These final values of $D_0 = 130$ cGy and $D_q = 450$ cGy from Figure 13.5 are listed in Table 8.3, with further discussion of the radiation response of the gastrointestinal tract in Chapter 13.)

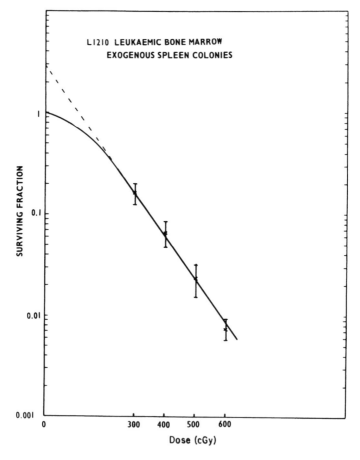

Figure 8.14. Survival curve for L1210 leukaemic bone marrow cells in DBA/2 mice irradiated with ^{137}Cs γ-rays. (Reproduced from Nias, 1988, by permission of Churchill Livingstone.)

Spleen colony assay

Figure 8.14 shows one of the most radiosensitive survival curves yet measured. This curve is included to illustrate two principles: that bone marrow stem cells are the most sensitive class of cells; and as a further illustration of the fact that survival curve data can be derived using cells assayed *in vivo* as well as *in vitro*. The data in Figure 8.14 were obtained using L1210 leukaemic cells, obtained from the femoral bone marrow of leukaemic DBA/2 mice irradiated with the doses as indicated. Leukaemic marrow cells were then injected into recipient mice, where some cells seed in the spleen. The mice were sacrificed after 7 days and their spleens examined for leukaemic colonies.

The assay system is analogous to that used for cells plated *in vitro* in most respects, but the irradiation of cells and their subsequent spleen colony formation is all undertaken *in vivo* – only the femoral marrow cells are counted *in vitro* to determine the correct number for injection into recipient mice. This is the method used by Till and McCulloch (1961) for normal haemopoietic cells and adapted by Bush and Bruce (1964) for leukaemic cells. It can be concluded that the same shape of survival curve is found by the *in vivo* method as is found *in vitro*, and that *in vitro* data are quite relevant to radiobiological problems that must ultimately be tested *in vivo*.

Another conclusion from the spleen colony method is that because similar survival curves are found for normal bone marrow, there is no difference in radiosensitivity between the normal and malignant bone marrow. If the radiotherapist is looking for an increased therapeutic ratio between the response of malignant and normal tissues, it is unlikely to be found in any difference in intrinsic radiosensitivity of cells of the same histological group. On the other hand, it is not often possible to make the same precise comparison between normal and malignant cells of the same histological type, using the same assay, as it is with the spleen colony method for bone-marrow stem cells. It would be a mistake, however, to draw general conclusions as to the relative radiosensitivity of different cell types, particularly when there are differences in cellular environment. The radiation response of bone marrow will be discussed further in Chapter 13.

The D_0 values of the survival curves do not vary very much (see Table 8.1) but there is a much larger variation in values for D_q (i.e. shoulder size). The survival curves for cell populations assayed in their own physiological environment tend to have larger shoulders, as is seen with the intestine.

THE SIGNIFICANCE OF SURVIVAL CURVES

Single-dose survival curves seem to show relatively small differences between the intrinsic radiosensitivity of different cell populations, certainly in terms of the D_0 values shown in Table 8.3. Table 8.3 lists the parameters

Table 8.3. Comprehensive list of survival curve parameters

Cell population	Assay	D_0 (cGy)	D_q (cGy)	N	Fig. no.
HeLa	*In vitro*	100	65	2	8.1
Chinese hamster (ovary)	*In vitro*	200	210	3	8.5
Chinese hamster (lung)	*In vitro*	170	400	10	8.8
Chinese hamster	*Spheroid*	170	900	200	8.8
Mouse leukaemia	*In vivo*	100	115	3.0	8.14
Rat rhabdomyosarcoma	*In vitro*	120	300	10	12.10
Mouse sarcoma	*In vivo*	134	290	9.5	12.11
Mouse skin	*In vivo*	135	350	–	13.3
Mouse small intestine	*In vivo*	115	430	40	13.5
Mouse marrow	*In vivo*	100	100	2.5	13.8
Mouse marrow	*In vitro*	105	95	2.5	13.8
Rat capillary endothelium	*In vivo*	170	340	7	
Mouse capillary endothelium	*In vitro*	200	160	2.3	13.10
Rat thyroid	*In vivo*	190	263	4	13.14

of the X-ray survival curves for the experimental cell populations mentioned in this book. They provide very little explanation for the differences in the radiosensitivity of both tumours and normal tissues that are found in clinical practice. Furthermore, while the D_0 values of the curves provide some indication of the radiosensitivity of the different cell populations, they only provide a measure of the final slope of the curve, usually over a dose range in excess of 2 Gy. In most cases the radiotherapist is only interested in the sensitivity of cells to fraction doses of around 2 Gy, so it is the initial portion of the survival curve that is of clinical interest.

The values for D_0 in Table 8.3 show a fairly narrow range, mostly between 100 and 200 cGy, but there is a much larger variation in values for D_q, which reflects the size of the shoulder portion of the curves. This was seen for the spheroid cultures in Figure 8.8. Figure 8.7 also showed the differences in the initial portions of survival curves of different tissues that may be found in practice. The final slopes may not vary very much but the D_q and N values cover a wide range. The D_q values of mouse cells given in Table 7.1 of Chapter 7 ranged from 100 to 550 cGy. The extrapolation numbers of V79 cell survival curves in Table 8.2 also show a wide range, depending on the conditions in which the cells were irradiated.

There is evidence for a wide variation in the extrapolation numbers of the curves derived from human tumour cell populations (Table 8.4) The values range from 1.1 for Burkitt lymphoma to 163 for adenocarcinoma of the rectum. Fertil and Malaise (1981) suggested an alternative parameter of radiosensitivity that would be more relevant to the doses used in fractionated radiotherapy and would take into account the variation in the size of the shoulders of these various curves. The surviving fraction is noted

Table 8.4. Human tumour cell survival

Tumour type	D_0 (Gy)	N	Survival at 2 Gy
Melanoma	1	40	0.77
Melanoma	1.05	23	0.61
Colon	1	5.5	0.40
Colon	0.88	30	0.57
Rectum	0.70	163	0.54
Cervix	1.3	3.8	0.48
Cervix	1.07	4.4	0.42
Pancreas	1	1.5	0.22
Burkitt	1.25	1.1	0.18

Reproduced from Fertil and Malaise, 1981, by permission of Elsevier Science Inc., 655 Ave. of the Americas, New York NY 10010-5107.

at the 2 Gy level (SF_2) and this is then used as a basis for comparison between different human tumours. Their study of 59 tumour cell lines showed that survival levels varied between 0.18 and 0.77 (Table 8.4). This is more than a fourfold range in 'radiosensitivity' and it seems to be much more in accord with clinical experience (Nias, 1988). A more recent review of 694 human cell lines found an even larger variation in SF_2 values from 0.03 to 0.81 Gy (Deschavanne and Fertil, 1996), but these included cells from people with genetic disorders such as ataxia telangiectasia, who are abnormally radiosensitive ($SF_2 = 0.03$). For the 271 tumour cell lines, the SF_2 values were similar to those in Table 8.4 and ranged from 0.21 to 0.81.

Because treatment seldom involves single doses of radiation, survival curves must be interpreted with care. However, they are useful when comparing the sensitivities of two or more cell types (compared in Table 8.3). Cell survival will also be modified by changing the quality of radiation (e.g. fast neutrons, see Chapter 9) and the environment of treatment (e.g. hypoxia, see Chapter 10). The purpose of this chapter has been to show the effects of single doses of radiation, where the biological effects are relatively simple and the usual shape of the cell survival curve can be established. The general principle of an initial shoulder followed by an exponential response to dose serves to illustrate the obvious truism that the larger the tumour cell mass, the larger the dose of radiation required to eradicate it.

SUMMARY OF CONCLUSIONS

(1) Mammalian cell survival curves show an exponential response to higher doses of X-radiation with a 'shoulder' over the low dose range.
(2) The exponential slope is defined in terms of the mean lethal dose, D_0, which is a measure of the intrinsic radiosensitivity of cells.

(3) The shoulder can be defined in terms of the extrapolation number, N, or the quasi-threshold dose, D_q.

(4) The shoulder is larger when cells are irradiated *in vivo*, in spheroid culture and later in the S phase of the cell cycle, but the D_0 values for all types of mammalian cell are similar.

(5) The mean inactivation dose, $\overline{D}$, is an alternative parameter.

(6) Mathematical models have been used to describe the shape of survival curves to conform with theories of hits and targets, but the shape is best described by the interaction of lesions produced by ionization tracks.

(7) The repair model provides an alternative explanation for the shoulder of such curves.

(8) The initial slope of an X-ray survival curve may show hypersensitivity to low doses.

(9) The surviving fraction after 2 Gy (SF$_2$) is a useful parameter for clinical radiotherapy.

REFERENCES

Bush, R. S. and Bruce, W. R., 1964. The radiation sensitivity of transplanted lymphoma cells as determined by the spleen colony method. *Radiation Research*, **21**, 612–621.

Coggle, J. E., 1983. *Biological Effects of Radiation*, 2nd edn. Taylor and Francis, London.

Deschavanne, P. J. and Fertil, B., 1996. A review of human cell radiosensitivity *in vitro*. *International Journal of Radiation Oncology, Biology, Physics*, **34**, 251–266.

Fertil, B. and Malaise, E. P., 1981. Inherent cellular radiosensitivity as a basic concept for human tumor radiotherapy. *International Journal of Radiation Oncology, Biology, Physics*, **1**, 621–629.

Fertil, B., Dertinger, H., Courdi, A. and Malaise, E. P., 1984. Mean inactivation dose: a useful concept for intercomparison of human cell survival curves. *Radiation Research*, **99**, 73–84.

Gordon, A. T. and McMillan, T. J., 1997. A role for molecular radiobiology in radiotherapy. *Clinical Oncology*, **9**, 70–78.

Joiner, M. C., Lambin, P., Malaise, E. P., Robson, T., Arrand, J. E., Skov, K. A. and Marples, B., 1996. Hypersensitivity to very-low single radiation doses: its relationship to the adaptive response and induced radioresistance. *Mutation Research*, **358**, 171–183.

Nias, A. H. W., 1988. *Clinical Radiobiology*, 2nd edn. Churchill Livingstone, Edinburgh.

Nias, A. H. W. and Gilbert, C. W., 1975. Response of HeLa and Chinese hamster cells to low doses of photons and neutrons. In *Cell Survival after Low Doses of Radiation*, edited by T. Alper. Wiley, Chichester, pp. 93–99.

Peters, L. J., Withers, H. P., Cundiff, J. F. and Dicke, K. A., 1979. Radiobiological considerations in the use of total-body irradiation for bone-marrow transplantation. *Radiology*, **131**, 243–247.

Puck, T. A. and Marcus, P. I., 1956. Action of X-rays on mammalian cells. *Journal of Experimental Medicine*, **103**, 653–684.

Sinclair, W. K., 1967. Radiation effects on mammalian cell populations *in vitro*. In *Radiation Research*, edited by G. Silini. North-Holland, Amsterdam, pp. 607–631.

Sinclair, W. K., 1972. Cell cycle dependence of the lethal radiation response in mammalian cells. *Current Topics in Radiation Research*, **7**, 264–285.

Sinclair, W. K. and Morton, R. A., 1966. X-ray sensitivity during the cell generation cycle of cultured Chinese hamster cells. *Radiation Research*, **29**, 450–474.

Sutherland, R. M. and Durand, R. E., 1976. Radiation response of multicell spheroids – an *in vitro* tumour model. *Current Topics in Radiation Research*, **11**, 87–139.

Till, J. E. and McCulloch, E. A., 1961. A direct measurement of the radiation sensitivity of normal mouse bone marrow cells. *Radiation Research*, **14**, 213–222.

Withers, H. R., 1975. Cell cycle distribution as a factor in multifraction irradiation. *Radiology*, **114**, 199–202.

Withers, H. R., Chu, A. M., Reid, B. O. and Hussey, D. H., 1975. Response of mouse jejunum to multifraction radiation. *International Journal of Radiation Oncology*, **1**, 41–52.

9 Densely Ionizing Radiation

The majority of this book is concerned with the effects of X-rays and γ-rays, which are sparsely ionizing types of radiations. This chapter will deal with α particles, neutrons, negative pions and atomic nuclei (such as helium, carbon or argon), which can be accelerated in nuclear physics machines. Their biological effects show important differences from those of X-rays and this depends on the intensity of the ionization, which is measured in terms of linear energy transfer (LET).

One of the biological effects of using more densely ionizing radiation is that the dose-modifying effect of oxygen is much less. (This is the subject of Chapter 10.) Another important difference is that the capacity of cells to shed sublethal and potentially lethal radiation damage is much reduced after exposure to high-LET radiation. This is manifest in cell survival curves described in Chapter 8, with the parameters D_0 (final slope) and N (shoulder size). All mammalian cells show a greater sensitivity to high-LET radiations with smaller values of D_0 and N; the latter therefore have a higher relative biological effectiveness (RBE) than X-rays. There is also much less variation in the radiosensitivity of cells during the different phases of the cell cycle.

Before these differences are discussed, the various particles will be described and how they interact with cells and tissues. The dosimetry of these high-LET radiations will also be outlined. The first task, however, is to define what is meant by LET and RBE.

LINEAR ENERGY TRANSFER

Linear energy transfer (LET) is the energy transferred per unit length of track, expressed in terms of kiloelectron-volts per micrometre (keV/μm). The importance of LET is that, as the intensity of ionization increases, there is an increasing probability that radiation energy will be deposited directly in a biological molecule so that damage will occur; the higher the intensity of ionization, the more the biological damage.

Figure 9.1 was used in Chapter 4 to explain the linear distribution of X-rays and γ-rays across the diameter of a biological target. More intensely ionizing radiation, such as α particles, is seen to have a greater probability of interacting with the target as it traverses it. Less intensely ionizing radiation, such as X-rays or γ-rays, is less likely to do this and the target

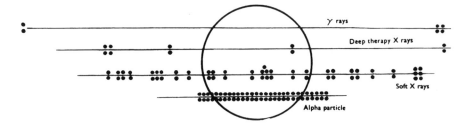

Figure 9.1. Separation of ion clusters in relation to the size of a biological target. (Reproduced from Gray, 1946, *Br. Med. Bull.*, by permission of the author.)

may suffer no ionizations at all, or perhaps one or two. If the 'target' is as complex as a mammalian cell then some critical part of the cell, such as the nucleus, needs to be hit before any damage will be achieved in the biological sense (see Chapter 5), and this becomes more likely as the intensity of the ionizations increases.

Figure 9.2 shows survival curves for cells exposed to three types of radiation: it is clear that neutrons are relatively more effective than X-rays, and α-rays are even more effective. The D_0 values are 50, 80 and 150 cGy for α-rays, neutrons and X-rays, respectively, and the dosages required to reduce the fraction of cells surviving to 10^{-2} are about 300, 450 and 900 cGy. This enables us to calculate the *relative biological effectiveness* (RBE) of α-rays

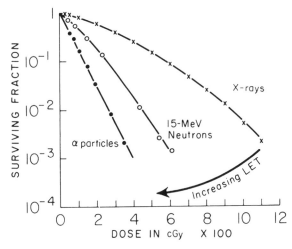

Figure 9.2. Survival curves for human cells treated with X-rays, neutrons or α particles. (Reproduced from Hall, 1988, by permission of Lippincott-Raven.)

and neutrons compared to X-rays, and the values are 3 and 2, respectively, at that value of survival. As LET increases, so does RBE (discussed later).

Unfortunately, LET can only be expressed as an average quantity because nearly all types of ionizing radiation have a range of energies and therefore a range of LET. It can either be expressed as a track average or energy average. Thus, for 15 MeV neutrons the track-average LET is about 12 keV/μm and the energy-average LET is about 75 keV/μm. (For X-rays, the two values are very similar at about 3 keV/μm.) The values quoted for high-LET radiations in this chapter may sometimes seem to be contradictory because different authors use the different definitions. The general principles will hold true, however, and these are summarized in Figure 9.3, which shows that as LET increases, RBE also increases but the oxygen enhancement ratio (OER) falls; this is related to the oxygen effect (see Chapter 10).

Figure 9.3 shows that after rising to a peak the RBE begins to fall with very high-LET radiation above 100 keV/μm. This is attributable to an 'overkill' effect, based on the fact that once a cell has received a lethal number of ionizing events, any more will have no further effect. This was shown by the very densely ionizing radiation depicted in Figure 9.1 for α particles. There were obviously more than enough ion clusters to kill a cell. Clearly, the most radiobiologically efficient radiation has a LET of 100 keV/μm, but no higher. Clusters were discussed in Chapter 5. Compared with the small clusters from low-LET radiation, the lethal damage from high-LET radiation involves a higher energy deposition of about 400 eV (15 ionizations) within large clusters of 5–10 nm. Such lesions are much less repairable (Goodhead, 1994).

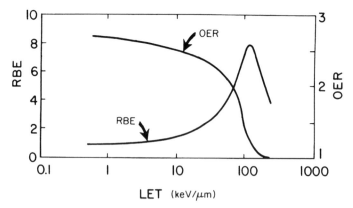

Figure 9.3. Variation of OER and RBE with LET. (Reproduced from Hall, 1988, by permission of Lippincott-Raven.)

TYPES OF RADIATION

Alpha particles

Gamma rays and β particles (electrons) were described in Chapter 4. They are both of low LET. Alpha particles are positively charged because they consist of two protons and two neutrons (i.e. they are helium nuclei without the two associated electrons). Because α particles are relatively massive (8000 times heavier than an electron), they move more slowly through tissue and penetrate only a short distance – a few hundred micrometres at most. Outside the body, α-radiation is of little importance. If such radiation is deposited internally (e.g. as 'hot' particles in the lung) it can be very damaging, and because the mixed emission from some radionuclides includes α particles (such as radon, Chapter 19) their mode of action merits description. Furthermore, they are produced by fast neutrons and negative pions in tissue.

As with electrons, the greatest intensity of ionization occurs at the end of the α-ray track, but it will be short and straight because it is massive and not easily deflected (in contrast to an electron track, which is very light and easily deflected). The low velocity and double charge of an α particle make it very densely ionizing. In terms of LET, the average value along the track would be about 165 keV/μm, compared to 3.0 for X-rays and 0.3 for Co γ-rays.

The ionization density for α particles varies considerably along their tracks, short though they are. This is shown in Figure 9.4, which also illustrates the same phenomenon for other types of charged particle. Both helium and hydrogen nuclei (i.e. α particles and protons) and negative pions ($-\pi$) are seen to deliver a relatively higher dose at 10 cm depth than at the surface, in contrast to the steady fall in dose with depth for X-rays and ^{60}Co γ-rays (after the initial build-up). The charged particle dose falls to zero when all the energy has been dissipated. At that point, all α particles will have attracted two electrons to themselves and come to rest in the tissue as helium atoms. This depth–dose relationship is relevant in radiotherapy, although α particles cannot be used because they have such poor penetrative power in tissues; protons have greater penetration, and the pattern of dose distribution for negative pions shows an even larger ratio between the dose in the initial plateau region and that at the peak.

Neutrons

Neutrons include slow (or thermal) neutrons generated in nuclear reactors, and fast neutrons that can be produced by accelerating deuterons onto a tritium target, resulting in a fusion reaction from which mono-energetic

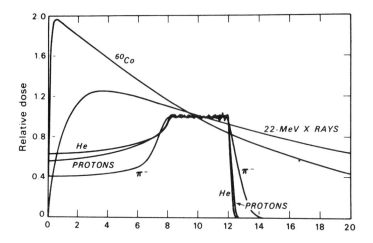

Figure 9.4. Central-axis depth–dose distributions of ^{60}Co γ-rays, 22 MeV X-rays, protons, helium ions and negative pions normalized to 50% dose at 10 cm. (Reproduced from Raju and Richman, 1972, by permission of Elsevier Science-NL, Sara Burgerharstraat 25, 1055 KV Amsterdam, The Netherlands.)

14.7 MeV neutrons are ejected. This reaction may be produced in specially designed D–T neutron generators. Alternatively, fast neutrons may be produced in a cyclotron, usually by the bombardment of a beryllium target with deuterons of 16–50 MeV. In this reaction the neutrons are stripped from the deuterons and a spectrum of neutron energies is produced whose mean energy is just under half that of the deuteron beam.

Because these particles have no electric charge, they will not interact with positively or negatively charged material as they pass through it, so no ionization is produced directly. Interaction can only result from direct collisions with atomic nuclei. Slow or thermal neutrons, with energies less than 100 eV, enter atomic nuclei and are 'captured'. (Boron neutron capture therapy is described below.)

Fast neutrons, with energies greater than 20 keV, interact mainly by elastic collisions with the nuclei. The most efficient interaction will occur when there is a head-on collision with a proton (i.e. a hydrogen nucleus), because protons and neutrons have equal mass. All the neutron energy will be transferred to the proton, which will recoil (or be 'knocked on').

Elastic scattering also occurs with nuclei of oxygen, carbon and nitrogen, from which densely ionizing recoil particles are produced. Inelastic scattering of fast neutrons may result from interaction with heavier atomic nuclei in tissues, with the production of γ-rays. A final form of attenuation may take place: nuclear disintegration (or fission). Neutrons are absorbed into nuclei, resulting in such instability that they explode, releasing fission fragments and other neutrons. Radiotherapists use beams of fast neutrons that have sufficient energy to achieve a useful depth–dose distribution. Boron neutron capture therapy (BNCT) has been used to treat brain tumours. A relatively high concentration of ^{10}B-enriched compounds can be achieved in such tumours and the fission products of neutron capture will selectively irradiate the tumour with high-LET radiation (Morris et al, 1997).

These interactions with tissues are quite different from the attenuation of X-rays and γ-rays described in Chapter 4. Because of this, the relative absorption of energy in the tissues is not the same as with X-rays. At a rough approximation, the absorption of neutrons is proportional to the concentration of hydrogen in the tissues. Fat, which is rich in hydrogen, will absorb much more energy from neutrons than from X-rays (Figure 9.5). By contrast, bone, which contains a high proportion of the higher atomic number elements calcium and phosphorus, will absorb proportionately less energy from neutrons than from low-LET radiation. Accordingly, neutrons will have a relatively smaller effect on bone than on (for example) subcutaneous tissues, which may be expected to absorb some 15–20% more energy from neutron radiation than from X-rays.

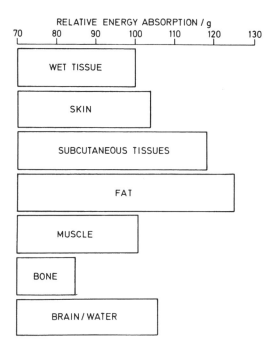

Figure 9.5. The relative absorption of fast neutrons in tissues. (Reproduced from Nias, 1988, by permission of Churchill Livingstone.)

Negative pi mesons (pions)

Negative pi mesons (or pions) are subatomic particles with a mass 276 times that of an electron, but with the same negative charge. They are produced by accelerating protons of extremely high energy (500–750 MeV) in a synchrocyclotron onto a graphite or lead target. Negative pions are interesting because the deposition of energy occurs mainly in the Bragg ionization peak, where the pions slow down and are captured by nuclei present in tissues. Pions produce densely ionizing particles when they are attenuated in tissues. This is the result of nuclear disintegrations releasing alpha particles, neutrons and protons following their capture in the nuclei of carbon, oxygen and nitrogen. The entrance, or plateau, region of the depth–dose curve is produced by the much less densely ionizing fast particles, so in this region the RBE of the pion beam is much lower. Figure 9.6 shows this diagrammatically for the physical distribution of dose, which is similar to that shown for pions in Figure 9.4 except that the plateau region is shown to extend over 10 cm. The diagram also shows the biological consequence of this physical distribution over the Bragg peak from 10 cm

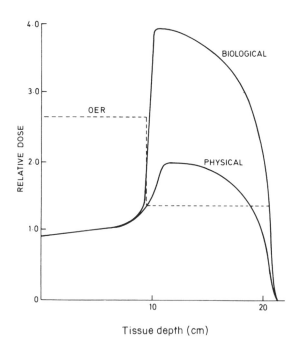

Tissue depth (cm)

Figure 9.6. Schematic representation of the relative physical and biological dose distribution of negative pions in tissues. The change in value of the OER is also of prime importance. (Reproduced from Nias, 1988, by permission of Churchill Livingstone.)

Table 9.1. Radiation weighting factors recommended by the ICRP

Type and energy range	Radiation weighting factor
Photons, all energies	1
Electrons and muons, all energies	1
Neutrons, energy < 10 keV	5
> 10–100 keV	10
> 100 keV–2 MeV	20
> 2–20 MeV	10
> 20 MeV	5
Protons, energy > 2 MeV	5
Alpha particles, fission fragments, heavy nuclei	20

onwards. At this depth, the RBE will rise and, as a consequence, the OER will fall.

The RBE values in the plateau region are about 1.0, but in the peak region a range of 'peak' RBE values from 1.6 to 3.0 has been demonstrated; the RBE of pions, however, is much less than that of neutrons and there is also much less variation with the size of dose than there is for neutrons. Nevertheless, pion beams present the practical possibility of delivering radiation with a reasonably low OER (about 1.8) to a well-circumscribed volume of tissue. Protons offer the same dose-localization potential but, because they have a relatively low LET, they do not have any radiobiological advantage in terms of OER and RBE (see Table 9.1).

Accelerated charged particles

It was mentioned above that fast neutrons may produce recoil protons by elastic collisions with hydrogen nuclei, and that collisions between neutrons and carbon, nitrogen, oxygen and other nuclei in a tissue will produce charged particles that will also be densely ionizing. Such charged particles can be produced externally by a very high-energy machine (e.g. a synchrotron) with enough energy to penetrate a tissue to a useful depth for therapeutic purposes before ionization reaches a peak (Figure 9.4). Of additional importance is the fact that the dose delivered at such a depth by these charged particles is more effective than orthodox radiation (i.e. has a higher RBE) because the particles are more densely ionizing.

Atomic nuclei of carbon, neon, argon and other elements have been the subject of experimental evaluation with a view to clinical application. These high-energy charged particles have physical and biological properties somewhat similar to those of negative pions. The particles produce good dose distributions, similar to protons, and the OER in the peak region may be slightly lower. High-energy heavy nuclei offer theoretical improvements in both the biological and physical characteristics of the treatment beam. Various RBE values have been reported at both plateau and peak positions, but what is important is the peak/plateau ratio in each case. These ratios range from 1.9 for carbon down to 1.0 for argon. The OER values range from 1.7 to 1.2. The depth–dose distribution, however, may not be as circum-scribed as that obtained with protons, which have a much wider Bragg peak. In the case of heavy ions, the addition of multiple peaks to produce an adequate high-dose volume may result in a smaller peak/plateau ratio.

NEUTRON DOSIMETRY AND WEIGHTING FACTOR

The dosimetry of ionizing radiations was discussed in Chapter 4. However, neutrons are uncharged and so do not directly ionize matter. For this reason indirect methods have to be used to measure neutron doses. Fast neutrons interact with hydrogen atoms to produce recoil protons, and it is these that cause ionization. For this reason fast neutron detectors use a hydrogenous material such as polythene, which is incorporated in the volume of the ionization chamber. For slow neutron measurements the ionization chambers are lined with boron. Boron captures slow neutrons with the emission of α particles, and these cause an ionization that can be detected.

The same unit of absorbed radiation dose as is used for X-rays, the gray (Gy), is used for neutrons, as well as for negative pions and the other charged particles described in this chapter. Where these different types of radiation are concerned, however, a multiplication or *weighting factor* has to be used to take into account the increased RBE (discussed next) of these types of radiation, which have a higher LET. Table 9.1 lists some examples of such weighting factors. The highest fractor is 20 for the most densely ionizing radiations, such as α particles and neutrons of energy between 100 keV and 2 MeV. Other neutrons have lower factors, depending on their LET, and protons have a factor of 5. These factors can be used to calculate the 'biologically effective' dose, whose unit is the sievert (discussed in the context of radiation protection in Chapter 20).

RELATIVE BIOLOGICAL EFFECTIVENESS

An important effect is seen when survival curves are compared after irradiation of cells with X-rays and fast neutrons. Figure 9.7 shows two survival curves of HeLa cells irradiated in air with 300 keV X-rays and 14.7 MeV monoenergetic neutrons from a D–T generator. The curves are obviously different in both final slope (D_0) and size of shoulder (N), as was seen in Figure 9.2. The D_0 values are 150 cGy and 80 cGy and the extrapolation numbers (N) are 3.2 and 1.6 for X-rays and neutrons,

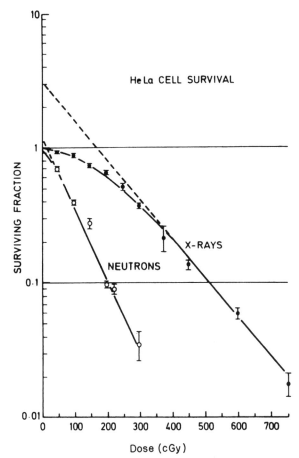

Figure 9.7. Survival curves for HeLa cells irradiated with 300 kV X-rays or 14.7 MeV neutrons in air. (Reproduced from Nias et al, 1967, by permission of *Int. J. Radiat. Biol.*, Taylor & Francis)

respectively. This provides an example of variation in biological response to different types of radiation over the range of doses used for fractionated radiotherapy. The parameter that varies is the RBE of fast neutrons compared with medium-voltage X-rays.

The data in Table 9.2 were obtained from the curves in Figure 9.7 and they illustrate the *definition of RBE*: the ratio of doses needed to produce a given amount of biological damage (i.e. survival). In this example it was convenient to use 300 keV X-rays as the reference radiation. Strictly speaking, ^{60}Co γ-rays should be used for comparison because they have an RBE value of unity (compared with a value of 1.15 for medium-voltage X-rays). The RBE rises from 2.3 to 4.3 when the neutron dose falls from 305 to 15 cGy.

Table 9.2. Variation of RBE with cell survival

Survival (%)	Neutron dose (cGy)	X-ray dose (cGy)	RBE
90	15	65	4.3
80	30	115	3.8
70	45	160	3.6
60	60	200	3.3
50	80	240	3.0
40	100	280	2.8
30	125	335	2.7
20	160	400	2.4
10	210	515	2.4
3	305	695	2.3

Reproduced from Nias et al, 1967, by permission of *Int. J. Radiat. Biol.*, Taylor & Francis.

The explanation for the considerable variation in the value of RBE with neutron dose lies in the difference in the size of the shoulder of the X-ray and neutron survival curves. This in turn is attributable to the difference in the capacity of the cells to recover from sublethal damage from the two types of radiation. Figure 9.8 shows how the amount of recovery is reduced to a very small value with neutrons compared to the typical pattern for X-rays. These data were obtained by a standard split-dose experiment (see Chapter 7) using doses that produced the same amount of cell killing for both types of radiation. As usual, the total dose was divided into two equal

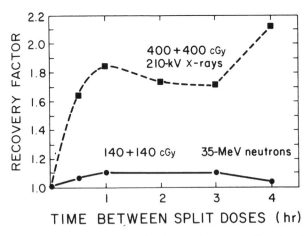

Figure 9.8. Split-dose experiments with Chinese hamster cells using X-rays and fast neutrons. (Reproduced from Hall et al, 1975, **117**, 173–178, by permission of Radiological Society of North America.)

fractions separated by 1–4 h and the relative increase in survival is plotted as a recovery factor. With X-rays there is a prompt repair of sublethal damage after 1 h but with neutrons there is almost none. This is because the damage from small clusters of ionizing events with low-LET radiation is repairable, but the lesions from the large clusters with high-LET radiation are not (Goodhead, 1994).

The problem is that the value of RBE changes considerably over just that range of dosage most commonly employed in fractionated radiotherapy. When fast neutron therapy has been used (perhaps because of the reduced OER), this variability has had to be remembered whenever a fractionated treatment was being prescribed, especially if it was proposed to choose a regime equivalent to one used for standard X-ray therapy. Different tissues prove to have differences in the exact values for RBE, but the fact that RBE varies with different doses has been shown to be generally applicable (Chapter 12).

PHASE SENSITIVITY

It has already been noted (Figure 9.3) that the absolute value of OER falls to unity with high-LET radiation (see Chapter 10). A similar reduction occurs in the cyclic pattern of radiosensitivity as higher LET radiation is used. This is shown in Figure 9.9, where the amount of variation in cell survival through the cycle is plotted against LET. The largest variation is for X-rays, which have a LET value of about 2 keV/μm; the smallest is for α particles (such as are emitted by polonium), which have a LET value of 165 keV/μm.

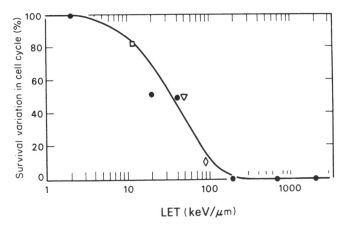

Figure 9.9. Dependence of cell cycle survival variation on the LET of the irradiation. (Reproduced from Bird and Burki, 1975, by permission of *Int. J. Radiat. Biol.*, Taylor & Francis.)

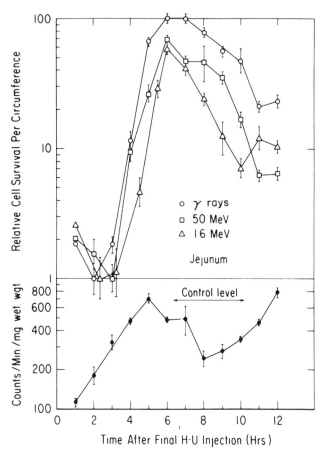

Figure 9.10. Response of synchronized jejunal crypt cells to irradiation with γ-rays or 50 MeV or 16 MeV neutrons at different stages of the cell cycle. The lowest curve shows the uptake of tritiated thymidine in aliquots of jejunum after synchronization at G_1/S by hydroxyurea. (From Withers et al, 1974, *Cancer*, **34**, 39–47. © (1974) American Cancer Society. Reprinted by permission of Wiley-Liss, Inc., a subsidiary of John Wiley & Sons, Inc.)

Such α particles are largely of academic interest because of their very low penetrability through matter (although they were used for the experiments illustrated in Chapter 5, Figure 5.3). Of more practical importance are fast neutrons of 16 and 50 MeV energy, which have a mean LET value of about 20 keV/μm. Figure 9.9 shows that there will be less variation in radiosensitivity through the phases of the cell cycle with such radiation.

This is indeed shown by the patterns in Figure 9.10, where mouse jejunum was irradiated *in vivo* at various time intervals after injection of hydroxyurea as a synchronizing agent. The data have all been normalized so that the lowest survival value for each type of radiation is at the same value of unity and other survival values can be compared. After 1100 cGy of γ-rays there is a 100-fold fluctuation in survival, but after equivalent doses of fast neutrons the fluctuation is reduced to 60–70-fold. This difference could be important in a clinical situation governed by radio-resistant cells in the late-S phase. Such cells will be relatively more sensitive to fast neutrons than to X-rays or γ-rays.

After irradiation with very much higher LET, the cyclic variation in radiosensitivity is absent altogether, as shown in Figure 9.9. The gradual flattening of the pattern is seen in Figure 9.11, which shows the response to three types of radiation of V79 Chinese hamster cells synchronized by mitotic selection. The doses were chosen to give a relatively equivalent biological effect, as seen by the survival data at 2–3 h when the cells would be at the beginning of the S phase: doses of 950 cGy of X-rays (LET = 1.9 keV/μm) provided the top line; 600 cGy doses of helium ions (LET = 19 keV/μm) gave the middle line, from two cohort populations; and 250 cGy doses of ^{12}C ions (LET = 191 keV/μm) were used for the bottom line. As the LET is increased, first tenfold and then 100-fold in value, the cyclic pattern is progressively flattened and is effectively absent with the accelerated charged carbon ions.

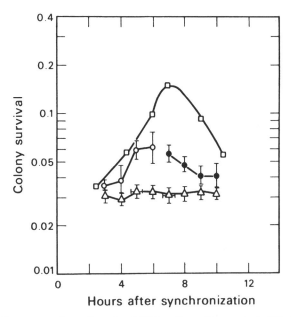

Figure 9.11. Response of synchronized V79 cells to X-rays ($\square$), ^{4}He ions ($\bigcirc$, $\bullet$) or ^{12}C ions ($\triangle$) at different stages of the cell cycle. (Reproduced from Bird and Burki, 1975, by permission of *Int. J. Radiat. Biol.*, Taylor & Francis.)

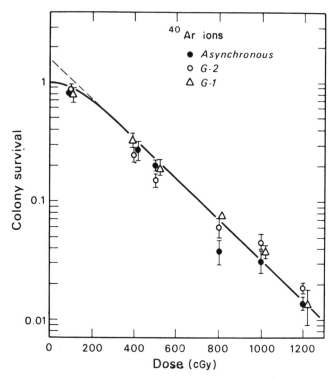

Figure 9.12. Survival curve for V79 cells irradiated with ^{40}Ar ions. (Reproduced from Bird and Burki, 1975, by permission of *Int. J. Radiat. Biol.*, Taylor & Francis.)

With such densely ionizing radiation the difference that has been noted between the response of an asynchronous cell population and cells from G_1 and S phases (see Figure 8.9 in Chapter 8) will finally disappear. This is shown for the extreme case of irradiation with ^{40}Ar (LET = 2000 keV/μm) in Figure 9.12; the survival data all fit the same dose–response curve. This is the only example in this book of a complete absence of variation in response to irradiation throughout the cell cycle.

SUMMARY OF CONCLUSIONS

(1) Some types of radiation are more densely ionizing than X-rays or γ-rays: they transfer more energy per unit length of track. This linear energy transfer (LET) is measured in keV/μm.
(2) The higher the LET, the more the relative biological effectiveness (RBE) compared to γ-rays.

(3) The RBE is also called the weighting factor, for radiation protection purposes. The factor may be as high as 20 for very high-LET radiation.
(4) After such radiation the cell survival curve will be steeper, i.e. with a smaller D_0. Because there is less recovery from sublethal damage, the curve will also have a smaller shoulder (i.e. smaller extrapolation number, N).
(5) Because of this, the RBE is larger for smaller doses of radiation and smaller for larger doses.
(6) The higher the LET, the lower the OER and the less the variation in radiosensitivity throughout the phases of the cell cycle.

REFERENCES

Bird, R. P. and Burki, H. J., 1975. Survival of synchronized Chinese hamster cells exposed to radiation of different linear-energy transfer. *International Journal of Radiation Biology*, **27**, 105–120.
Goodhead, D. T., 1994. Initial events in the cellular effects of ionizing radiations: clustered damaged in DNA. *International Journal of Radiation Biology*, **65**, 7–17.
Gray, L. H., 1946. Comparative studies of the biological effects of X-rays, neutrons and other ionizing radiations. *British Medical Bulletin*, **4**, 11–18.
Hall, E. J., 1988. *Radiobiology for the Radiologist*. Lippincott, Philadelphia.
Hall, E. J., Roizin-Towle, L., Theus, R. B. and August, L. S., 1975. Radiobiological properties of high-energy cyclotron-produced neutrons used for radiotherapy. *Radiology*, **117**, 173–178.
ICRP, 1991. 1990 Recommendations of the International Commission on Radiological Protection. ICRP Publication 60. *Annals of the ICRP*, **21** (nos 1–3).
Morris, G. M., Coderre, J. A., Hopewell, J. W., Micca, P. L. and Fisher, C. D., 1997. Response of the central nervous system to fractionated boron neutron capture irradiation: studies with borocaptate sodium. *International Journal of Radiation Biology*, **71**, 185–192.
Nias, A. H. W., 1988. *Clinical Radiobiology*, 2nd edn. Churchill Livingstone, Edinburgh.
Nias, A. H. W., Greene, D., Fox, M. and Thomas, R. L., 1967. Effect of 14 MeV monoenergetic neutrons on HeLa and P388F cells *in vitro*. *International Journal of Radiation Biology*, **13**, 449–456.
Raju, M. R. and Richman, C., 1972. Negative pion radiotherapy: physical and radio-biological aspects. *Current Topics in Radiation Research*, **8**, 159–233.
Withers, H. R., Mason, K., Reid, B. O., Dubravsky, N., Barkley, H. T., Brown, B. W. and Smathers, J. B., 1974. Response of mouse intestine to neutrons and gamma rays in relation to dose fractionation and division cycle. *Cancer*, **34**, 39–47.

10 The Oxygen Effect

The majority of the tissues of the body are nourished by a blood supply that provides an adequate concentration of oxygen for their metabolic requirements. There are some tissues, such as cartilage and skin, that are slightly less well oxygenated but as a general rule normal tissues are well vascularized so that the partial pressure of oxygen exceeds 40 mmHg. This is shown in Figure 10.1, which relates such partial pressures to radiosensitivity. The curve is almost horizontal over the physiological range of partial pressure between arterial and venous blood.

Figure 10.1 shows that when the partial pressure of oxygen begins to fall below 20 mmHg, radiosensitivity also begins to fall at a faster rate than before. Eventually, with complete anoxia, radiosensitivity will fall to unity, but half this final fall in radiosensitivity occurs over the last 5 mmHg. This 5 mmHg partial pressure of oxygen is referred to as the K value, i.e. the oxygen concentration that will give half of the possible enhancement of radiosensitivity that oxygen can provide. (The K value is discussed later.)

The full enhancement of radiosensitivity will only be possible in a tissue where the cells are completely anoxic and yet still viable. This condition applies to some solid tumours. Many such tumours have regions of inadequate nutrition because they have outgrown their blood supply. The

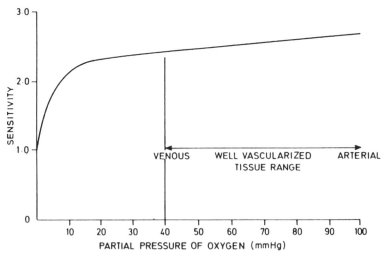

Figure 10.1. Relationship of radiosensitivity to oxygen tension. (Reproduced from Deschner and Gray, 1959, by permission of Academic Press, Inc.)

normal physiological control of blood supply is disorganized as part of the pathological conditions of solid tumours, so at any one moment there will be cells under a range of oxygen tension from zero up to the normal limits. Figure 10.2 shows pictures of the consequence of this process, with complete necrosis in the centre of a tumour in human lung and the same pattern developing in the centre of cultured spheroids (Chapter 8). These are formed when cells are cultured *in vitro* in such a way that they grow in three dimensions, like nodules of cancer *in vivo*. As the spheroids increase in size a critical radius is reached at which central necrosis forms, very similar in appearance to that seen in the tumour.

Just as the nutritional requirements of spheroids depend upon the culture medium in which they are growing, so the requirements of tumours depend upon the vascular stroma in which they grow. In the case of squamous cell carcinomas the tumours grow as 'cords' that, although surrounded by stroma, have no capillaries penetrating between the individual cells. As a result there is a falling gradient in oxygen tension between the periphery and the centre of each tumour cord.

OXYGEN DIFFUSION DISTANCE

The oxygen diffusion distance, or gradient, is illustrated by the diagrams in Figure 10.3, which show the distribution of partial pressure of oxygen through cylinders of radius 100, 145 and 300 μm. The middle diagram applies to a tumour cord with a critical radius where anoxia will begin to occur in those cells in the centre. The three diagrams depict what will apply to the three spheroids shown in Figure 10.2. The middle spheroid has a small number of necrotic cells, the left one has none at all but the right one has a large necrotic centre.

Thomlinson and Gray (1955) calculated the critical radius to be 145 μm and this is the distance often assumed in subsequent literature. However, they commented that the diffusion constant used in their calculations could differ by 30% in either direction, and the respiratory quotient could be an even less certain value in their calculations. They had not been able to find any measurements relating to the human lung cancers used to derive the diagrams in Figure 10.3.

The critical radius will depend upon the metabolic status of the cells and the oxygenation of the blood supply, but 145 μm seems to apply to the examples shown in Figure 10.2. Because of their lower oxygen concentration, the innermost viable cells in a tumour cord will be much more radioresistant than those at the periphery of the cord. Radiosensitivity will also be influenced by the particular metabolic conditions of the innermost cells.

This is shown by the radiosensitivity of the cells from a spheroid of 349 μm diameter. This is larger than the critical size for complete oxygenation from

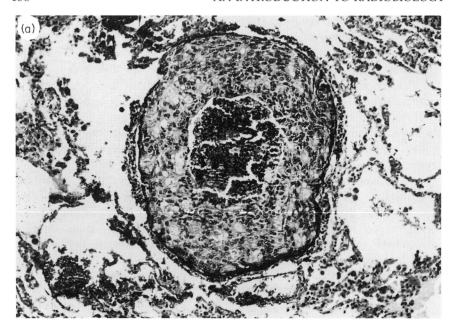

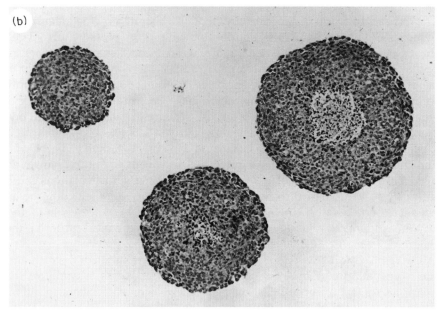

Figure 10.2. Photomicrographs of (a) a human lung metastasis from a primary adenocarcinoma of the colon (×190) and (b) sections through three spheroids (×185). (Reproduced from Sutherland and Durand, 1976, by permission of Elsevier Science-NL, Sara Burgerhartstraat 25, 1055 KV Amsterdam, The Netherlands.)

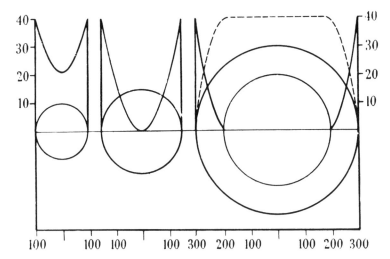

Figure 10.3. Distribution of partial pressure of oxygen (in mmHg) through cylinders of respiring tissue of increasing diameter (in μm). (Reprinted from *Br. J. Cancer*, **9**, 539–549, Thomlinson and Gray, The histological structure of some human lung cancers and the possible implications for radiotherapy. © 1955, by permission of the publisher Churchill Livingstone.)

the surrounding medium when the spheroids are cultured at 37 °C. Figure 10.4 shows that a biphasic survival curve applies to such cells, reflecting the hypoxic state of the innermost cells. (Survival curves for fully oxic and fully hypoxic cells at 37 °C are shown for comparison.) If the temperature is reduced to 24 °C, however, the metabolic requirements of the cells are reduced and the diffusion distance of oxygen is increased. As a result, the survival curve for such spheroid cells loses its biphasic shape and follows that of fully oxygenated cells.

Under normal conditions *in vivo* the tumour will grow as a result of proliferation of the outer cells, and then the innermost cells will be further removed from blood vessels than the critical distance compatible with survival. If the tumour is irradiated, however, the radiation will kill the more radiosensitive outer cells of a tumour cord but not the more resistant inner cells. As a result, there will be an increase in the supply of nutrients to those inner cells, which may once again start proliferating if they have retained their reproductive integrity.

The two processes of growth of the outer cells and necrosis of the inner cells result in a constant proportion of tumour cells that are hypoxic but viable. In terms of the histological pictures in Figure 10.2, this represents a relatively small proportion of the tumour cell population, of the order of 10%. In terms of the radiation response, however, this 10% of anoxic cells plays a very important part.

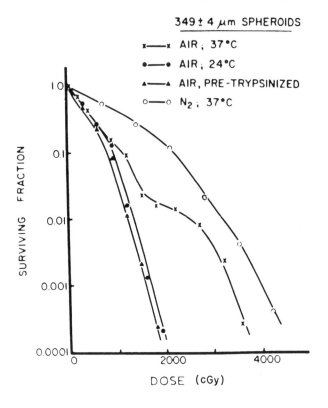

Figure 10.4. Survival of cells from spheroids irradiated under various conditions and then trypsinized. (Reproduced from Sutherland and Durand, 1973, by permission of *Int. J. Radiat. Biol.*, Taylor & Francis.)

The explanation can be obtained from Figure 10.5, which shows the biphasic shape of the survival curve of a tumour cell population in which 10% of the cells are anoxic. The initial part follows the shape of the curve for the well-oxygenated proportion of the cell population. At higher doses, however, the radioresistant anoxic cells predominate and the survival curve has a much shallower slope. Even a very small tumour will contain at least 10^6 cells and, because of the usual exponential nature of the dose–response curve, if all these are to be eradicated then the majority of the radiation dosage will be that required to reduce the surviving fraction along this radioresistant 'tail'. In the case of a surviving fraction of 10^{-6} a dose of 2400 cGy will be required, and not merely the 1000 cGy dose that would be sufficient for oxygenated cells.

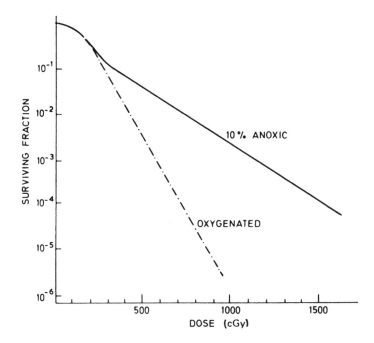

Figure 10.5. Schematic cell survival curve of a tumour cell population with a proportion of anoxic cells that produce the radioresistant 'tail' at higher dose levels. (Reproduced from Nias, 1988, by permission of Churchill Livingstone.)

OXYGEN ENHANCEMENT RATIO (OER)

The fundamental reason for this oxygen effect was outlined in the section on 'Radiation chemistry' in Chapter 4. Radiation–induced free radicals are either 'fixed' by oxygen or repaired by sulphydryl compounds in the absence of oxygen, and there will be competition between these two processes, depending upon the environment at the time.

With low-LET radiation the addition of oxygen increases radiosensitivity two or three times. The precise value is called the oxygen enhancement ratio (OER), which is a ratio of the doses of radiation required to produce a given level of cell killing when delivered under anoxic or aerated conditions. Although the ratio can be derived from a comparison of the exponential slopes of the two phases of the curve in Figure 10.5, it is more satisfactory to use data obtained from cells irradiated *in vitro* when the conditions can be controlled. The upper two curves in Figure 10.6 show the dose–response of HeLa cells treated with X-rays either in air or in nitrogren with oxygen excluded. Because both of the survival curves extrapolate to the same number ($N = 3$), the effect of oxygen is equally dose modifying at all survival levels and the value of OER can therefore be derived from a

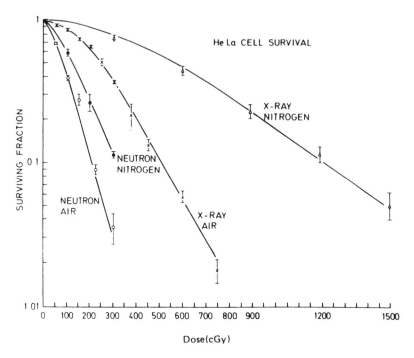

Figure 10.6. Survival curves for HeLa cells irradiated in air and nitrogen with 14 MeV neutrons and 250 kV X-rays. (Reproduced from Nias et al, 1967, by permission of *Int. J. Radiat. Biol.*, Taylor & Francis.)

comparison of the values of D_0, which are 150 cGy in air and 360 cGy in nitrogen, i.e. the OER for X-irradiated HeLa is 2.4. This is a typical value for mammalian cells, which show a range of OER from 2 to 3.

The OER for cells irradiated with higher LET radiations is lower, as shown by the difference between the final slopes of the two neutron curves in Figure 10.6. Fast neutrons have a higher relative biological effectiveness than X-rays (Chapter 9), so both neutron survival curves are much steeper than the X-ray curves and have a smaller extrapolation number ($N = 1.6$). More noteworthy, however, is that the difference between the two slopes is much less. For neutron irradiation of aerated cells the D_0 is 77 cGy, and for cells irradiated in nitrogen it is 116 cGy. Thus, the OER value is only 1.5, compared with 2.4 for X-rays. If radiotherapists use such neutrons instead of X-rays to treat hypoxic tumours, there should be a *therapeutic gain factor* of 1.6 (derived from the neutron/X-ray ratio of the two values of OER). The value for OER falls even further with higher LET radiations (see Figure 9.3 in Chapter 9).

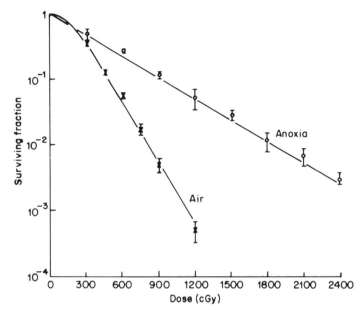

Figure 10.7. Survival curves for HeLa cells irradiated with 300 kV X-rays in air or under anoxic conditions. (Reproduced from Nias et al, 1973, by permission of *Int. J. Radiat. Biol.*, Taylor & Francis.)

THE OXYGEN EFFECT AT LOW DOSES

Figure 10.7 shows another pair of HeLa cell X-ray survival curves. The curve for aerated cells is very similar in shape to that shown for X-rays in Figure 10.6, although it spans an extra decade in survival because it extends over a wider range of single doses. The curve for anoxic cells, on the other hand, is quite different in shape from the 'nitrogen' curve in Figure 10.6. As well as extending over a wider range of dosage, it shows a purely exponential shape with an extrapolation number of unity. While the nitrogen curve in Figure 10.6 could be fitted to the same extrapolation number as its corresponding aerated curve, the two curves in Figure 10.7 cannot.

The two curves appear to overlap near their origin but this is not significant because the lowest dose measured was 300 cGy in air and so the low-dose hypersensitivity (HRS) phenomenon would not have been observed. Both HRS and the relationship to induced radioresistance (IRR) were mentioned in Chapter 8 (see Figure 8.4). The HRS/IRR phenomenon applies to low radiation doses of below 30 cGy in air; it also applies to hypoxic cells, but at a higher dose level (Marples et al, 1994).

The difference in shape between the hypoxic curves in Figures 10.6 and 10.7 can be attributed to the fact that the hypoxic environment of the cells in

Table 10.1. Variation of OER with survival level

Survival level (%)	Dose in air (cGy)	Dose under hypoxia (cGy)	OER
60	200	200	1.00
45	250	325	1.30
35	300	425	1.42
20	400	625	1.56
10	500	950	1.90
3	650	1450	2.23
1	800	1900	2.37
0.3	1000	2400	2.40

Reproduced from Nias, 1988, by permission of Churchill Livingstone.

Figure 10.6 had been obtained by gassing with very pure (white spot) nitrogen, which reduced the oxygen tension to a low level (<10 ppm) but not complete anoxia. The data shown in Figure 10.7 were obtained with cells in a crowded cell suspension, which respired itself to such a low oxygen tension that it amounts to complete anoxia.

The survival data in Figure 10.7 have been listed in Table 10.1, where values for OER are shown at different survival levels. The OER is assumed to be unity at a survival level of 60% and above. At lower survival levels, the value of OER rises progressively and the ultimate value would reach 2.93 at doses so high that the contribution of the D_q of the aerated curve becomes negligible, so that the ratio of the D_0 values of the two curves is then applicable.

The important conclusion to be drawn from Table 10.1 is that the OER may be considerably lower over the range of single doses customarily used for fractionated radiotherapy, i.e. oxygen is not equally dose modifying at all survival levels. Such data apply to the extreme cases where the cells are completely anoxic. These cells may not be of importance in clinical radiotherapy because they will not retain viability unless they are reoxygenated within a short period. Such reoxygenation may not be so uncommon, however. By contrast, cells that are hypoxic rather than completely anoxic may not show the lower values of OER shown in Table 10.1. It seems likely, however, that a single value for OER cannot be applied to all tumour cell populations over the range of fraction doses used in radiotherapy.

Indeed, there is evidence that when cells are in a state of chronic hypoxia, they become slightly more radiosensitive, probably because of depletion of sulphydryl. The effect of oxygen upon the variation in radiosensitivity through the cell cycle (Chapter 8) is minimal, however. Figure 10.8 shows how the survival pattern of synchronized cells is very similar after equivalent doses of 3 Gy in air and 9 Gy under hypoxic conditions. (There does appear to be a smaller OER for mitotic cells, where the value falls from 3 to 2, but this may be a technical problem.)

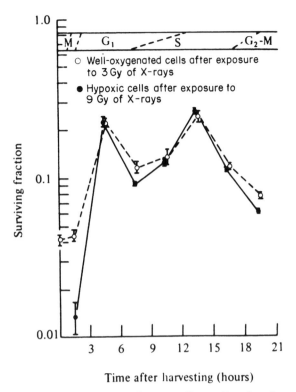

Figure 10.8. Response of synchronized HeLa cells irradiated under well-oxygenated or hypoxic conditions at different stages of the cell cycle. (Reproduced from Sapozink, 1977, by permission of Academic Press, Inc.)

HYPOXIC FRACTION

The two curves in Figure 10.7 show the radiation dose–response for cells at the two extremes of complete aeration and complete anoxia. In many tumour tissues, however, the cell population will be a mixture of these two extremes and the actual dose–response curve will be biphasic. This was shown by Figure 10.5, and Figure 10.9 illustrates this in more detail for a mouse tumour studied by the endpoint dilution assay technique (described in Chapter 12). If the donor animal is alive at the time of irradiation, then its tumour cells are oxygenated and the lowest curve is obtained. If the animal is killed long enough beforehand, all the cells will be anoxic and the uppermost curve is found. With intermediate time intervals the other curves will be obtained, which are biphasic, starting with an aerated slope and changing to the anoxic slope when all the aerated cells have been sterilized.

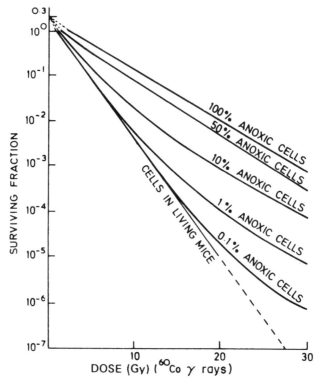

Figure 10.9. Survival curves for cell populations with various proportions of anoxic cells. (Reprinted from *Br. J. Cancer*, **13**, 675–684, Hewitt and Wilson, The effect of tissue oxygen tension of the radiosensitivity of leukaemia cells irradiated *in situ* in the livers of leukaemic mice. ©1959, by permission of the publisher Churchill Livingstone.)

The relevant curve for radiotherapy is probably the 10% anoxic cell example used for Figure 10.5, although information on the degree of hypoxia of human tumours is very inadequate and a broad range of values can be presumed to apply. The main conclusion from this is that hypoxia may not represent a clinical problem when small fraction doses are used over the range where the biphasic curve approaches the aerated slope. It follows from this that any benefit from the use of hypoxic cell radio-sensitizers, such as hyperbaric oxygen, is more likely to be found with larger fraction doses used in radiotherapy.

K VALUE

It is by no means certain that the OER is a constant value with photons. A range of values from 2 to 3 has been found from experimental systems.

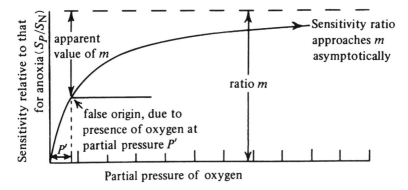

Figure 10.10. Relationship of oxygen enhancement ratio (m) to oxygen concentration. (Reproduced from Alper, 1979, by permission of Cambridge University Press.)

Nor is the K value a constant – again, a range of values has been found: 2–7 mmHg. Different tumours may well have different values for these two parameters and this information will determine the likely response to a regime such as hyperbaric oxygen radiotherapy.

The K value is the concentration of oxygen that gives 50% of the sensitivity obtained in fully oxygenated conditions, and it depends on the rate of fixation of radiation damage by oxygen. It is the inverse of the slope of the curve that shows the rate of increase in radiosensitivity with the rate of increase in O_2 tension. Figure 10.10 uses another version of Figure 10.1 to show the consequence of starting the curve at a false origin due to the existence of oxygen at a partial pressure p'. The OER (designated m in Figure 10.10) will then appear smaller and K will appear larger than the true value.

The shapes of the curves may also differ: that for chronic hypoxia is more like that of the full range shown in Figure 10.10 with a low K value; that for acute hypoxia is 'flatter', similar to the shape drawn from the false origin in Figure 10.10 with a high K value. In fact, the extent of the types of curve will be the same, and comparisons of the response of different tumours need to consider the consequence of such differences in K value over the particular range of partial pressure of oxygen that is relevant to the clinical situation.

Figure 10.11 illustrates the relationship of K value and OER (which is again designated m in the figure). It shows how a tumour that has a low K value will derive less benefit from hyperbaric oxygen than one with a high K value, and a tumour with a higher OER (or m) will also show more benefit in terms of an increase in effective dose. If the two parameters are put together, there may then prove to be a more rational basis for using regimes such as hyperbaric oxygen on certain types of tumours with a high OER and where the K value is high. More research is needed to establish these values of K and OER.

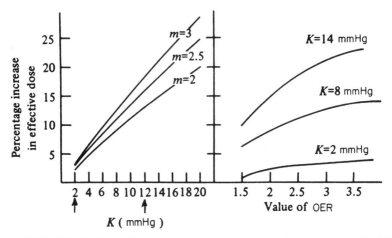

Figure 10.11. Relative benefit of using hyperbaric oxygen for tumours with different *K* value or different OER. (Reproduced from Alper, 1979, by permission of Cambridge University Press.)

Cullen and Walker (1980) found that the *K* value for mouse Ehrlich ascites tumour cells was 1.7 times greater for cells in the exponential phase of growth than for those in plateau phase. If these conditions are equated to acute and chronic hypoxia, respectively, then there may be a therapeutic advantage for the use of hyperbaric oxygen or carbogen for treating tumours in which a state of acute hypoxia occurs. It has been suggsted that chronic hypoxia does not present a therapeutic problem because cells in that state are doomed to die anyway. It has also been suggested that radiosensitizing and radioprotecting drugs may be most effective in cells with an intermediate level of oxygen tension around the *K* value.

HYPERBARIC OXYGEN (HPO)

If the supply of oxygen to tumour cells is insufficient to ensure their radio-sensitivity, then the obvious solution to the problem is to increase the oxygen supply. The most widely used technique has been the administration of oxygen at high pressure, which saturates the plasma and tissue fluids with oxygen during irradiation. The amount of oxygen available is greatly increased in this way by the increased diffusion gradient from the capillaries to the hypoxic tumour cells. Normally oxygen at 3 atm of pressure is employed, which will allow diffusion to a distance of about 1000 μm instead of the usual 100–200 μm.

Unfortunately there are two major problems concerning the clinical use of HPO techniques in radiotherapy. The first problem is the uncertainty of whether the oxygen dissolved at high pressure in the plasma does actually

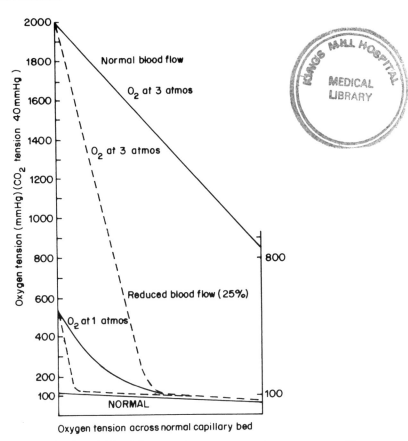

Oxygen tension across normal capillary bed

Figure 10.12. Effect of reduced blood flow on the oxygen tension across a capillary bed when oxygen is breathed at one or three atmospheres. (Reproduced from Nias, 1988, by permission of Churchill Livingstone.)

reach the hypoxic cells in tumours. Any obstruction of the vascular tree will greatly reduce the oxygen available to the related tissues, and vaso-constriction is a known response to high oxygen tension. Figure 10.12 illustrates the effect of reduced blood flow, which may largely negate the advantage of breathing high-pressure oxygen. Solid tumours may not only outgrow their blood supply but also compress the vascular network. The gradients shown in Figure 10.3 will still apply even though the initial oxygen tension may start at a higher level with HPO.

Some experimental work has shown that it may not be necessary to raise the oxygen pressure as high as 3 atm to achieve the maximum radiation response of a tumour. These studies had first showed that the vaso-constrictive effect of oxygen can be opposed by anaesthesia so long as the

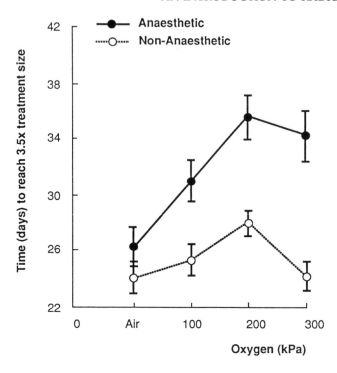

Figure 10.13. Growth delay of C$_3$H mouse mammary tumours irradiated with 25 Gy in air or various pressures of oxygen with or without anaesthesia. (Reproduced from Perry and Nias, 1992, by permission of BIR.)

optimal time interval is used. Then it was shown (Figure 10.13) that the maximum regrowth delay occurred when 25 Gy was delivered to tumours in mice exposed to only 2 *atm* (200 kPa oxygen), with a 25-min interval after anaesthesia. A shorter time interval was less effective. Figure 10.13 shows that there was less benefit from 300 kPa oxygen (3 atm) as well as from lower oxygen pressures, and no anaesthesia.

The second disadvantage of HPO is the possibility that some normal tissues may be sensitized to a small extent. Figure 10.1 showed that this is less likely to occur with the majority of normal tissues that are well vascularized with a partial pressure of oxygen above 40 mmHg. It can be a problem with tissues such as cartilage, which are less well oxygenated, and then the therapeutic ratio between tumour and normal tissue responses will be reduced (see Chapter 16).

Even using 3 atm of oxygen, several clinical trials have shown that HPO can improve the results of radiotherapy under certain circumstances. The most convincing result was reported by Henk (1986) for head and neck tumours. The tumour cure rate was increased from 30% in air to 55% in hyperbaric oxygen at 5 years. This trial exploited the advantage of using larger doses of X-rays for each treatment. Figure 10.5 illustrated the cell survival curve for a mixed population of well-oxygenated and hypoxic cells. In the initial part of the survival curve the response is predominantly determined by the proportion of well-oxygenated cells. With smaller fraction doses of 200 cGy, therefore, no differential effect might be expected unless there was some change in the shape of this cell survival curve (such as occurs due to reoxygenation). It is only when larger dose fractions are given in hyperbaric oxygen that a reduction of the oxygen effect might be demonstrated in some cancers.

CARBOGEN

Carbogen, – a gas mixture of 5% carbon dioxide and 95% oxygen – increases tumour oxygenation by improving blood flow. It is of particular benefit in acute hypoxia caused by the transient occlusion of blood vessels in tumours, in contrast to the chronic hypoxia that results from tumours outgrowing their blood supply (see earlier discussion of K values). Carbogen is a convenient alternative to hyperbaric oxygen because it is effective at normal pressure. Figure 10.14 shows the result obtained when the mouse mammary carcinoma CaNT was given 40 fractions of X-ray treatment over 26 days. The tumours in mice that breathed carbogen were controlled by a much lower dose than those in mice breathing air. At the TCD_{50} level (50% tumour control) there was an enhancement ratio of 1.44. It has been found that further enhancement can be obtained if a small dose of nicotinamide is added to this form of treatment, and it is now in clinical trial with the CHART fractionation regime (Chapter 16) under the title ARCON.

RECOVERY IN HYPOXIC CELLS

The detailed pattern of recovery from sublethal damage (SLDR) was described in Chapter 7. The question arises whether hypoxic cells can recover from sublethal damage to the same extent as oxygenated cells. Table 10.2 applies to HeLa cells that were made hypoxic by the same technique of nitrogen gassing as used for Figure 10.6. Under such conditions the two-dose experiment shows less recovery from sublethal damage by hypoxic cells 1 and 2 h after the first dose. This might mean only that hypoxic cells recover more slowly and that, after a longer time interval, recovery might reach the same level as shown by oxygenated cells at the earlier time. It is shown by Figure 10.15, which shows the pattern of recovery curves as they applied to mouse ascites tumours *in vivo*, that this is

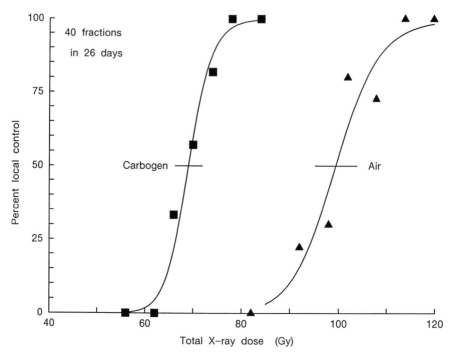

Figure 10.14. Dose–effect curves for mouse mammary tumours given 40 fractions of radiotherapy in 26 days to CBA mice breathing either (▲) air or (■) carbogen. (Redrawn from Rojas et al, 1996, by permission of Elsevier Science Inc., 655 Ave. of the Americas, New York NY 10010-5107.)

not so. These provide models of clinical situations because an ascites tumour cell population is well oxygenated on the first day but poorly oxygenated by the sixth day. Quite obviously, from Figure 10.15 there is less recovery in the hypoxic than in the oxygenated tumour at all time intervals.

Recovery from sublethal damage in cells exposed to different conditions of oxygenation during and after irradiation has been the subject of much study and it can be concluded that cells that are hypoxic during and after irradiation show less recovery from damage than aerated ones. Survival curves for cells irradiated under hypoxic conditions can often be drawn with extrapolation numbers significantly less than those for aerated cells, particularly when statistical analysis is applied. While the survival curves in Figure 10.6 showed that a full shoulder was maintained when the cells were given X-rays under moderately hypoxic conditions, the anoxia curve in Figure 10.7 had no shoulder and was purely exponential. Two-dose experiments under conditions of more severe hypoxia showed no recovery from SLDR at all. It would appear therefore that the biochemical repair mechanism (Chapter 7) is depleted by the metabolic consequence of

Table 10.2. Relative survival (divided dose/single dose[a]) for HeLa cells maintained in air or in nitrogen between divided doses

Time between doses (h)	Relative survival when maintained in:	
	Air	Nitrogen
1	1.4 + 0.2	1.09 + 0.08
2	2.52 + 0.36	1.44 + 0.25

[a]Single dose = 1200 cGy in nitrogen ($\sim$ 8% survival). Divided dose = 600 cGy first dose in nitrogen; 200 cGy second dose in air (200 cGy in air is equivalent to 600 cGy in nitrogen).
Reproduced from Fox and Nias, 1970, by permission of Elsevier Science-NL, Sara Burgerhartstraat 25, 1055 KV Amsterdam, The Netherlands.

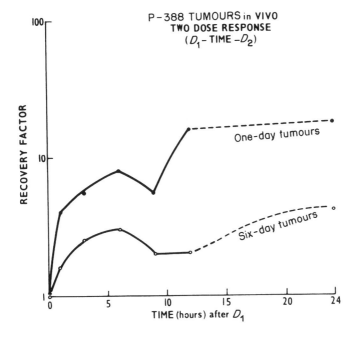

Figure 10.15. Two dose–response curves of ascites tumours. (Reproduced from Belli et al, 1967, by permission of Oxford University Press.)

hypoxia. While there may still be some repair when hypoxia is acute, repair seems to be absent altogether under conditions of chronic hypoxia.

By contrast, hypoxic cells may be the ones that *do* recover from potentially lethal damage (PLDR) (Chapter 7). Potentially lethal damage is repaired by cells that are not proliferating for some reason, and this applies to hypoxic cells. The distinction between PLDR and SLDR may not be a true one under certain conditions and, clearly, the fact that SLDR is reduced and PLDR is increased by hypoxia in some cells leads to a complicated situation with perhaps no net effect unless recovery has been perturbed by some drug combination (Chapter 11).

SUMMARY OF CONCLUSIONS

(1) Due to inadequate blood supply, some tumours contain hypoxic regions because oxygen cannot diffuse much more than 145 μm.
(2) The oxygen diffusion distance may be increased when hyperbaric oxygen is used. It will also increase when the metabolic requirement for oxygen is reduced, e.g. in spheroids cultured at 24°C.
(3) When the partial pressure of oxygen falls below 20 mmHg, radio-sensitivity also falls by up to a factor of 3.
(4) Thus, the presence of oxygen enhances the biological effect of radiation. The difference in radiosensitivity is called the oxygen enhancement ratio, OER.
(5) The oxygen concentration that will give half this enhancement is called the K value. This is larger with acute hypoxia than chronic hypoxia.
(6) The OER appears to be smaller with lower doses of X-rays, perhaps because there is less recovery from sublethal damage in hypoxic cells.
(7) Because solid tumours may contain 10% hypoxic cells, larger fraction doses of radiation are needed if hyperbaric oxygen is to be effective. Anaesthesia may be advantageous.
(8) Carbogen plus nicotinamide is an effective radiosensitizer.

REFERENCES

Alper, T., 1979. *Cellular Radiobiology*. Cambridge University Press, Cambridge.
Belli, J. A., Dicus, C. J. and Bonte, F. J., 1967. Radiation response of mammalian tumor cells. I. Repair of sub-lethal damage *in vivo*. *Journal of the National Cancer Institute*, **38**, 673–682.
Cullen, B. M. and Walker, H. C., 1980. Variation of the radiobiological oxygen constant, *K*, with the proliferative activity of the cells. *International Journal of Radiation Biology*, **38**, 513–524.
Deschner, E. E. and Gray, L. H., 1959. Influence of oxygen tension on X-ray induced chromosomal damage in Ehrlich ascites tumor cells irradiated *in vitro* and *in vivo*. *Radiation Research*, **11**, 115–146.
Fox, M. and Nias, A. H. W., 1970. The influence of recovery from sub-lethal damage on the response of cells to protracted irradiation at low dose rate. *Current Topics in Radiation Research*, **7**, 71–103.

Hewitt, H. B. and Wilson, C. W., 1959. The effect of tissue oxygen tension of the radiosensitivity of leukaemia cells irradiated *in situ* in the livers of leukaemic mice. *British Journal of Cancer*, **13**, 675–684.

Marples, B., Joiner, M. C. and Skov, K. A., 1994. The effect of oxygen on low-dose hypersensitivity and increased radioresistance in Chinese hamster V79 cells. *Radiation Research*, **138**, S17–S20.

Nias, A. H. W., 1988. *Clinical Radiobiology*, 2nd edn. (Suppl.) Churchill Livingstone, Edinburgh.

Nias, A. H. W., Greene, D., Fox, M. and Thomas, R. L., 1967. Effects of 14 MeV monoenergetic neutrons on HeLa and P388F cells *in vitro*. *International Journal of Radiation Biology*, **13**, 449–456.

Nias, A. H. W., Swallow, A. J., Keene, J. P. and Hodgson, B. W., 1973. Absence of a fractionation effect in irradiated HeLa cells. *International Journal of Radiation Biology*, **23**, 559–569.

Perry, P. M. and Nias, A. H. W., 1992. The optimum pressure of oxygen for radiotherapy of a mouse tumour. *British Journal of Radiology*, **65**, 784–786.

Rojas, A., Hirst, V. K., Calvert, A. S. and Johns, H., 1996. Carbogen and nicotinamide as radiosensitizers in a murine mammary carcinoma using conventional and accelerated radiotherapy. *International Journal of Radiation Oncology, Biology, Physics*, **34**, 357–365.

Sapozink, J. D., 1977. Oxygen enhancement ratios in synchronous HeLa cells exposed to low LET radiation. *Radiation Research*, **69**, 27–39.

Sutherland, R. M. and Durand, R. E., 1973. Hypoxic cells in an *in vitro* tumour model. *International Journal of Radiation Biology*, **23**, 235–246.

Sutherland, R. M. and Durand, R. E., 1976. Radiation response of multicell spheroids – an *in vitro* tumour model. *Current Topics in Radiation Research*, **11**, 87–139.

Thomlinson, R. H. and Gray, L. H., 1955. The histological structure of some human lung cancers and the possible implications for radiotherapy. *British Journal of Cancer*, **9**, 539–549.

11 Radiosensitizers and Radioprotectors

In the not too distant future, gene therapy techniques will be available for increasing the radiation response of cells and tissues by modifying their intrinsic radioresistance. One example would be the transfection of wild-type p53 into p53 mutant cells, so as to increase radiation-induced apoptosis (Chapter 6). Another example would be the transfer of antisense oligo-nucleotides to knock out DNA damage repair genes such as DNA–PK (Chapter 7). It has been estimated that the number of surviving cells in a 1 g tumour (10^9) would then decrease from 2.24×10^4 to 2.24×10^3 after thirty 2 Gy fractions, which is the equivalent of giving an extra six fractions (Gordon and McMillan, 1997). With all such strategies, however, it is important to maintain a therapeutic ratio between the sensitivity of normal and tumour cells. It would be no use knocking out the repair mechanism in tumour cells unless it was maintained in the relevant normal cells.

The most effective radiosensitizing agent, up to now, has been oxygen, which will only affect tumours that have a hypoxic fraction of cells. Conversely, the most effective radioprotection occurs when oxygen is absent at the time of irradiation. Radiation chemistry was discussed in Chapter 4 and methods of modifying oxygen levels were discussed in Chapter 10, but there are alternative approaches, which will be discussed later (see later section on *hypoxic cell radiosensitizers*). There are various other drugs that can modify the effect of radiation to produce a net increase or decrease in biological effect. The problem arises of how to separate the chemical effects of such drugs from the physical effects of the radiation. Some drugs will indeed potentiate or reduce radiobiological effects, but only at a dose level that is toxic to cells and tissues. Oxygen is not toxic under physiological conditions, and so the ideal chemical sensitizer should also be effective at a non-toxic dose. In practice, however, some toxicity is unavoidable and that is why this chapter will discuss the interactions with radiation of a wide range of drugs.

When a cell is treated with ionizing radiation the damage follows directly or indirectly from physical events that actually occur during exposure to the beam. When the beam is switched off, no more energy is absorbed, no more molecules are ionized and any molecular lesions will either be expressed or repaired during the next few minutes. Metabolic processes will be involved but these will utilize the normal enzymatic complement of the cell. No chemical has been added. The time scale is short.

By contrast, treatment with a chemical agent implies the introduction of a foreign substance into the environment of the cell for a variable period of time and at a variable concentration. Before any intracellular interaction can occur, the chemical must travel to the exterior of the target cell. It must then diffuse actively or passively across the cell membrane and may then affect the cytoplasm and its organelles before crossing the nuclear membrane. This may occur quickly or slowly and there may be metabolic interaction to change either the chemical or the biochemical targets in the cell, or both. Unlike irradiation, which can be switched on and off and is uniformly distributed throughout the cell volume, a chemical agent cannot be 'switched off' and is subject to concentration gradients in the passive sense and specific biochemical interactions that result in a non-uniform distribution of damage in the cell.

BIOCHEMICAL SENSITIZERS

The biochemical approach to radiosensitization is to use anti-cancer compounds, which affect DNA structure and function, e.g. by an alteration or delay in DNA synthesis. Reduced recovery from sublethal damage (Chapter 7) and a reduction in the size of the shoulder of the cell survival curve (Chapter 8) may explain increased radiosensitivity, but toxic concentrations of the compounds are usually necessary to achieve this. There is often no difference in their effect between normal and malignant cells, although the usual clinical problem of achieving a favourable therapeutic ratio between normal tissue and tumour damage still applies to these compounds.

There are many different types of anti-cancer agent. Many of their sites of action are shown in Figure 11.1 at different points along the synthetic pathway of cellular macromolecules (although not all anti-cancer agents affect synthetic pathways directly). The end result of such action will depend upon the extent to which DNA is damaged, because this is the principal target molecule for cytotoxic agents used in cancer chemotherapy. This is the basis for the classification of cancer chemotherapy agents:

(1) *Antimetabolites* (such as methotrexate, 5-fluorouracil and cytosine arabinoside), which inhibit DNA synthesis.
(2) *Alkylating agents* (such as nitrogen mustard and cyclophosphamide) which cross-link strands of DNA.
(3) *Antibiotics* (such as actinomycin D and bleomycin), which intercalate between DNA base pairs and block RNA production.
(4) *Miscellaneous* (such as platinum drugs and the *Vinca* alkaloids), which have different mechanisms of action.

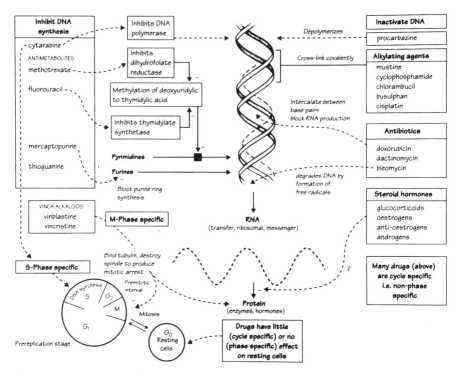

Figure 11.1. Drugs used in cancer treatment. (Reproduced from Neal, 1997, by permission of Blackwell Science Ltd.)

The period of time during which such a chemical may react with sensitive cellular targets depends on a large number of factors relating to drug disposition. This will be the result not only of the duration of exposure (i.e. before the chemical is naturally diluted) but also of the original concentration in the extracellular environment and upon the stability of the chemical. Thus the half-life of the bifunctional alkylating agent nitrogen mustard in aqueous solution at 37 °C is 45 min, so this drug is chemically unstable. By contrast, the half-time for clearance from the blood of *cis*-platinum is 89 h. Platinum can be given in a slow infusion but nitrogen mustard must be injected as soon as the solution has been made up, if it is to be effective.

DRUG–RADIATION COMBINATIONS

The nitroheterocyclic compound misonidazole was the subject of detailed laboratory research in the 1970s and a clinical trial in the 1980s, so its mode of action and efficacy as a radiosensitizer are relatively well understood (see

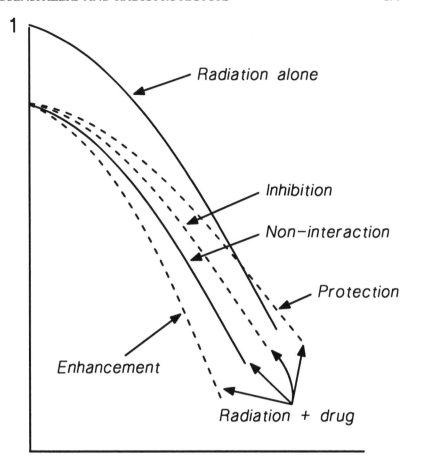

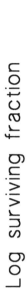

Figure 11.2. Terminology for drug–radiation interactions. Reprinted from *Int. J. Radiat. Oncol. Biol. Phys.*, Steel, Terminology in the description of drug-radiation interactions, **5**, pp. 1145–1150, 1979, with permission from Elsevier Science.

later section on hypoxic cell sensitizers). It is regrettable that the same degree of detailed study has not been made of all the other chemotherapeutic agents available for cancer treatment in combination with radiotherapy. The extent of the problem is illustrated by the scheme of dose–response curves in Figure 11.2. The topmost curve is for radiation alone, while the other curves show the various possibilities when a drug combination is used. The solid line applies to a combination where the drug simply lowers the radiation dose–response curve with no change in its shape, i.e. there is no interaction between the two modalities of treatment.

The dashed line shows how the radiation dose–response curve may be steepened by the drug; this is called enhancement. If it is made shallower, this is called inhibition. Figure 11.2 also shows the extreme case where the combination gives less effect than radiation alone at a high dose level. This is called protection.

This schematic diagram illustrates the terminology used in the description of drug–radiation interactions. If an agent is completely inactive when used by itself, then evidence from sensitization or protection can be obtained without more detailed study. This requirement is usually satisfied for radiosensitization by oxygen, because this substance is non-toxic under normal conditions.

In nearly every other combination of drug and radiation, both agents show an effect that is dose dependent. Figure 11.3 shows this for the platinum coordination complex CHIP (cis-dichloro-trans-dihydroxy-cis-bis(isopropylamine) platinum IV). There are dose–response curves for both CHIP (1) and X-rays (2), plus a curve for the combination of a drug dose and then radiation doses (3). The difference between the final slope of the second and third curves shows enhancement. Dose–response curves for both agents were necessary for this information to be obtained. In nearly every example in the literature this requirement is not satisfied, and conclusions are reached with insufficient data.

The combination of radiation and drug may be more effective because of one or more of the following mechanisms: (i) interaction may occur with the drug present during irradiation; (ii) the drug may interfere with repair of radiation damage; and (iii) there may be some differential effect upon the proliferation kinetics of tumour and/or normal cells.

The presence of the drug during radiation should ideally be demonstrated by standard biochemical and pharmacological techniques. If the active moiety of the drug molecule can be labelled with a radioactive isotope, this demonstration is relatively simple (although invasive methods of sampling, such as biopsies, are not always possible or ethically desirable with human subjects). If the active moiety cannot be labelled or tissue samples cannot be studied, then indirect evidence of drug binding will have to suffice, but doubt must then remain as to if or how the drug interacted with the radiation. It will also be important to know whether the drug binds to the target molecules in the cell following passive diffusion or some mechanism of active transport.

The large amount of literature describing the mechanism of radiation damage is not matched by equivalent knowledge of the various drugs in common use. Only a few examples can be given in this book. Radiation dosimetry, for example, is a relatively very precise physical technique where the distribution in treated tissues can be measured precisely and the clinician can repeat a treatment in the confident knowledge that the prescribed dose will be faithfully delivered. For most drugs it is almost

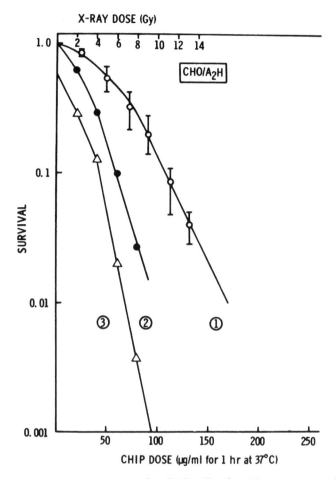

Figure 11.3. Dose–response curves for CHO cells after (1) treatment with CHIP, (2) treatment with X-rays and (3) treatment with CHIP 58 μg/ml for 1 h and then with X-rays after a 1 h interval. (Reprinted from *Br. J. Cancer*, **42**, 292–296, Szumiel and Nias, Isobologram analysis of the combined effects of anti-tumour platinum complexes and ionizing radiation on mammalian cells. ©1980, by permission of the publisher Churchill Livingstone.)

impossible to emulate this precision. Certain minimal information should nevertheless be available before a drug is used. What is the mode of action at the cellular level? Does the drug reach the intracellular target molecules by passive diffusion or active transport? Is the drug active in its original form or as some degradative product (e.g. after cyclization in the case of cyclophosphamide)? What is the rate of degradation and loss of activity of the drug (e.g. the half-time of hydrolysis in water or preferably in some medium relevant to the *in vivo* milieu at 37 °C)? Does the drug degrade to a

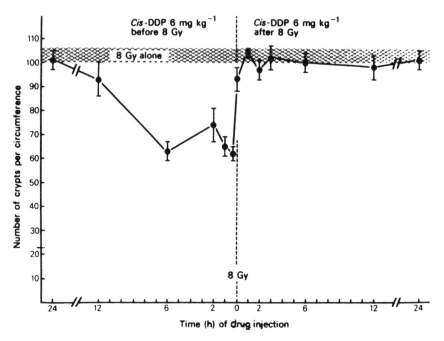

Figure 11.4. The effect of *cis*-platinum and irradiation on intestinal crypt cells. (Reprinted from *Br. J. Cancer*, **49**, 779–786, von der Maaser, Interactions of radiation and adriamycin, bleomycin, mitomycin C or *cis*-diaminedichloroplatinum II in intestinal crypt cells. ©1984, by permission of the publisher Churchill Livingstone.)

final product that is non-toxic? What are the pharmacokinetics? What is the role of liver metabolism? Solubility of the drug is another consideration – is it soluble in aqueous media and (apart from temperature effects) is its activity influenced by pH? Does any other change in the substrate influence drug activity?

The terms in Figure 11.2 should only be used when dose–response data are available for both drug and radiation effects used separately. The combinations can then be tested for the most effective interaction, which may be described as synergistic when the result is much more than would be expected from the sum of the cytotoxic effects of each dose of each agent used alone. For this test three dose–response curves are needed, as shown in Figure 11.3 for a clone of CHO cells treated with the platinum drug CHIP.

Figure 11.3 features the result of the study of only one time interval between drug and radiation. Other examples are available in the literature, where different time intervals were used as well as variations in dose levels of the drug and radiation. Figure 11.4 shows a time-line for the interaction of *cis*-platinum (*cis*-DDP) and radiation on the response of small intestinal crypt cells (see Chapter 8 for the assay). The maximum effect occurs when

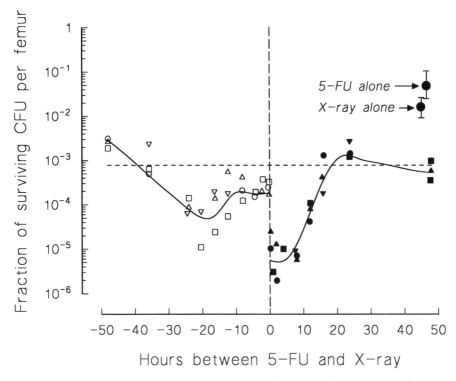

Figure 11.5. The effect of 5-fluorouracil (5-FU) and X-rays in the treatment of mouse leukaemia. (Reproduced from Viette et al, 1971, by permission of Oxford University Press.)

the drug is injected up to 6 h before irradiation. The drug has no effect upon intestinal crypt cells when given after irradiation. By contrast, Figure 11.5 shows an older time-line for the interaction of 5-fluorouracil (5-FU) and radiation. The surviving fractions with either 5-FU alone or X-ray alone are shown and the dashed line shows the reduction in survival that would occur simply with both effects added together. When combined in sequence, survival falls below the dashed line at various time intervals but the maximum effect on leukaemic cells occurred when 5-FU was given up to 8 h *after* irradiation. (The CFU assay is also described in Chapter 8).

RECOVERY

After radiation, the shoulder portions of cell survival curves can be correlated with recovery but there is no reason for this as far as most drug survival data are concerned. Not all drug dose–response curves have a shoulder (e.g. nitrogen mustard curves are purely exponential). Even with those drugs where there is an initial shoulder to the survival curve (e.g. Figure 11.3), tests for recovery from sublethal drug damage fail to reveal the sort of increase in survival found with radiation (Chapter 7). This may be due to the problem of continued drug activity during the fractionation interval.

Damage to DNA may be repaired by removal of bound molecules by an excision process. If such excision repair is not completed before the DNA is used as a template for DNA replication, some cells can circumvent the damage by a process called post-replication repair. Both excision and post-replication repair processes facilitate the recovery of cells from DNA damage introduced by chemical agents. Inability to synthesize past lesions in the DNA is associated with mitotic delay, chromosome damage and eventually cell death.

Following radiation, it is known that the timing of events within a cell attempting to recover from damage to its DNA will depend upon four factors: (i) the nature and number of lesions produced in its DNA; (ii) the ability of the cell to perform those different types of repair required by such lesion; (iii) the growth conditions at the time, which may help or hinder the cell's repair mechanism; and (iv) the efficiency of each repair event in restoring the full competence of the original DNA in both its transcriptional and replicative roles.

The same sort of information should be sought for each drug before the repair mechanism can be expected to be understood in drug–radiation combinations. At the present time there is a relative dearth of information, but such data as are available show that many drugs may reduce repair capacity following radiation. It is not clear if and how the molecular biological evidence for the repair of DNA strand breakage can be correlated with the biological phenomenon usually termed 'recovery from sublethal damage', but it is known that the drug actinomycin D, which inhibits RNA synthesis, also inhibits recovery from sublethal radiation damage (SLDR). Other drugs that are known to reduce the amount of SLDR include 5-fluorouracil, BUdR and IUdR, vinblastine and platinum coordination complexes. A difference in the cellular environment at the time of irradiation may influence the degree of recovery from potentially lethal damage independently from such effects on sublethal damage.

Figure 11.6 shows the evidence for recovery from potentially lethal drug damage for the three drugs cyclophosphamide (an alkylating agent), 5-fluorouracil (a pyrimidine analogue that is an anti-metabolite) and bleomycin (an antibiotic that causes single- and double-strand breaks). For comparison, the top left box shows the extent to which potentially lethal radiation damage can be repaired in Chinese hamster cells held in plateau phase for 6 h or more after irradiation before subculture; survival increases more then tenfold. The other three boxes in Figure 11.6 compare the response of EMT-6 mammary sarcoma cells excised from the mouse 2 h

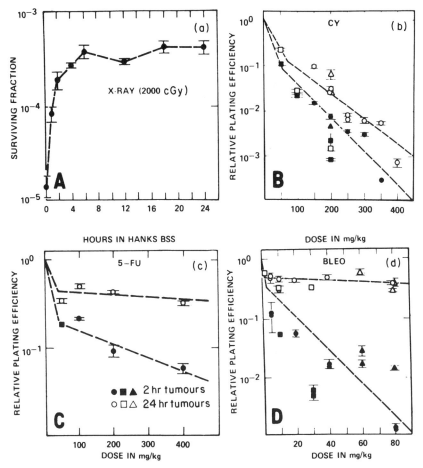

Figure 11.6. Repair of potentially lethal damage following X-ray treatment of plateau-phase Chinese hamster cells *in vitro* (a) and treatment of EMT-6 mouse mammary sarcoma *in vivo* with cyclophosphamide (b), 5-hydroxyurea (c) and bleomycin (d). (Reproduced from Hahn, 1975, by permission of Radiological Society of North America.)

(closed symbols) or 24 h (open symbols) after drug administration and then plated out *in vitro*. The survival curves differ markedly in all three cases, with the result for bleomycin being the most striking; approximately 99% of the cells are able to deal with potentially lethal damage after high drug doses if they are left in the tumour for 24 h.

PHASE-SPECIFIC DRUGS

The dose–response curves for the three drugs in Figure 11.6 were biphasic in shape. This suggests that the tumour contained two cell populations of

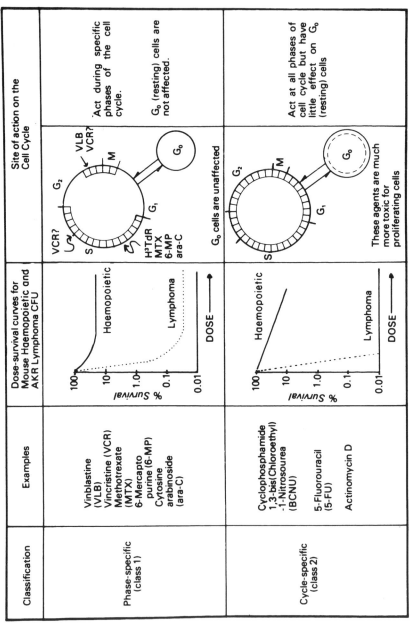

Figure 11.7. Phase-specific and cycle-specific drugs. (Reproduced from Bruce et al, 1966, by permission of Oxford University Press.)

differing chemosensitivity. Such a pattern is carried to an extreme in the response of cells to drugs that are classified as phase-specific (Figure 11.7). This means that a drug is cytotoxic during certain phases of the cell cycle and has a minimal effect during other phases. As a result, the survival curve only falls to a certain level and then becomes horizontal with no further killing of cells from any higher drug dosage. This applies to drugs such as the *Vinca* alkaloids vinblastine and vincristine, which are active in the mitotic phase, and the anti-metabolites methotrexate, 6-mercaptopurine and cytosine arabinoside, which are active in the DNA synthetic phase of the cell cycle. By contrast, drugs that are classified as cycle-specific are cytotoxic throughout the cell cycle, so that the dose–response curves have a simple shape; the higher the dose, the lower the survival. This applies to drugs such as cyclophosphamide, 5-fluorouracil and actinomycin D.

Both of the schematic diagrams in Figure 11.6 show a systematic difference between the dose–response of normal haemopoietic cells and malignant lymphoma cells. The malignant cells are more sensitive to the action of both classes of drugs than are normal cells. This would provide a therapeutic advantage if the scheme applied to clinical situations but, unfortunately, this laboratory model has only a restricted application. Furthermore, the 'protective' mechanism of cycle-specific drugs will only apply if such drugs are given over a period of time that is short relative to the phases of the cell cycle (e.g. by injection). If drug administration is protracted over a longer period (e.g. by infusion, then the cells that were in resistant phases will have time to progress into the sensitive phases. If this process is continued, then the dose–response curve will lose its biphasic shape and become similar to that of a cycle-specific drug.

RECALL

Recall is a phenomenon that is sometimes observed in clinical practice, when the effect of radiation is enhanced by the addition of a chemo-therapeutic agent. The classical example involves a radiation skin reaction that was not evident after the original course of radiotherapy but develops in the irradiated area when a dose of drug is administered *subsequently*. The skin reaction is then more severe than would be expected from the radiation dose. Actinomycin D is a drug that may lead to the recall reaction. The phenomenon is quite different from sensitization, which occurs when the drug is administered before or during the radiation. With recall, the drug is delivered several months after the radiation and so the mechanism of interaction is different.

PROTECTION AND SENSITIZATION

Clinical trials have shown that the best radiation sensitizer is oxygen dissolved in the tissues at a physiological concentration. With normal tissues, of course, oxygen is usually present in the cellular environment, so sensitization can only be demonstrated by comparison with solid tumours, when the tissues may be hypoxic. If the concentration of oxygen molecules in the vicinity of the irradiated tissue is reduced, this will swing the radiation chemical competition in favour of the endogenous hydrogen donors in that tissue.

The balance may be effected in the opposite direction by the addition of protective compounds such as those containing the sulphydryl group, —SH (e.g. cyteamine and cysteine). In terms of reactions, then, while oxygen is more damaging because of the effect already discussed in Chapter 4:

$$R^{.} + O_2 \longrightarrow RO_2^{.}$$

a compound containing an —SH group will have the following effect:

$$R^{.} + -SH \longrightarrow RH + -S^{.}$$

The sulphydryl group has enabled the ionized molecule to be restored to its normal state. In practice, most —SH compounds investigated so far have proved toxic in the concentrations necessary to be effective in clinical use. The thiophosphates are less toxic, however, but are not protective until they are transformed by enzymes inside living cells. The best example of this is WR-2721 (see Figure 11.13). Most cells contain measurable amounts of —SH groups, but the concentrations are not high enough to compete successfully with atmospheric O_2 for the $R^{.}$. As well as protection by the mechanisms discussed, there are also several other ways by which protective compounds may operate (see later).

HYPOXIC CELL SENSITIZERS

Alternative sensitizers to oxygen must not only act by intracellular binding of naturally occurring radioprotectors (such as the —SH compounds) but may also act by swinging the radiation chemical competition in favour of the oxidative pathway and against the reductive. The main products of the irradiation of water are the $OH^{.}$ radicals, which are oxidative, and the hydrated electrons (e_{aq}^{-}), which are powerful reducing agents (Chapter 4). Any compound that is affinic for such electrons will therefore tend to be radiosensitizing. This is the mechanism of action of the nitroimidazole compounds, which have been used clinically on the assumption that they mimic the oxygen effect in those hypoxic tissues to which they can diffuse.

Because oxygen is the most effective radiosensitizer (Chapter 10), the most effective radiosensitizing drugs will be those compounds that mimic the effect of oxygen and only sensitize hypoxic cells. The potentiation shown in Figure 11.3 by CHIP was obtained using aerated cells and, although this drug also sensitizes hypoxic cells, this effect on aerated cells is a serious disadvantage. The ideal hypoxic cell radiosensitizer will be completely non-toxic at the dose level needed for effective sensitization.

The most effective agents are the electron-affinic compounds and the bioreductive drugs. The latter are compounds that are activated in hypoxic cells by reductive metabolism to form substances that are toxic to such cells. Some compounds combine both the electron-affinic property of hypoxic cell sensitization and the bioreductive property. The main examples are nitro-heterocyclic agents (Adams et al, 1991) such as the nitroimidazoles, including metronidazole (Figure 11.8) and misonidazole (Figures 11.8 and 11.9). Less toxic analogues include pimonidazole, nimorazole and RSU 1069. The latter is an active bioreductive drug (Figure 11.10).

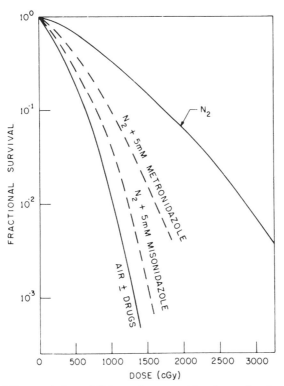

Figure 11.8. Effects of the addition of metronidazole and misonidazole to the medium on the survival curves of mammalian cells irradiated in air or nitrogen. (Redrawn from Chapman and Urtasun, *Cancer*, **40**, 484–488. ©(1977) American Cancer Society. Reprinted by permission of Wiley–Liss, Inc., a subsidiary of John Wiley & Sons Inc.)

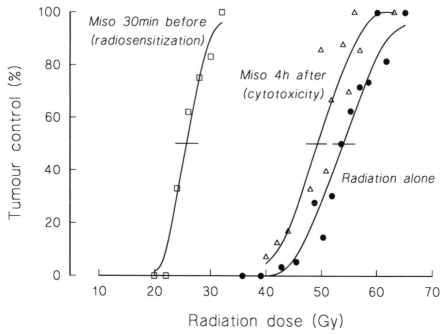

Figure 11.9. Tumour control in C$_3$H mouse mammary tumours measured 120 days after irradiation. Misonidazole (1 g/kg) was given either 30 min before or 4 h after irradiation. (Reproduced from Overgaard and Horsman, 1993, by permission of Edward Arnold.)

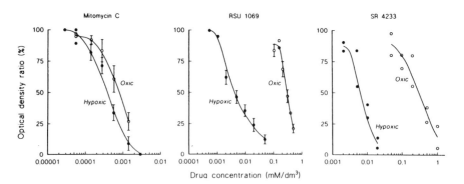

Figure 11.10. Dose–effect curves for V79 cells treated under oxic or hypoxic conditions with three different cytotoxic agents. The optical density of the cell cultures provides a measure of the surviving fraction. (Reproduced from Stratford and Stephens, 1989, by permission of Elsevier Science Inc., 655 Ave. of the Americas, New York NY 10010-5107.)

Figure 11.8 shows results with two of the nitroimidazoles added for 1 h and then removed immediately after irradiation of cells *in vitro*. The oxygen enhancement ratio (OER) of 2.8 is reduced to some extent by metronidazole, and even more so by misonidazole. In both cases it is the nitrogen curves that are affected. The survival curve of cells irradiated in air is unaffected by either of the drugs. Because there was no toxicity from the drugs, these results show true hypoxic cell radiosensitization *in vitro*.

This has also been demonstrated *in vivo* with tumour control data. Figure 11.9 shows dose–effect curves comparing the effect of radiation given alone or with misonidazole. If the drug was administered 30 min *before* radiation, there was a significant reduction in the dose required to control half of the tumours (TCD_{50}): from 54 Gy to 26 Gy (an OER of 2.1). If the drug was given *after* radiation, there was a very small reduction of TCD_{50} to 49 Gy (an OER of only 1.1). In the latter case the drug had only a cytotoxic effect, but the drug is a very effective radiosensitizer of mouse tumours such as C_3H mammary tumour, without toxicity. The OER of 2.1 is not far below the OER that can be obtained with mammalian cells. Unfortunately, that dose level of misonidazole would lead to neurotoxicity in clinical practice and lower dosage is not very effective. More than 7000 patients have been included in 50 clinical trials (Overgaard, 1994). With epithelial carcinomas only a small benefit was found with misonidazole and metronidazole. Pimonidazole and nimorazole were more effective.

Agents such as misonidazole are *bioreductive drugs*, which are activated by metabolic reduction in tumour cells to form highly effective cytotoxins; this mechanism will therefore be an additional factor to their radiosensitization of hypoxic cells. There are three different classes of these drugs: heterocyclic nitrocompounds such as misonidazole and RSU-1069; N-oxides such as tirapazamine (SR 4233); and quinones such as mitomycin C (Adams and Stratford, 1994). Figure 11.10 shows dose–effect curves for the three types of bioreductive drug and illustrates how much more effective they are against hypoxic cells. They would clearly be expected to be less active against oxic normal cells than against hypoxic cells found in tumours, and are obviously a useful adjunct to radiotherapy.

Tirapazamine shows the largest effect of the three drugs in Figure 11.10 and is now in clinical trial. It has been shown that the preferential killing of hypoxic cells by the drug restores the oxic fraction of an experimental tumour with the same kinetics as occurs after irradiation. Kim and Brown (1994) call this drug effect 'rehypoxiation', to contrast with the well-established phenomenon of reoxygenation after irradiation (to be described in Chapter 16, Figure 16.3). As an alternative to its use as a hypoxic cell radiosensitizer, tirapazamine can be combined with other types of cytotoxic chemotherapy, e.g. with platinum (*cis*-DDP), thus combining a hypoxic and an oxic cytotoxin (Durie and Brown, 1993).

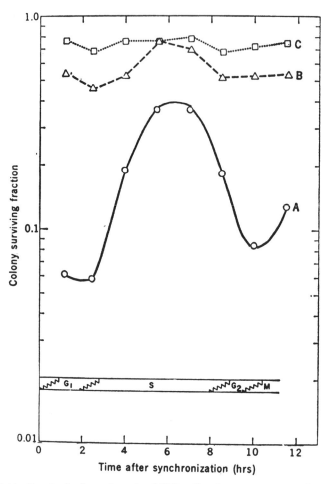

Figure 11.11. Survival of synchronized V79 cells after treatment with 710 cGy of X-rays alone (A) or in the presence of cysteamine, 5 mM (B) or 50 mM (C), at different times during the cell cycle. (Reproduced from Sinclair, 1968, by permission of *Science,* ©1968 American Association for the Advancement of Science.)

PROTECTION

Figure 11.11 shows the converse effect when V79 hamster cells are treated with the radioprotective drug cysteamine (an —SH-containing agent whose mode of action was discussed in Chapter 5). The cells were synchronized by mitotic selection and their radiation response through the cell cycle is shown in curve A. Curves B and C show the effect of treatment with 5 mM and 50 mM cysteamine immediately prior to irradiation (these two concentrations of the drug were non-toxic during the 15–20 min period

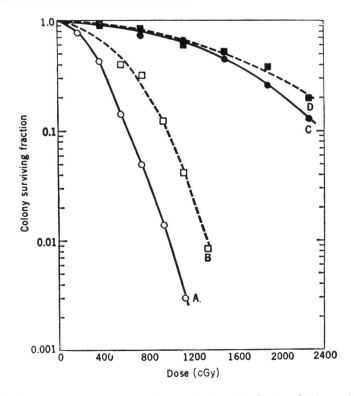

Figure 11.12. Survival curves of synchronized V79 cells after irradiation at 1½ h (G$_1$) or 7 h (late S) after mitotic selection. Curves A and B for G$_1$ and S cells irradiated alone. Curves C and D for G$_1$ and S cells irradiated in the presence of 50 mM cysteamine. (Reproduced from Sinclair, 1968, by permission of *Science*, © 1968 American Association for the Advancement of Science.)

required for addition, irradiation and removal of the agent). Not only do the cells show much higher survival to the radiation dose of 710 cGy but also the differential response in curve A is reduced and is almost completely removed in curves B and C, respectively.

The results with 50 mM cysteamine are shown in the form of radiation dose–response curves in Figure 11.12 for cells irradiated in G$_1$ or in late S-phase. Curves A and B show the sort of dose–responses that were illustrated in Chapter 10, Figure 10.5, with the difference being primarily in terms of the larger shoulder of the survival curve for S-phase cells. When the cells are irradiated in the presence of cysteamine, however, there is not only a large measure of protection but also a reduction in the difference between the radiation response of G$_1$ and late-S cells (curves C and D). These patterns can be expressed in terms of the dose-modifying factors for cysteamine, which are 4.2 for G$_1$ cells and 2.7 for S cells.

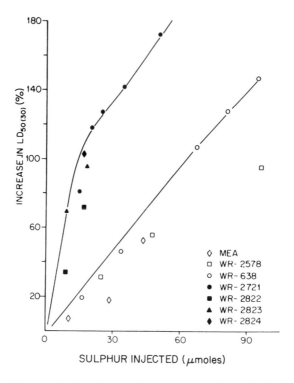

Figure 11.13. Dose reduction factors for haematopoietic death in the C57BL/6J mouse as a function of the number of μmoles of sulphur injected in the form of various radioprotective drugs. (Reprinted from Yuhas, 1980, by permission of John Wiley & Sons, Inc.)

This protective effect of cysteamine, which levels off the variations in X-ray sensitivity throughout the cell cycle, indicates that at least part of the reason for such variations is the level of naturally occurring radioprotective constituents that mammalian cells possess at different phases in their cycle. Whatever their nature, it is clear that these constituents are not present in saturation quantities at any stage of the cycle, because cysteamine provides protection even at the most resistant stage. Evidence for the fact that the protective action of cysteamine is not dependent upon the state of oxygenation of the cell was discussed in Chapter 10, where it was shown (in Figure 10.8) that the variations in X-ray sensitivity throughout the cell cycle are the same for both fully oxygenated and hypoxic cells.

What is important is the concentration of sulphydryl groups. Figure 11.13 shows how the dose of radiation required for haemopoietic death (see Chapter 14) can be increased by various radioprotective drugs in relation to the amount of sulphur injected. Drugs such as WR-2721 (Ethiofos) are obviously more effective in this respect and have now been given clinical trial (McDonald et al, 1994) to protect the salivary glands in patients receiving radiotherapy for head and neck tumours. It is important to find a dose level that is not too toxic, and also to ensure that the tumour is not protected as much as the normal tissues. As an alternative, the use of pharmacological agents to protect normal tissues against radiation will be described in Chapter 13.

SUMMARY OF CONCLUSIONS

(1) The most effective radiosensitizing agent is oxygen if it is present at the cellular target at the time of irradiation. Oxygen is non-toxic at physiological concentration.

(2) Radioprotection occurs in the absence of oxygen and/or the presence of endogenous hydrogen donors, such as those containing the sulphydryl group —SH, but these may be toxic.

(3) Electron affinic compounds such as the nitroimidazoles mimic the effect of oxygen but they may also be toxic.

(4) Bioreductive drugs provide an effective cytotoxic action against hypoxic drugs.

(5) Other drugs enhance the effect of radiation in aerated cells because of the additional biochemical toxicity; they are usually toxic at an effective dose level.

(6) Sulphydryl-containing drugs are radioprotective, but often toxic.

REFERENCES

Adams, G. E. and Stratford, I. J., 1994. Bioreductive drugs for cancer therapy: the search for tumor specificity. *International Journal of Radiation Oncology, Biology, Physics*, **29**, 231–238.

Adams, G. E., Bremner, J., Stratford, I. J., et al, 1991. Nitroheterocyclic compounds as radiosensitizers and bioreductive drugs. *Radiotherapy and Oncology*, **20** (Suppl. 1), 85–91.

Bruce, W. R., Meeker, B. E. and Valeriote, F. A., 1966. Comparison of the sensitivity of normal haematapoietic and transplanted lymphoma colony forming cells to chemotherapeutic agents administered *in vivo*. *Journal of the National Cancer Institute*, **37**, 233–245.

Chapman, J. D. and Urtasun, R. C., 1977. The application in radiation therapy of substances which modify cellular radiation response. *Cancer*, **40**, 484–488.

Durie, M. J. and Brown, J. M., 1993. Tumor-specific, schedule-dependent interaction between Tirapazamine (SR 4233) and Cisplatin. *Cancer Research*, **53**, 4633–4636.

Gordon, A. T. and McMillan, T. J., 1997. A role for molecular radiobiology in radiotherapy. *Clinical Oncology*, **9**, 70–78.

Hahn, G. M., 1975. Radiotherapy and chemotherapy: some parallels and differences. *Radiology*, **114**, 203–211.

Kim, I. H. and Brown, J. M., 1994. Reoxygenation and rehypoxiation in the SCCV11 mouse tumour. *International Journal of Radiation Oncology, Biology, Physics*, **29**, 493–497.

McDonald, S., Meyerowitz, D. D. S., Smudzin, T. and Rubin, P., 1994. Preliminary results of a pilot study using WR-2271 before fractionated irradiation of the head and neck to reduce salivary gland dysfunction. *International Journal of Radiation Oncology, Biology, Physics*, **29**, 747–754.

Neal, M. J., 1997. *Medical Pharmacology at a Glance*, 3rd edn. Blackwell Science, Oxford.

Overgaard, J., 1994. Clinical evaluation of nitroimidazoles as modifiers of hypoxia in solid tumours. *Oncology Research*, **6**, 509–518.

Overgaard, J. and Horsman, M. R., 1993. Overcoming hypoxic cell radioresistance. In *Basic Clinical Radiobiology*, edited by G. G. Steel. Edward Arnold, London.

Sinclair, W. K., 1968. Cysteamine: differential X-ray protective effect on Chinese hamster cells during the cell cycle. *Science*, **159**, 442–444.

Steel, G. G., 1979. Terminology in the description of drug–radiation interactions. *International Journal of Radiation Oncology, Biology, Physics*, **5**, 1145–1150.

Stratford, I. J. and Stephens, M. A., 1989. The differential hypoxic toxicity of bioreductive drugs determined *in vitro* by the MMT assay. *International Journal of Radiation Oncology, Biology, Physics*, **16**, 973–976.

Szumiel, I. and Nias, A. H. W., 1980. Isobologram analysis of the combined effects of anti-tumour platinum complexes and ionizing radiation on mammalian cells. *British Journal of Cancer*, **42**, 292–296.

Viette, T., Eggerding, F. and Valeriote, F., 1971. Combined effect of X-radiation and 5-fluorouracil on survival of transplanted leukemic cells. *Journal of the National Cancer Institute*, **47**, 865–870.

von der Maase, H., 1984. Interactions of radiation and adriamycin, bleomycin, mitomycin C or *cis*-diaminedichloroplatinum II in intestinal crypt cells. *British Journal of Cancer*, **49**, 779–786.

Yuhas, J. M., 1980. On the potential application of radioprotective drugs in solid tumor radiotherapy. In *Radiation–Drug Interactions in the Treatment of Cancer*, edited by G. H. Sohal and R. P. Maickel. Wiley, New York, pp. 113–135.

12 Normal and Malignant Cells

This chapter will ask the question whether there is any difference between normal and malignant cells in their response to radiation. If we disregard the cell cycle, cell population kinetics and the pathological organization of malignant cell populations, then the simple answer would be no! This is because the radiosensitivity of an asynchronous normal cell population and its exact malignant counterpart is often found to be the same. Certainly, dose–response curves are similar for survival of the colony-forming ability of the individual cells cultured *in vitro* (Chapter 8). Normal and malignant cells do not usually live in such an artificial state, however, because they are part of their respective tissues. In these circumstances their response to radiation will often show differences. Such differences are nearly all the consequence of a variety of cell population kinetic and histopathological factors that are the essence of malignancy and normality in the respective tissues. Gene mutations such as those in the tumour suppressor gene p53 may also affect radiosensitivity. (The differences due to cell population kinetics will be discussed later.)

The sort of evidence for the earlier statement concerning the similar response of normal and malignant cells is obtained from studies where a normal cell population is transformed into a malignant cell population by treatment with a carcinogenic chemical or radiation. This is illustrated by Figure 12.1. The upper part shows a survival curve for C_3H mouse embryo cells (10 $T\frac{1}{2}$ cells) with the usual shoulder portion for doses up to 500 cGy; thereafter, the curve is exponential with $D_0 = 150$ cGy. The lower part shows a curve for malignant transformation, which rises to a maximum at 500 cGy and then falls, with a final slope parallel to that of the cell survival curve. So with higher doses cell killing exceeds malignant transformation and the relative incidence of malignant change is much lower at higher doses (see Chapter 19).

The cells then show various changes in the morphology of their colonies and in their response to various chemicals and surface-acting agglutinating agents. The ultimate test of malignancy is the formation of a metastasizing tumour when such cells are inoculated into the same genetic strain of animal from which the normal cells were derived. At the single-cell level, however, the differences can only be tested *in vitro*. For Figure 12.2 the malignant transformation was achieved by using the carcinogenic chemical NMU (methyl nitrosourea). Figure 12.2 shows how both the original normal

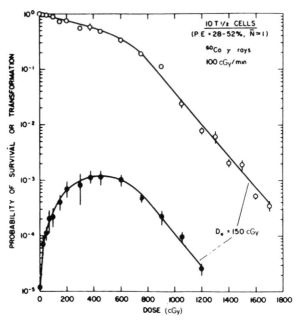

Figure 12.1. Survival and malignant transformation of 10 T$\frac{1}{2}$ cells exposed to ^{60}Co γ-rays. (Reproduced from Han et al, 1980, by permission of American Association for Cancer Research.)

and the transformed cells from such a procedure have identical radio-sensitivity, although they differ in all the other respects described above.

The other sort of evidence comes from a comparison of cells derived from a tumour with cells taken from the equivalent normal tissue. One of the most common tumour cell systems used for the testing of new anti-cancer drugs is the L1210 leukaemia. Leukaemia is a tumour of bone marrow and such L1210 cells can therefore be compared with normal bone marrow cells. This can be done in the same strain of mouse using the spleen colony assay system (described in Chapter 8). Leukaemic bone marrow is a rapidly proliferating cell population so it is necessary to stimulate the normally quiescent normal bone marrow into a similar state of rapid proliferation to enable the comparison of radiosensitivity to be made under identical conditions. All this was done by Hendry (1972), who found that the parameters of the X-ray dose–response curves of normal and malignant bone marrow cell populations had similar values when the marrow was irradiated in the femur. The D_0 values were 82 cGy. Only the extrapolation numbers differed, being 1.3 and 3.4 for normal and leukaemic cells respectively.

This comparison confirmed *in vivo* the earlier *in vitro* evidence that there may be no difference between the *intrinsic* radiosensitivity of malignant and normal cells of the same histological type. Both the environment of the cells

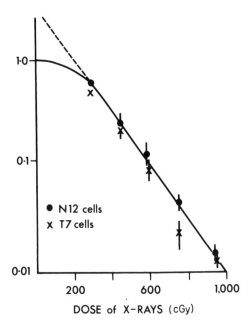

Figure 12.2. X-ray dose–response curves of normal (N12) and transformed (T7) Chinese hamster cells. (Reproduced from Wilkinson, 1971, by permission of Manchester University.)

and their proliferative state had to be matched before this comparison could be made properly. Under the physiological conditions of normal cell populations and the pathological conditions of malignant cell populations in their respective *tissues* such requirements are rarely met, so the radiation responses of such cell populations *will* be different.

RADIOSENSITIVITY OF TUMOUR CELL POPULATIONS

Changes in the environment and proliferative state of tumour cells are not the only factors to be considered. Molecular biological techniques have also shown changes in tumour cells that might affect their radiosensitivity. The p53 tumour suppressor gene, which is activated following radiation, should provide time at the G_1 checkpoint for DNA repair (Chapter 2). Cells carrying mutant p53 alleles or no p53 alleles might therefore be expected to be more radiosensitive than cells carrying the wild-type p53 gene. Unfortunately, Figure 12.3 shows that very little correlation has been

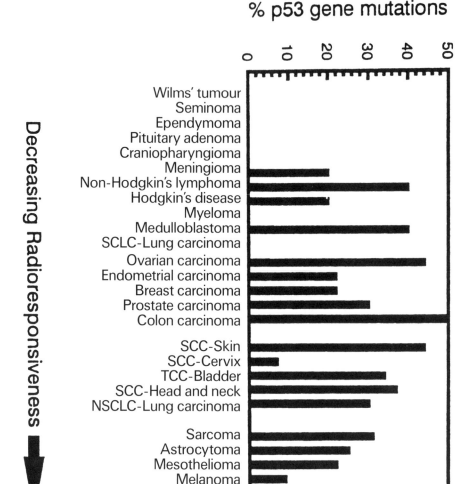

Figure 12.3. The incidence of p53 gene mutations and the radioresponsiveness of various types of human tumour. (Reproduced from Bristow et al, 1996, by permission of Elsevier Science Ireland Ltd, Bay 15K, Shannon Industrial Estate, Co. Clare, Ireland.)

found so far between the p53 status of different types of human tumour and the response of their cells to radiotherapy. The use of clonogenic assays to assess human tumour radiosensitivity is discussed later.

As far as tumour cell environment is concerned, the most important factor is that such tissues have escaped from the physiological growth

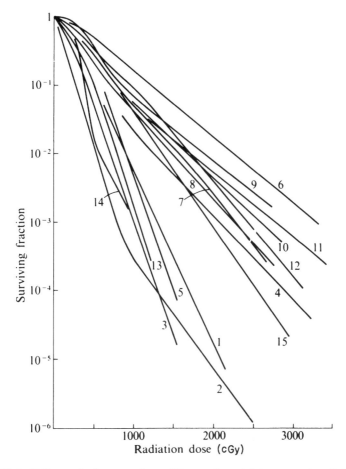

Figure 12.4. Cell survival curves from 15 experimental tumours irradiated in air-breathing animals. (Reproduced from Steel, 1977, by permission of Oxford University Press.)

control mechanisms and show abnormalities in architecture. As far as radiation response is concerned, the most important abnormality concerns the vascular supply of such abnormal tissues. The simplest statement is that 'tumours outgrow their blood supply'. As a consequence there are regions in tumours that are undernourished in general and hypoxic in particular. The radiobiological consequence of hypoxia was discussed in Chapter 10, where the architecture of hypoxic regions in tumours and the spheroid culture model of tumours were illustrated.

The proportion of hypoxic cells at the time of irradiation will obviously affect the radiosensitivity of a tumour. This is seen in Figure 12.4, where the survival curves for 15 different experimental tumours are shown. It is clear that these curves fall into two groups: six show more radiosensitivity, with most D_0 values between 105 and 165 cGy; the other nine show more radioresistance, with D_0 values averaging 370 cGy. The explanation for the difference rests quite simply upon the fact that most of the sensitive tumours had much less than 1% hypoxic cells and the resistant tumours all had more than 10%. (The details are described by Steel, 1977.) The two anomalous curves, 2 and 14, in the sensitive group had 1% and 2% hypoxic cells, respectively. The curves are biphasic (as was seen in Chapter 10, Figure 10.5), with a steep initial slope for the well-oxygenated proportion of the tumour cell population and a shallower final slope over the higher doses where the radioresistant hypoxic cells predominate.

All the survival curves were obtained by removing the tumours from the animal immediately after irradiation in order to perform the clonogenic assays (Chapter 6). If the cells had been left in the animal for a few hours after treatment they would have been able to repair potentially lethal damage, especially when the tumours contain a stationary cell population (Chapter 7). These curves therefore underestimate the survival in tumours that are left intact (see last edition on 'Human tissues' for the use of the PCC and FISH techniques for assaying human tumour radiosensitivity).

Two of the curves are from the same tumour system but at different stages of development. P388 leukaemia cells grow as ascites tumours in the peritoneal cavity of mice. After 1 day there are only a small number of cells and these are well oxygenated by contact with the two layers of peritoneum. The cells are radiosensitive, as shown by curve 5 in Figure 12.4 ($D_0 = 131$ cGy). By 6 days, however, the leukaemic cell number has increased to such an extent that the peritoneal cavity is distended and a proportion of the cells are so distant from the peritoneal blood vessels that they are hypoxic. The cells are then much more radioresistant, as shown by curve 6 ($D_0 = 458$ cGy). This P388 ascites tumour system was used to show the effect of hypoxia upon recovery from sublethal radiation damage, described in Chapter 10.

The first thing that happens to a cell population after it becomes hypoxic is that it slows down and then stops growing altogether, i.e. it becomes stationary. Subsequently, the cell number decreases and with it the viability of the cells. This is shown in Figure 12.5 for a population of Chinese hamster cells grown *in vitro*. The effect of hypoxia, induced by gassing with nitrogen, is shown in the lower solid lines in comparison with the upper dotted line, which is the exponential growth curve of cells grown under aerated conditions. All three of the hypoxic curves show a brief period of growth and then curve 2 shows an apparent plateau or stationary cell population, but these cells include those that have detached from the glass surface and are floating in the culture medium. Curve 3 shows those cells that have remained attached, but curve 4 shows only the cells that have passed the eosin dye exclusion test of viability.

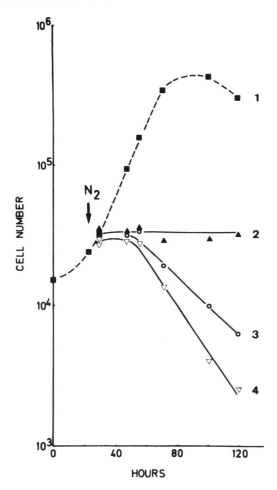

Figure 12.5. Growth curves of Chinese hamster cells under normal (1) and hypoxic (2–4) conditions. (Reproduced from Born et al, 1976, by permission of Elsevier Science Inc., 655 Ave. of the Americas, New York, NY 10010-5107.)

Tumours with hypoxic cells that remain viable will be less radiosensitive by the usual oxygen enhancement ratio of 2.5–3. Different repair mechanisms will have opposite effects: on the one hand, hypoxic cells are less able to recover from sublethal radiation damage; on the other hand, stationary-phase tumour cells will be more likely to recover from potentially lethal radiation damage but there will be a small number of more sensitive G_1–S cells. Many of these opposing factors depend upon the kinetics of the cell populations: the growth fraction, cell loss, total cell cycle time and the lengths of the phases of the cycle (Chapter 3).

Table 12.1. Labelling index and turnover time for mouse cell populations

	Labelling index (%)	Turnover time (h)
Carcinoma cells	35.1	22
Capillary endothelial cells	11.4	55
Fibroblasts	9.1	75

Reproduced from Tannock, 1970, by permission of American Association for Cancer Research.

KINETICS OF NORMAL AND MALIGNANT CELL POPULATIONS

The most realistic method of comparing normal and malignant cell populations is to study a tumour and its associated stroma, i.e. the vascular and fibrous cells that are closely associated with the malignant cells in such a tumour tissue. This has been done with transplanted C_3H mouse mammary tumours such as the serially transplanted one whose growth kinetics were described in Chapter 3. An earlier, third-generation, transplant had kinetic values as shown in Table 12.1. Clearly the tumour cell population had a much shorter turnover time (or potential doubling time) than the vascular and fibrous cell populations.

These different rates of proliferation may be a major cause of the slowing of tumour growth exemplified in Chapter 3, Figure 3.1. In a small well-nourished tumour the growth fraction is high and the turnover time is low. As the tumour grows the relatively slow proliferation of vascular endothelial cells leads to an increase in the intercapillary distance and a decrease in the nutrition of those regions of the tumour that are further from blood vessels. Table 12.2 shows the mitotic index, labelling index and grain count of tumour cells all fall between the regions nearest to the blood vessels and those furthest away near the necrotic regions. In such regions

Table 12.2. Kinetic values in three regions of mouse tumours

	Mitotic index (%)	Labelling index (%)	Grain count
Region near blood vessel	4.3	50	40
Intermediate region	2.5	30	27
Region near necrosis	0.6	10	10

Reproduced from Tannock, 1970, by permission of American Association for Cancer Research.

the growth fraction will be much lower, cell loss much higher and the turnover time of the tumour cells will be as long as that for endothelial cells.

Quite obviously such a comparison of the kinetics of tumour and endothelial cell populations is complicated by these changing conditions but such changes apply more to the tumour than its stroma. This is shown by the histograms in Figure 12.6 for another tumour system. The stromal elements do not show any change between 7.5 and 11.5 days but the proportion of viable carcinoma cells decreases from 65% to 24% and the necroses increase from 9% to 49%. The kinetics of such viable carcinoma cells are hardly changed but the number is much reduced in relative terms. (The total number will increase, but at a slower rate as the tumour becomes larger.) These factors all complicate the response of tumours to radiation.

These are other reasons why the growth kinetic parameters of malignant and normal cell populations are usually different. Almost by definition, the cell loss factor of a tumour cell population is less than the 100% of an adult normal cell population (otherwise the tumour would not have grown abnormally in the first place). On the other hand, the cell cycle times and

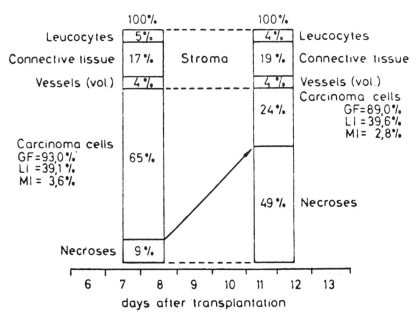

Figure 12.6. Changes in the histological and kinetic indices of Walker carcinoma 256 with time after transplantation. (Reprinted from *Eur. J. Cancer*, **5**, 1329–1336 from Brammer et al, 1979, Changes of histological and proliferative indices in the Walker carcinoma with tumour size and distance from blood vessel. With kind permission from Elsevier Science Ltd, The Boulevard, Langford Lane, Kidlington, OX5 1GB, UK.)

growth fractions of normal and tumour cell populations vary widely and show no systematic difference. Before a first dose of X-ray treatment, the actual doubling times of the two cell populations will usually be different: the tumour will be growing, but the normal tissue will not. Thereafter the positions may be reversed, with repopulation of normal cells eventually exceeding that of normal cells. Shrinkage of the irradiated tissue volume will also be associated with reoxygenation of hypoxic tumour regions. What started out as an apparently unfavourable therapeutic ratio between the likely radiation responses of the tumour and its associated normal tissues, can change with time into a favourable ratio.

RADIATION RESPONSE OF TUMOURS

The radiation response of tumours has to be distinguished from the *radiosensitivity* of the tumours. Radiosensitivity was shown in terms of the survival curves in Figure 12.4, but such measurements do not predict the rate at which a tumour shrinks after irradiation nor the rate at which it regrows, unless the radiation dose has been sufficient to sterilize the whole population. The size of that dose can be predicted from the shape of the survival curves together with a knowledge of the total number of viable tumour cells that must be eradicated. The rate at which such cells are eradicated depends upon their kinetics.

Such a response is shown in Figure 12.7 in terms of the volume of a tumour before and after a dose of radiation. After treatment the tumour slows down and then stops growing for a time and begins to regress. The rate of regression is similar to the rate of growth because of the kinetics of the cell population. If the radiation dose has been large enough the regression continues until the tumour is eradicated. After a smaller dose, however, enough viable cells will remain for the tumour to regrow.

After the X-ray dose the solid line represents the composite effect of three cellular processes: cells that are dying, surviving cells that are dividing and some injured cells that go through some abortive divisions and then die. The rate of decrease and the subsequent rate of increase of the total cell population is determined by its kinetics. A short cell cycle time will be associated with a more rapid fall and rise pattern rather than a long cycle time, but the pattern also depends upon other kinetic parameters: growth fraction and cell loss factor. The latter is obviously increased by a damaging agent such as the radiation dose, whose effect is illustrated in Figure 12.7.

All these kinetic parameters were compared between the five different tumour cell populations listed in Chapter 3, Table 3.1. These same tumour types are included now in Table 12.3, to illustrate how the rate of response of a tumour depends upon its actual doubling time, which is the end result of all the kinetic parameters considered in Chapter 3. The longer the

TUMOUR GROWTH BEFORE AND AFTER TREATMENT

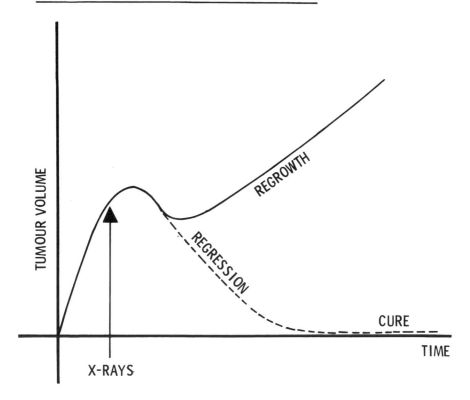

Figure 12.7. The growth pattern of a tumour before and after a dose of radiation. (Reproduced from Tozer, 1982, by permission of London University.)

doubling time of the tumour, the slower it grows and the longer the patient survives.

The extent of the descending portion of the tumour response shown in Figure 12.7 will be dependent on the size of the radiation dose, but only to a limited extent. The gross response of the mouse mammary tumour (described in Chapter 3) is shown in Figure 12.8 after single doses of X-rays in the range 0–80 Gy. In this case the volume of the tumour is plotted with an arithmetical scale (Figure 12.9 uses a logarithmic scale). The lower doses lead only to some slowing of tumour growth with no shrinkage at all. It is only when doses of 50 Gy or more are delivered that shrinkage occurs, and then the pattern is similar for all the higher doses. This is because this sort of response is determined only by the kinetics of the tumour. The extent of the subsequent shrinkage depends upon the size of the radiation dose. Half of the tumours will be cured altogether by a dose of 67.5 Gy, but the

Table 12.3. Prognostic significance of doubling times of human tumours

Pathological groups	Doubling time of lung metastasis (days)	Survival time of the patients (months)
Embryonal	19.5	9.5
Reticulosis	29.5	10.5
Sarcoma	35.6	15.5
Squamous cell carcinoma	51.0	15.6
Adenocarcinoma	90.4	20.4

Reproduced from Tubiana and Malaise, 1976, by permission of the authors.

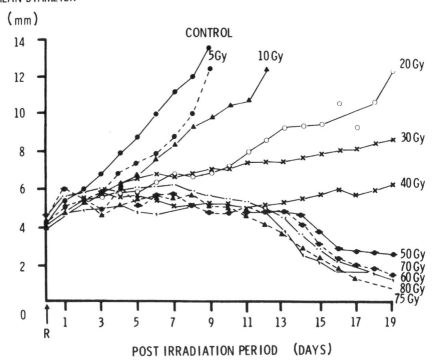

Figure 12.8. Response of C_3H mouse mammary tumours to single doses of X-rays (R = day of irradiation). (Reproduced from Abdelaal and Nias, 1979, by permission of Royal Society of Medicine.)

remainder will grow back again after a time that will be much longer than that shown diagrammatically in Figure 12.7 but with the same sort of pattern. After a dose as high as 80 Gy, all the tumours will be cured and there will be no regrowth at all.

CLONOGENIC ASSAYS

Animal tissues

Many of the tumours studied in animals as transplantable tissues can also be examined in tissue culture. The R1 rhabdomyosarcoma was one of the first animal tumour models to be investigated in this way. Figure 12.9 combines observations on the tumour measured as it grows in the animal (A) and in its cells assayed *in vitro* (B). The sort of shape of the upper growth curve (1) of an untreated tumour was discussed in Chapter 3 (Figure 3.1). The lower growth curve (2) shows the response of the tumour to a single dose of 2000 cGy (and has a similar shape to that shown in

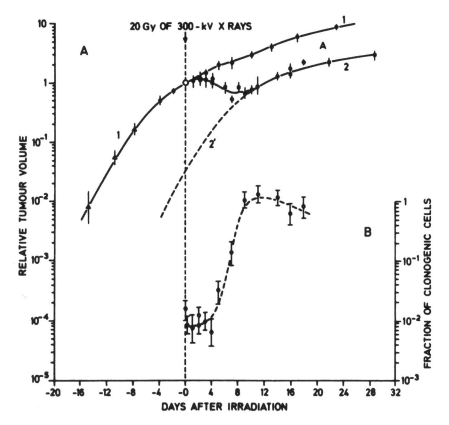

Figure 12.9. (A) Growth curves of a transplanted rhabdomyosarcoma (1) without treatment, (2) after 20 cGy, measured *in vivo*. (B) Survival of cells from the irradiated tumour assayed *in vitro*. (Reprinted from *Eur. J. Cancer*, **5**, 173–189, from Hermens and Barendsen, 1969, Changes in cell proliferation in a rat rhabdomyosarcoma before and after X-irradiation, with kind permission from Elsevier Science Ltd, The Boulevard, Langford Lane, Kidlington, OX5 1GB, UK.)

Figure 12.7). The tumour first stops growing and then shrinks, but by the 12th day after treatment growth resumes at a rate similar to that of the untreated tumour. During this period the viability of cells taken from the treated tumour was assayed by a clonogenic test *in vitro*. The results of this are shown in the lowest curve in Figure 12.9.

The fraction of clonogenic cells falls to 10^{-2} (or 1%) immediately after irradiation and remains at this level during the 4-day period when the tumour has stopped growing in the animal and has begun to shrink. Thereafter the clonogenic fraction begins to rise but the tumour continues to shrink because of death and removal of that 99% of the cells whose viability was destroyed by the radiation dose. By the 12th day, however, the clonogenic fraction has returned to unity, all the cells in the tumour are now viable and the tumour resumes the growth rate that would be expected from the other measurements. This *in vitro* assay provides a clear explanation of the radiation response of the tumour *in vivo*. The *in vitro* assay can also be used to test cellular radiosensitivity in terms of survival curves.

The question arises whether tumours are less radiosensitive when they recur than they were initially. Using the word in its strict sense to mean the sensitivity of clonogenic tumour cells to further treatment, evidence such as that shown in Figure 12.10 shows no change in radiosensitivity *in vitro*. This is a further example of the use of the rat rhabdomyosarcoma (R1), which was shown in Figure 12.9. On the other hand, although the cells from recurrent tumours were not less radiosensitive, the actual recurrent tumours did show a reduced response to radiation in terms of the regrowth delay. The difference is attributable to the *tumour bed effect* (Chapter 15). Radiation damages the vascular stroma in which the tumour cells are growing and this damage is expressed when the stromal tissue is stimulated into proliferation by the implanted tumour cells. The damaged stroma is less able to support the needs of the growing tumour. If such cells are implanted into an unirradiated bed, they will grow at the normal rate; conversely, if unirradiated cells are implanted in an irradiated bed, they will grow more slowly.

Alternative methods of assaying the radiation sensitivity of tumour cells include two *in vivo* techniques. The first of these is the endpoint dilution assay of Hewitt and Wilson (1959) (used for Figure 10.9 in Chapter 10). Leukaemic cells infiltrate the liver of the donor mouse and a cell suspension is then made. After increasing doses of radiation to the donor mice, increasing numbers of cells must be inoculated into the groups of recipient mice if tumours are to develop. By suitable variation of the cell dilution, an average of one viable cell is inoculated into each mouse and the usual exponential dose–response is established; but the method takes a long time and many animals.

A second and faster alternative is the lung colony assay illustrated in Figure 12.11, where the suspensions of single cells from tumours irradiated

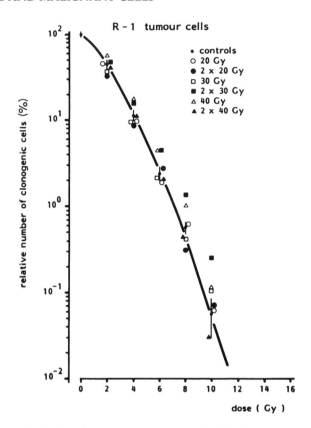

Figure 12.10. Radiation dose–response curves of cells from untreated R1 tumours and from tumours that recurred once or twice after treatment with various doses of radiation. (Reproduced from van Rotterdam et al, 1987, by permission of Elsevier Science Ireland Ltd, Bay 15K, Shannon Industrial Estate, Co. Clare, Ireland.)

in donor mice are injected intravenously into recipient mice. A proportion of the cells proliferate in the lungs, and macroscopic tumour nodules appear after about 20 days. These lung 'colonies' can be counted and the dose–response curve derived in terms of the surviving fraction of irradiated tumour cells. The curve shown in Figure 12.11 has similar parameters to that obtained with the same KHT mouse sarcoma using the endpoint dilution assay. These *in vivo* tumour cell assay methods both involve an *in vitro* cell-counting step, but the important irradiation and cell proliferation steps occur *in vivo* (as in the spleen colony assay). Thus, the sort of curve shown in Figure 12.11 confirms that an initial shoulder and a final exponential dose–response relationship can be presumed to apply to the X-irradiation of tumours *in vivo* as well as *in vitro* (Chapter 8).

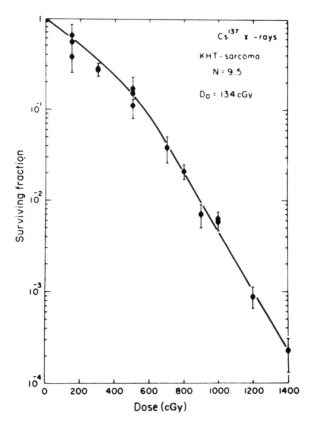

Figure 12.11. Survival curve for KHT sarcoma cells irradiated with ^{137}Cs γ-rays assayed by the lung colony technique. (Reproduced from Hill and Bush, 1969, by permission of *Int. J. Radiat. Biol.*, Taylor & Francis.)

Human tissues

The radiation sensitivity of the cells in human tissues cannot usually be assayed *in vivo* because of ethical objections. Long-term tissue cultures can be used but the biological properties of tumour cells are known to change after they are explanted and grown *in vitro*. A similar criticism applies to data obtained from xenografts where human tumours are grown in immune-deprived mice. Under these conditions the human tumour material is represented only in the parenchymal cells; the mouse provides the stroma.

The solution is to use short-term clonogenic assays *in vitro*. A 70% success rate can now be achieved and the data can be used to predict the response of a patient to radiotherapy (West, 1995). The surviving fraction after a 2 Gy dose (SF2) is a convenient parameter (see Chapter 8, Table 8.3). This parameter was used for Figure 12.12, which shows a difference of 10^5 in the

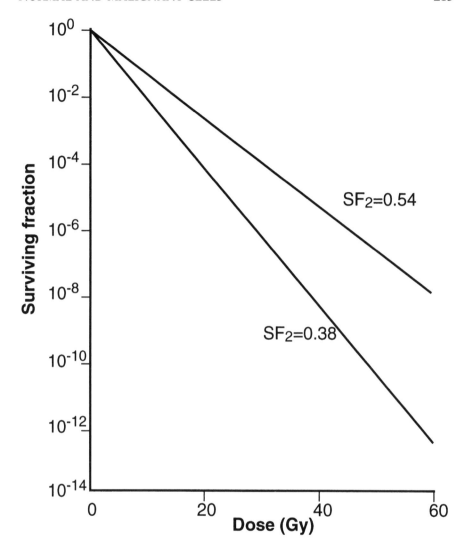

Figure 12.12. The effect of small differences in SF2 on the response of tumours to a full course of radiotherapy in women free of disease (0.38) or with recurrence (0.54). (Reproduced from West, 1995, by permission of BIR.)

final survival of cells from patients who suffered local recurrence of their radioresistant cervix tumours (SF2 0.54) and those with sensitive tumours (SF2 0.38) who were free of disease after 30 fractions of radiotherapy. This provides another example of the variation in intrinsic radiosensitivity that can be found in human tumour cells (see Figure 12.3).

Table 12.4. Radiosensitivity of human lymphocytes

Source	D (Gy)
Normal	2.98
AT	0.69
Breast OR	1.65
Breast NOR	2.36

Reproduced from West et al, 1995, by permission of Taylor & Francis.

A similar variation can be found in the radiosensitivity of the normal tissues of patients. Clonogenic assays of fibroblasts have been used but these take time, and a faster alternative is to assay peripheral blood lymphocytes. Table 12.4 shows the D values (i.e. mean activation dose; see Chapter 8) from normal individuals, patients who suffer from ataxia–telangiectasia (A–T) and patients with breast cancer who either suffered severe reactions to radiotherapy (OR) or did not (NOR). The data show how very radiosensitive the patients are who have A–T, while the OR patients were only slightly more sensitive than the NOR patients.

An alternative method of predicting the radiosensitivity of human tumours is to score chromosome aberrations by the premature chromosome condensation (PCC) and fluorescence *in situ* hybridization (FISH) techniques (Chapter 5). This method has the advantage that it removes the problem of a possible *in vitro* modification of cellular radiosensitivity during the clonogenic assays described above. With this method the tumour cells are irradiated *in situ* and left there for sufficient time to allow all repair to have been completed before they are removed (by biopsy) and assayed for chromosome aberrations. The method has been found to correlate with the results of clonogenic assay (Sasai et al, 1994).

The final conclusion is that the radiosensitivity of normal and malignant cells *can* be distinguishable. Although there may sometimes be no difference when the comparison is made under the same conditions, differences are observed when such cells form particular tissues. Genetic abnormalities will also alter radiosensitivity. The radiation responses of tumour tissues have been described in this chapter and normal tissues will be described in the next.

SUMMARY OF CONCLUSIONS

(1) There may be no difference in the intrinsic radiosensitivity between normal and malignant cells of the same histological type unless genetic changes occur, such as p53 mutation.

(2) This can be shown by comparing the survival curves of cells before and after malignant transformation.

(3) Tumour cell populations will show decreased radiosensitivity, however, when a proportion of the cells are hypoxic.

(4) Tumours also differ from normal tissues in their cell population kinetics. Before treatment the turnover time of a tumour may be shorter than that of the surrounding normal tissue, but the reverse may apply after radiation.

(5) The rate of response of a tumour to radiation depends upon its growth kinetics and not upon its radiosensitivity.

(6) Clonogenic assays show no change in the radioisensitivity of cells taken from primary or recurrent tumours. The proportion of clonogenic cells in a tumour may be quite low.

(7) Clonogenic assays can be used to predict the radiosensitivity of human tumours. Chromosome aberrations can also be assayed by the PCC and FISH techniques.

REFERENCES

Abdelaal, A. S. and Nias, A. H. W., 1979. Regression, recurrence and cure in an irradiated mouse tumour. *Journal of the Royal Society of Medicine*, **72**, 100–105.

Born, R., Hug, O. and Trott, K. R., 1976. The effect of prolonged hypoxia on growth and viability of Chinese hamster cells. *International Journal of Radiation Oncology*, **1**, 687–697.

Brammer, I., Zywietz, F. and Jung, H., 1979. Changes of histological and proliferative indices in the Walker carcinoma with tumour size and distance from blood vessel. *European Journal of Cancer*, **15**, 1329–1336.

Bristow, R. G., Benchimol, S. and Hill, R. P., 1996. The p53 gene as a modifier of intrinsic radiosensitivity: implications for radiotherapy. *Radiotherapy and Oncology*, **40**, 197–223.

Han, A., Hill, C. K. and Elkind, M. M., 1980. Repair of cell killing and neoplastic transformation at reduced dose-rates of [60]Cobalt gamma rays. *Cancer Research*, **40**, 1–18.

Hendry, J. H., 1972. The response of haemopoietic colony-forming units and lymphoma cells irradiated in soft tissue (spleen) or a bone cavity (femur) with single doses of X-rays, X-rays or D–T neutrons. *British Journal of Radiology*, **45**, 923–932.

Hermens, A. F. and Barendsen, G. W., 1969. Changes of cell proliferation in a rat rhabdomyosarcoma before and after X-irradiation. *European Journal of Cancer*, **5**, 173–189.

Hewitt, H. B. and Wilson, C. W., 1959. The effect of tissue oxygen tension on the radiosensitivity of leukaemia cells irradiated *in situ* in the livers of leukaemic mice. *British Journal of Cancer*, **13**, 675–684.

Hill, R. P. and Bush, R. S., 1969. A lung-colony assay to determine the radiosensitivity of the cells of a solid tumour. *International Journal of Radiation Biology*, **15**, 435–444.

Sasai, K., Evans, J. W., Kovacs, M. S. and Brown, J. M., 1994. Prediction of human cell radiosensitivity: comparison of clonogenic assay with chromosome aberrations scored using premature chromosome condensation with fluorescence *in situ* hybridization. *International Journal of Radiation Oncology, Biology, Physics*, **30**, 1127–1132.

Steel, G. G., 1977. *Growth Kinetics of Tumours*. Clarendon Press, Oxford, p. 255.

Tannock, I. F., 1970. Population kinetics of carcinoma cells, capillary endothelial cells and fibroblasts in a transplanted mouse mammary tumour. *Cancer Research*, **30**, 2470–2476.

Tozer, G. M., 1982. Hyperbaric oxygen and tumour response to radiation in the C3H mouse. PhD Thesis, London University.

Tubiana, M. and Malaise, E. P., 1976. Growth rate and cell kinetics in human tumours: some prognostic and therapeutic implications. In *Scientific Foundations of Oncology*, edited by T. Symington and R. L. Carter. Heinemann, London, pp. 126–136.

van Rotterdam, A., Barendsen, G. W. and Gaiser, G. R., 1987. Radiosensitivity of cells in recurrent experimental tumours and the effectiveness of tumour retreatment. *Radiotherapy and Oncology*, **8**, 171–176.

West, C. M. L., 1995. Intrinsic radiosensitivity as a predictor of patient response to radiotherapy. *British Journal of Radiology*, **68**, 827–837.

West, C. M. L., Elyan, S. A. G., Berry, P., Cowan, R. and Scott, D., 1995. A comparison of the radiosensitivity of lymphocytes from normal donors, cancer patients, individuals with ataxia–telangiectasia (A–T) and A–T heterozygotes. *International Journal of Radiation Biology*, **68**, 197–203.

Wilkinson, C. R., 1971. Characterisation of cloned populations of mammalian cells after chemical treatment *in vitro*. PhD Thesis, Manchester University.

13 Radiation Pathology

Normal tissues respond to radiation in patterns that depend upon the kinetics of the cell populations that are involved. When Bergonié and Tribondeau were looking into the effect of radiation on rat testes they discovered (1906) that the dividing (germinal) cells were markedly affected by the radiation, while the non-dividing (interstitial) cells appeared undamaged. On the basis of these observations they derived their 'law', which stated that actively dividing tissues are 'radiosensitive' and non-dividing tissues are 'radioresistant'. Thus, in mammals the liver was often classified under 'radioresistant tissues' because in the adult it exhibits little active cell division and is composed of specialized cells. In contrast, the cells of the epithelium of the intestine were classified under 'radiosensitive tissues'. Such generalizations are misleading because it is essentially the processes of cell division that are 'radiosensitive' and not the different types of cells in tissues.

The Law of Bergonié and Tribondeau should thus be restated more precisely: the cell populations with the higher rate of cell division show the earlier response to radiation. Skin, intestine and bone marrow are more responsive, vascular and connective tissue are intermediate and the central nervous system (CNS) is slowest to respond (Table 13.1). In each case the 'biological target' is a cell. Any cell has only a statistical probability of being damaged by the ionizing radiation and a proportion of cells will remain unscathed. Whether or not the damage becomes manifest as a significant depletion of the cell population depends to a large extent on the detailed characteristics of the renewal system of which that cell is a part. These characteristics will now be described for the

Table 13.1. Kinetic properties of various cell populations

No mitosis No cell renewal	Low mitotic index Little cell renewal	Frequent mitoses Cell renewal
Central nervous system	Liver	Epidermis
Sense organs	Thyroid	Intestinal epithelium
Adrenal medulla	Vascular endothelium	Bone marrow
	Connective tissue	Gonads

Reproduced from Bertalanffy and Lau, 1962, by permission of Academic Press, Inc.

normal tissues, together with such quantitative information as is known for their radioresponsiveness.

SKIN

Skin is a composite organ and consists of an outer epidermal layer, a cutaneous and subcutaneous connective-tissue layer and various accessory organs, such as hair, nails, exocrine glands and sensory receptors. All of these structures participate to varying degrees in the reaction of skin to radiation exposure.

The epidermal layer represents a cell renewal system that can be compared to intestinal epithelium, but cell replacement and transit times are slower. Only about 2% of all cells are renewed daily in the epidermis, in contrast to 50% in the intestine. The epidermal cells divide in the germinal stratum, differentiate by keratinization and finally are shed from the surface of the skin. The length of the cell cycle and the transit time depend largely on the anatomical site, age, species and functional state of the skin. Thus, transit time in the epidermis varies from about 14–17 days in humans and 8–12 days in mice and rats. The cell cycle times are about 7 and 5 days, respectively, and the transit times are related simply to cell cycle times because the epidermal layer is normally two to three cells thick, except on plantar and palmar regions.

One to two days after exposure to 800 cGy or more, the skin may redden temporarily. During this early erythema the blood vessels are congested and oedema occurs in the subcutaneous layer, whereas the epidermis appears normal except for mitotic arrest. This initial erythema increases during the first week but fades to a minimum on the 10th day. The main erythematous reaction then becomes maximal on the 15th day and lasts 20–30 days after exposure. Figure 13.1 shows this on the basis of skin reflectance, which provides a measure of the change in skin colour. The main erythema reaction involves not only the epidermis but also the underlying strata of skin, especially the blood vessels. When the basal layers of the epidermis regenerate, the erythema disappears, but it may reappear in a wave-like manner and lead to dry or moist desquamation.

Once desquamation occurs, erythema measurements, like those in Figure 13.1, become meaningless and a quantitative measure of skin reaction can only be obtained by the use of an arbitrary scale extending from mild erythema to moist desquamation of the entire irradiated area. Trained observers can make useful comparisons by using such a scale, and the observations on mouse skin have been used (Figure 13.2) to show that proliferation does not begin to influence the response to fractionated irradiation until the third week, i.e. at the same time as the skin reaction becomes obvious after a single dose of radiation. So, it is the normal

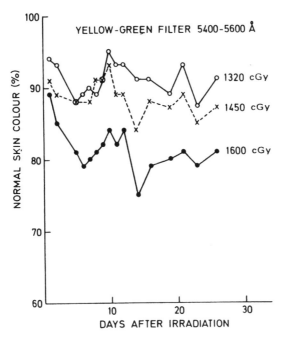

Figure 13.1. Erythema measurements of human skin. (Reproduced from Nias, 1963, by permission of BJR.)

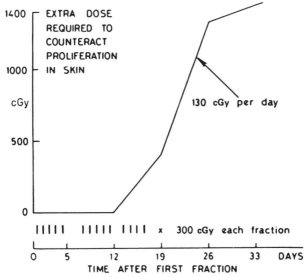

Figure 13.2. The extra dose required to counteract proliferation in mouse skin during fractionated irradiation. (Reproduced from Denekamp, 1973, by permission of BJR.)

turnover time of the basal layers of the epithelium that determines the pattern of radioresponsiveness. The reaction of skin to radiation can be reduced if essential fatty acids are administered during the expression of damage (Hopewell et al, 1994). The effect is greater for late damage (see the section on Late effects).

Turning to radiosensitivity, Figure 13.3 shows a dose–response curve for epidermal stem cells. This was obtained on the basis of the number of regenerating nodules formed in the denuded skin of mice after varying doses of irradiation. A special technique is used whereby increasing areas of skin are shielded from a lethal dose delivered first to a surrounding area to ensure that no stem cells can migrate into the area to be tested. Because only a limited number of nodules can be counted within a given area of skin, there is a lower limit of dose below which this method cannot be used to resolve the dose–response relationship. The curve in Figure 13.3 is limited to the exponential portion of what is presumed would be a 'shouldered' dose–response curve if the lowest dose range could be resolved. This presumption is justified by the results of split-dose experiments, which

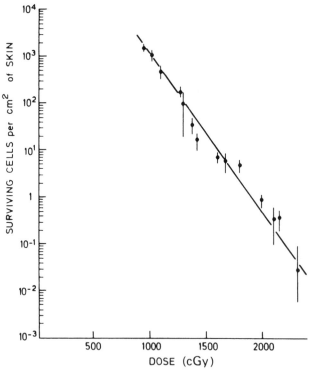

Figure 13.3. Dose–response curve for mouse epidermal cells. (Reproduced from Withers, 1967, by permission of BJR.)

show that recovery occurs and that the D_q amounts to 350 cGy (on the basis of a $D_2 - D_1$ calculation; see Chapter 7). This would be the extent of the shoulder of a complete curve.

The radiosensitivity of this mouse epidermal stem-cell population can thus be shown to be typical of many other cell populations (Chapter 8) when measured *in vivo* in this way. Under aerated conditions the D_0 value is 135 cGy; under hypoxic conditions D_0 is 350 cGy. The oxygen enhancement ratio is thus 2.6, which is also typical of other cell populations (Chapter 10), and this observation suggests that, in the mouse at least, skin is normally well oxygenated.

GASTROINTESTINAL TRACT

In the whole digestive tract (the mouth, pharynx, oesophagus, stomach, small intestine, large intestine and rectum) the small intestine is the most important site of radiation injury. All three regions, the duodenum, jejunum and ileum, are lined (Figure 13.4) by a columnar epithelium consisting of mucus and columnar or 'chief' cells. The crypts, which contain the generative cells for epithelial replacement, are found in the mucosa at the base of the villi. The cells of the crypts and of the related villi can be

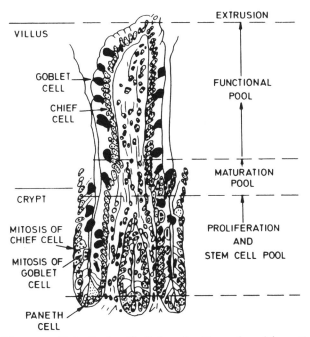

Figure 13.4. Diagram of intestinal epithelial pools. (Reproduced from Bond et al, by permission of Academic Press, Inc.)

considered parts of a cell-renewal system that is in a state of kinetic equilibrium. Cell renewal occurs in the mitotic areas in the crypts. From there, newly formed cells migrate out and move from the base of the villi to the top, designated as the extrusion zone.

In the past, radiobiological studies employed intestinal death as the endpoint, but nowadays such questions can be examined using the response of intestinal stem cells, which was described in Chapter 8 with a composite survival curve (Figure 8.13). The simple survival curve for mouse jejunum (Figure 13.5) has an apparently very large shoulder but the final exponential portion of that curve is 'real'. This is because the D_0 value of 115 cGy is based upon the number of regenerating crypts of Lieberkuhn, which can be counted around the circumference of a section of gut, when fixed and stained 3–4 days after single doses of radiation over the dose range above 1100 cGy.

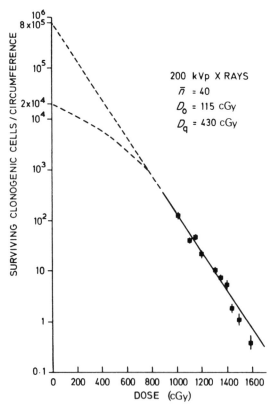

Figure 13.5. Cell survival curve for intestinal epithelial cells. (Reproduced from Withers and Elkind, 1969, by permission of Academic Press, Inc.)

The survival curve for epidermal stem cells (Figure 13.3) was also restricted to a middle range of doses. In both cases the number of surviving stem cells becomes higher than one per regenerating crypt or skin nodule when lower doses are administered. Estimation of the real size of the shoulder was described in Chapter 7 – split-dose experiments show a D_q value of 430 cGy for intestine after high doses. This is larger than the D_q value of 350 cGy for skin but, because the D_0 values for the skin and intestinal cell populations are very similar (135 cGy and 115 cGy, respectively), the more acute radiation response of intestine must be attributed to differences in the kinetics of the cell populations (the turnover time for mouse intestinal cells is 3 days; for skin it is 24 days).

The acute radiation effects on the intestine are readily explained by the cellular depletion of the epithelium. There is an immediate decrease in the numbers of dividing cells and early death of the cells in the crypts of Lieberkuhn. If the radiation dose is high enough, say 1000 cGy single exposure, there is rapid cell loss in the intestinal crypts and the intestinal villi become short and blunted. Absorption defects and bacterial invasion of the bowel wall may be detected, associated with excessive loss of fluid and electrolytes. Late effects are normally seen in patients who have had some degree of acute or subacute enteropathy and the lesion is a combination of epithelial damage associated with vascular deficiency and fibrosis.

BONE MARROW

This varies in structure and cellular composition with age and with anatomical location. In the young individual it is distributed through all bones and acts as one single organ system. In the rodent, active marrow persists in the adult, particularly in the long bones. In humans and larger animals, active marrow is confined to the flat bones (sternum, ribs, iliac crest) and the epiphyses of long bones. The haemopoietic bone marrow is composed principally of three cell renewal systems – erythropoietic, myelopoietic and thrombopoietic – but the morphological identity of the stem cells of the bone marrow and even the anatomical boundaries of their normal site of origin and their location are not known precisely. About 3×10^{11} blood cells are generated per day by an average human. This is achieved by a large amount of cellular proliferation in the bone marrow, which has a defined developmental hierarchy of cell categories.

This hierarchy starts with a stem cell that initiates a variable number of cell divisions, during which differentiation and maturation gradually supervene before the cells appear in the peripheral blood in a recognizable form. Figure 13.6 shows the sequence from primitive stem cells (P.S.C.), through precursor cells, which are spleen colony-forming units (CFU-S); then to colony-forming cells of mixed lineage (CFC-mix) and on to the four

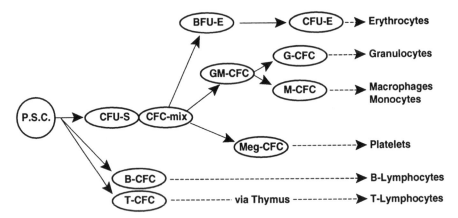

Figure 13.6. *In vitro* colony-forming cells generated from the pluripotent stem cell (P.S.C.) compartment in the bone marrow. (Reproduced from Lord, 1995, by permission of Taylor & Francis.)

main types of peripheral blood cell. Erythrocytes develop from erythroid burst-forming units (BFU-E) and erythroid colony-forming units (CFU-E). The granulocyte/macrophage colony-forming cells (GM-CFC) lead either to G-CFC for granulocytes or M-CFC for monocytes. Platelets are formed from megakaryocyte colony-forming cells (Meg-CFC). The B and T lymphocyte

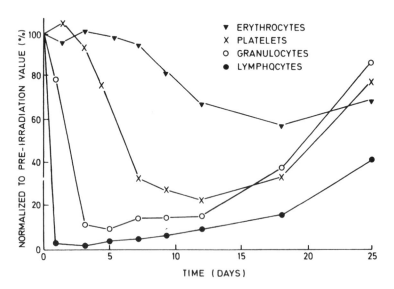

Figure 13.7. Peripheral blood counts of rats following 500 cGy whole-body irradiation. (Reproduced from Casarett, 1968, by permission of Prentice-Hall.)

precursors peel off at an earlier stage (before CFU-S) of the multipotent stem-cell population.

It is noteworthy that red cells have a relatively very long lifespan in the peripheral blood for all species (115 days for humans). The other cell types have both a shorter total lifespan and a shorter period in the peripheral blood. It is the total time, however, from start to finish, that determines the responses shown in Figure 13.7, which shows the peripheral blood counts of rats about 500 cGy of whole-body irradiation. After the bone marrow is irradiated there is an interval before maximum depression, followed by recovery to a normal level. This time interval depends upon the kinetics of the various types of stem-cell population. Each of the marrow populations has its own kinetics and the time scale of the perturbation in the peripheral blood count varies accordingly.

There are various *cytokines*, or growth factors, that can stimulate haemopoetic cell populations to recover from radiation. They are produced by recombinant technology and act on specific cell types. In addition to promoting cell proliferation, they may regulate differentiation, suppress apoptosis (and thereby increase survival of critical cell after irradiation) and promote the function of mature cells. The cytokines include GM-CSF, which promotes the recovery of granulocytes and macrophages, and G-CSF, which promotes granulocytes alone. In Chapter 14, Figure 14.7 shows how such cytokines can double the tolerable dose of radiation.

Figure 13.8 shows radiation survival curves for the various types of progenitor cells in mouse bone marrow. The cell types include many of those shown in Figure 13.7. In addition there are curves for colony-forming cells responding to granulocyte colony-stimulating factor (G), the most radiosensitive type, and for fibroblastoid colony-forming units (CFU-F), which are stromal cells and are the most radioresistant type. The other cell types have intermediate radiosensitivity. Survival of bone-marrow stem cells can be measured by a variety of methods, e.g. the spleen colony method (Chapter 8) and erythropoietin response. The values of D_0 varies between 60 and 125 cGy for the most part, but for CFU-F the value is as high as 232 cGy. Most of these values of D_0 overlap the range for cells cultured *in vitro*, although they fall at the lower end of the range.

THE IMMUNE SYSTEM

The immune system consists of a number of interacting components, which include the cell types shown in Figure 13.9, that can be identified by immunohistochemical markers. They are all derived from multipotential stem cells in the bone marrow (as were the other elements shown in Figure 13.6). The B cells primarily affect the humoral or antibody-mediated immune response. The precursors of that lineage develop in the bone

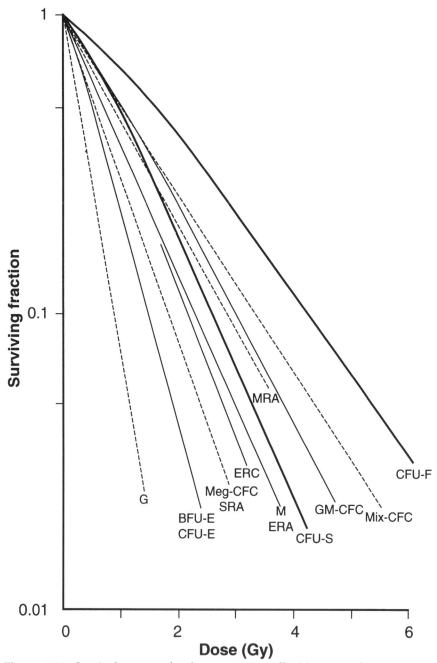

Figure 13.8. Survival curves for haemopoietic cells in mouse bone marrow. (Reproduced from Millar and Hendry, 1997, by permission of *Int. J. Radiat. Biol.*, Taylor & Francis.)

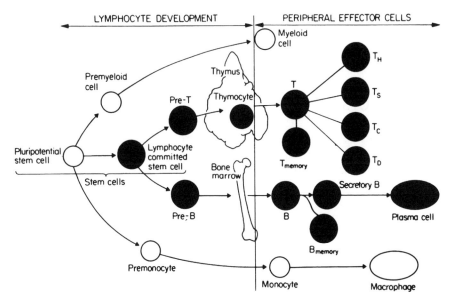

Figure 13.9. Cellular participants in the immune system. (Reproduced from Chapel and Haeney, 1988, by permission of Blackwell Science Ltd.)

marrow and B lymphocytes are then released into the bloodstream or lymph.

The T cells are responsible for various forms of cell-mediated immune response. The precursors of that lineage migrate to the thymus gland to mature. After their release into the blood or lymph, T lymphocytes become distinct biochemical and functional entities in the form of helper cells (T_H), suppresser cells (T_S), cytotoxic cells (T_C) or delayed hypersensitivity cells (T_D). These cells mount immune surveillance by detecting and then destroying virus-infected cells in the body within 1 or 2 days after infection. Suppressor T cells are more radiosensitive than helper T cells, and B cells have an intermediate sensitivity.

The immune system is obviously complicated and the effect of irradiation will depend not only upon the intrinsic radiosensitivity of each type of cell but also upon the functional consequence of suppressing the cytological and/or humoral activity of each component. Damage to effector activity could have the opposite effect. The time scale of radiation damage to the immune system will vary with the turnover time of a particular cell type and the half-life of a humoral component.

As usual in cellular radiobiology, mature cells are less radiosensitive than undifferentiated precursors. Thus, mature plasma cells continue to secrete antibody at a normal rate after doses as high as 100 cGy, whereas B-cell precursors are very radiosensitive, with a D_0 value of 40–90 cGy. Activated

T and B cells are also less sensitive to radiation-induced interphase cell death than are their precursors. Perhaps this is why delayed-type hypersensitivity and graft-versus-host responses are relatively radio-resistant.

LATE EFFECTS ON NORMAL TISSUES

The immediate cellular effects of radiation on living tissues have now been described. They are normally self-limiting and are repaired within 6 weeks. Late radiation changes in normal tissues and organs may be recognized usually no earlier than 3 months after irradiation, but in respect of other effects such as leukaemogenesis and the induction of cancer (described in Chapter 19) a latent period of 8–10 years or even longer may be observed. These late effects are the manifestation of progressive degenerative processes induced by the radiation, and their incidence increases with time to a maximum and then declines.

There is an indirect relationship between the degree of early reaction in a tissue and the probability of developing a late reaction, but the pathogenesis of early and late reactions is different. Tissues that show a response soon after radiotherapy do so because of the faster kinetics of their cell populations. It follows that the process takes longer in those tissues with slower kinetics. There will also be a latent period before the clinical appearance of the radiation damage in some tissues, e.g. 2–4 months for lung, 6–24 months for the CNS and more than 1 year for kidney. This latent period is shorter after higher doses because most of the target cells in those tissues are quiescent. Some of these quiescent cell populations may show an 'avalanche' effect after radiation:

> As the first radiation-sterilized cells attempt division and die, an increased number of quiescent cells are called into proliferation by the homeostatic control system, so precipitating the death of yet more sterilized cells and requiring a still higher proportion of quiescent cells to be called into the reproductive cycle. This gives rise to an exponentially increasing rate of depopulation which has been termed the avalanche effect. (Wheldon et al, 1982.)

The larger the radiation dose and the larger the volume irradiated, the more the likelihood that such an 'avalanche' will reduce the cell number below a level that is adequate for the function of that tissue, and the earlier the clinical appearance of the resultant radiation reaction. The majority of the late reacting cell populations (e.g. lung, CNS and kidney) show this 'flexible' type of response to radiation, in contrast to the hierarchical response of stem-cell populations such as bone marrow.

Although these radiation reactions depend predominantly on the number of parenchymal cells killed by radiation, the development of late reactions is

Table 13.2. Pathogenesis of early and late radiation effects

Early effects		
Differentiated cell	Cell depletion	Hypoplasia
Vascular endothelium	Increased permeability	Oedema
Late effects		
Differentiated cell	Cell depletion	Atrophy
Vascular endothelium	Increased permeability	Oedema
	Endarteritis	Fibrosis
		Ischaemia

Reproduced from Nias, 1988, by permission of Churchill Livingstone.

also influenced by two other processes associated with progressive secondary damage (Table 13.2). These changes are associated with ischaemia and fibrosis produced in the tissue. The ischaemia results from damage to the endothelial cells and walls of the blood vessels. Fibrosis may well also be directly related to the degree of cell killing in the vascular endothelium.

There is increasing experimental evidence that radiation-induced late normal tissue injury can be modified by pharmacological agents (Moulder et al, 1997). Post-radiation treatment with anti-inflammatory drugs is effective in reducing damage to kidney, CNS, lung and heart. Polyunsaturated fatty acids (PUFA) can be effective with skin and spinal cord. The angiotensin-converting enzyme (ACE) inhibitor captopril reduces radiation damage in long, skin and kidney (see Figure 13.6). The advantage of all these pharmacological agents is that they can be effective with non-toxic doses.

The radiation response of an organ can also be influenced markedly by the condition of other irradiated or non-irradiated tissues and cells in the body, owing to so-called *abscopal* effects. If certain parenchymal cells are removed but can be replaced by differentiation of more primitive cells or by migration of similar cells from a different tissue, the overall effect may be lessened. For example, bone-marrow cells from one part of the body can repopulate irradiated marrow in other parts of the body.

VASCULAR TISSUE

In functional terms the heart and the large arteries and veins appear to be less affected by radiation, whereas the capillaries seem to be more affected. This is because occlusion occurs in capillaries and small arteries after moderate doses of radiation. Capillary occlusion will block the blood supply not only to the tissues in the immediate vicinity of the occluded area but to all tissue further along the capillary. For this reason capillary endothelium is perhaps the most important tissue limiting the irradiation of

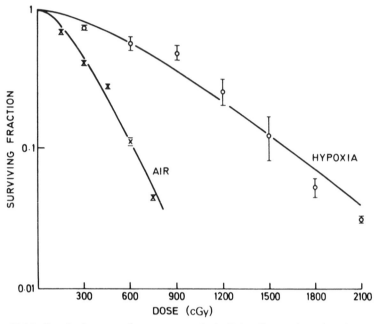

Figure 13.10. Survival curves for mouse endothelial cells irradiated with X-rays in air or under hypoxic conditions. (Reproduced from Nias, 1974, by permission of Charles C. Thomas.)

a patient. At a cellular level the endothelial lining of large vessels is probably as sensitive as that in capillaries but, because of the large diameter of those vessels, even if endothelial proliferation and swelling or blood clotting does occur, the vessels will not be occluded.

In terms of cellular response, studies of capillary endothelial cells from mouse kidney *in vitro* show 'typical' cell survival curves (Figure 13.10), with D_0 values of 200 cGy in air and 530 cGy under hypoxic conditions, the same extrapolation number (2.3) and thus an oxygen enhancement ratio of 2.65. It will be remembered that the turnover of these cells is rather slow, with a cycle time of 50 h, so they will not, in terms of an early reaction, appear to be highly radioresponsive. In the development of late effects, however, their response is of prime significance. If these results are relevant to human blood vessels, they show that vascular endothelial cells are just as *radiosensitive* as other cells.

By contrast, *radioresponsiveness* will depend upon a combination of the particular vascular architecture of the tissue and the complex interaction of the mechanisms of cell death, recovery and repopulation (and reoxygenation in the case of tumours), which were discussed as separate phenomena in earlier chapters. The results of such interactions and their modification by pharmacological agents will be discussed now for various late-reacting tissues.

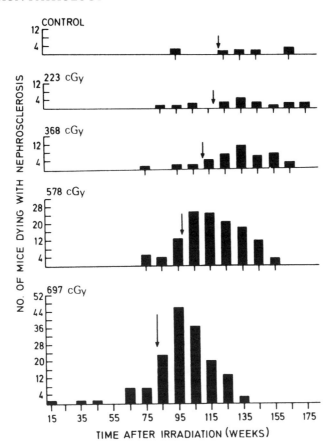

Figure 13.11. Age distribution of death with nephrosclerosis in male mice (arrows indicate mean age at death from all causes in each dose group). Reproduced from Upton, A. C., Kimball, A. W., Furth, J., Christenberry, K. W., and Benedict, W. H., *Cancer Res.* 20(8/2): 23 (1960), by permission of American Association for Cancer Research.

KIDNEY

The kidney is an organ with many highly specialized functions and in general its cell systems have very slow turnover rates. As a result, radiation injury is usually not seen until some months after exposure. However, the incidence of renal damage and its time of presentation after irradiation have been shown in mice to depend on the dose of irradiation (Figure 13.11). It also depends upon the volume of kidney irradiated. Following single doses of X-rays below 1000 cGy, few early changes can be seen in the kidney and it is usually only after higher doses that impairment of renal function is found. Doses in excess of 2000 cGy to both kidneys are likely to lead to renal failure in a high proportion of patients. The kidney is a good example of a flexible 'F'-type organ.

The clinicopathological types of renal damage may be classified as 'acute' and 'chronic' radiation nephropathy. Acute radiation nephropathy or progressive glomerular sclerosis has a latent period of 6–12 months and is associated with proteinuria, anaemia and hypertension. Patients rapidly become seriously ill after the onset of symptoms and about 30% will die in the acute illness. All who recover will have chronic radiation nephropathy, but in about half of patients the blood pressure may be brought under control.

Because hypertension plays a major role in radiation nephropathy, inhibition of the vasoconstrictor angiotensin II (A-II) production by ACE inhibitors should be effective in prevention of the syndrome. Figure 13.12 shows a comparison of the efficacy of various antihypertensive agents on the development of nephropathy in rats after bone-marrow transplantation (BMT). The animals received 17 Gy of total body irradiation (TBI) and the results show that a low dose of the ACE inhibitor captopril, or enalapril (a non-thiol ACE inhibitor), had a small effect. A larger dose of captopril was better but the A-II antagonist was the most effective in ameliorating BMT nephropathy. Other antihypertensive drugs had no effect. Captopril is most beneficial when given 3.5–9.5 weeks after TBI, which suggests that the effect of ACE inhibitors is related to the 'avalanche' effect described earlier.

An assay for the survival of renal tubule cells has been developed (Withers et al, 1986) that can be used to measure clonogenic cell survival. The radiation dose–response curve has a D_0 value of 150 cGy and is similar to that of stem cells in acutely responding tissues. The incidence of radiation nephropathy is believed to be due to depletion of such parenchymal cells in the tubules and those in the glomeruli, as well as to vascular injury. The later onset of nephropathy is due to the slower kinetics of the parenchymal cell populations, but they still seem to have the same intrinsic radio-sensitivity in terms of D_0 value as other mammalian cell populations.

Figures 13.11 and 13.15 (later) illustrate a general principle of the effects of radiation on tissues: namely that, while morbidity and mortality are increased by increasing doses of radiation, for the most part these effects are not a unique consequence of radiation. The syndrome occurs to a smaller extent anyway, but radiation increases the incidence and lowers the age when it occurs. It is for this reason that radiation can be said to have an *ageing* effect, although there is no evidence that radiation increases senility in general.

THORACIC ORGANS

The lungs and oesophagus will be considered under this heading because irradiation of the chest will usually involve all of these organs. The effects of thoracic irradiation can be contrasted with the lethal response to whole-body irradiation, which will be described in Chapter 14. A well-defined sequence of CNS, gut and bone-marrow syndromes will be shown to have a cellular basis in which the response to progressively higher dosage can be related to the shortening time scales associated with the three modes of death. Similarly, for thoracic irradiation, an early 'starvation death' occurs after higher dose levels that principally produce oesophageal damage, while a later mortality is seen to occur in experimental animals from lung fibrosis after lower doses. This will be described in Chapter 14 under partial body irradiation, which will show the relationship between radiosensitivity and the time span of radiation response, applied to thoracic irradiation. With a dose of about 30 Gy the mice die after 10–40 days from oesophageal damage. After a lower dose they may die of pulmonary damage, but not until much later. For thoracic irradiation, then, there are various syndromes, each of which can be shown to have a cellular basis.

LUNG

The adult lung is a stable tissue with a very slow cellular proliferation in its differentiated cells and in the endothelial cells. This contrasts with the oesophagus which has a very rapid cell-renewal system. It is for this reason that the effects of radiation appear early in the oesophagus, whereas the effects on the lung are seen much later.

Radiation pneumonitis follows damage to either or both of the cell populations found in the alveolar septa of the lungs: endothelial and alveolar cells. The response of capillary endothelial cells has already been mentioned. The alveolar cells include a type that are vacuolated and secrete lung surfactant. Radiation pneumonitis may be just as much the consequences of dose-dependent loss of these alveolar cells as the result of capillary endothelial cell loss. In either or both cases there will be damage to the lung stroma, characterized by oedema followed by hyalinization and fibrosis of the alveolar walls. Resulting impairment of ventilatory and diffusion capacities of the lung may be significant in the long-term effects of radiation (see Table 13.3). The ACE inhibitor captopril can ameliorate such

Table 13.3. The development of radiation pneumonitis

Phase	Sequence of events	Time span (days)
Exudative	Cell damage, inflammatory exudates	0–40
Pneumonitis	Desquamation, consolidation, organization	20–60
Fibrosis	Fibrosis, devascularization	60–200
Secondary changes	Calcification, metaplasia, neoplasia	>200

Reproduced from van den Brenk, 1971, by permission of Williams and Wilkins.

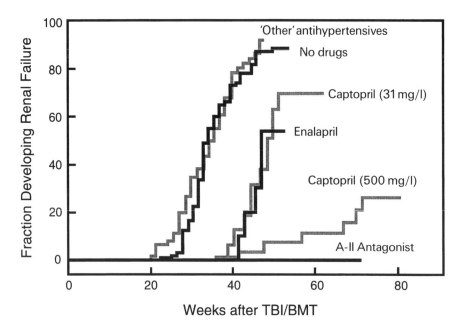

Figure 13.12. Effect of antihypertensive therapies on the development of nephropathy in rats after BMT. (Reproduced from Moulder et al, 1997, by permission of Kluwer Academic Publishers.)

damage, as can anti-inflammatory drugs such as dexamethasone and indomethacin.

CENTRAL NERVOUS SYSTEM

The CNS was considered at one time to consist of tissues of high radioresistance. It is now recognized that this false interpretation resulted from the commonly late manifestation of radiation injury, which is related to the slow turnover of cells in nervous tissue. There are two modes of radiation injury, depending on the dose and time after irradiation. The earlier mode affects white matter through damage to the supporting glia, and is most clearly seen with single exposures of 30–40 Gy. The later mode is vascular and predominates with single exposures of 20–30 Gy.

The two modes of damage can be explained in cellular terms and the earlier type is another example of the 'avalanche' phenomenon, with a latent period inversely related to dose followed by a rapid onset of the neurological syndrome. This is another syndrome where pharmacological agents can ameliorate the effect (Moulder et al, 1997); anti-inflammatory drugs such as dexamethasone and PUFAs have been tried. The syndrome is due to demyelination and necrosis of the white matter consequent upon loss of the oligodendrocyte population and may occur about 6 months after a radiation dose above the therapeutic range. The level of tolerance will obviously have been exceeded when the catastrophe of transverse myelitis occurs (see Chapter 16, Figure 16.13).

The incidence of paralysis, and the latent period before it develops, depends on both the radiation dose and the length of spinal cord that has been irradiated. Figure 13.13 shows the incidence for three different lengths of cord. A higher dose is needed for a shorter length, and vice versa. The study also showed that animals treated with methotrexate suffered a small increase in paralysis (an enhancement ratio of 1.2 with the 8 mm length of cord). By contrast, a small *delay* in the onset of paralysis can be produced when animals are treated with PUFA.

When the brain is irradiated to the high levels of dosage used in cancer therapy there is the risk of late brain necrosis. Chronic radiation encephalopathy usually presents 3–24 months after high-dose irradiation;

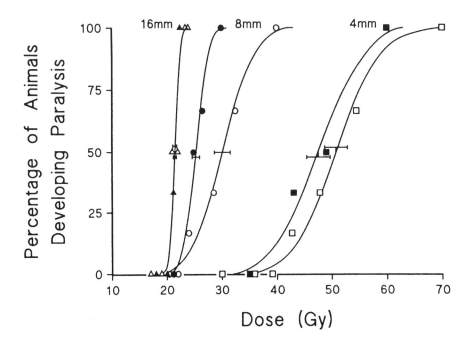

Figure 13.13. Dose-related changes in the proportion of rats developing paralysis after irradiation of different lengths of spinal cord: open symbols, radiation alone; closed symbols, MTX 4 mg/kg 30 min before radiation. (Reproduced from Morris et al, 1992, by permission of BIR.)

the higher the dose, the shorter the latent period. The injury is strikingly selective of the white matter, as indicated by widespread demyelinization. The cerebral cortex is least affected but the brainstem is particularly vulnerable. The blood vessels are also normally seen to be damaged, with all the degrees of degenerative change previously described, and may include complete thrombosis, which will have grave clinical consequences in the brain.

The effects of very high doses, of the order of 100 Gy single exposure, will be described in Chapter 14. This level of exposure leads rapidly to acute meningoencephalopathy. It is characterized by oedema of all intracranial structures and increased production of cerebrospinal fluid. Increased pressure and death in most cases is due to coning of the mid-brain. There is gross vascular damage, increased permeability of the blood–brain barrier and diffuse neuronal destruction.

THYROID GLAND

Morphology and function of the normal thyroid appear to be relatively resistant to direct effects of irradiation, whereas the hyperactive thyroid responds more readily and stimulated cell renewal in the thyroid is as radiosensitive as it is in other organs. High doses of radiation, however, can permanently damage normal thyroid and eventually cause hypothyroid- ism. The radiosensitivity of rat thyroid tissue has been determined by transplanting single cells and assaying the formation of morphologically and functionally normal thyroid follicles. This technique has been used to derive a thyroid cell survival curve for single doses of X-rays (Figure 13.14), with parameters that show that thyroid cells have a radiosensitivity within the usual range for mammalian cells.

LENS AND CATARACT FORMATION

The most prominent radiation effect on the eye is the development of lens opacities. Most of the experimental studies on radiation cataractogenesis used the murine lens as the model system, but it should be noted that the murine lens is particularly sensitive in this respect. The sensitivity of the lens is very much related to species, and in larger mammals, including human, the lens is much more resistant to radiation damage. The sensitivity of the lens is also age-dependent: the older the animal, the greater the radiation effect and the shorter the latent period after irradiation.

In most cases, lens opacities develop after a latent period between exposure and the appearance of the cataract, which is an inverse function of dose. While in humans the average latent period is 2–3 years, the time of

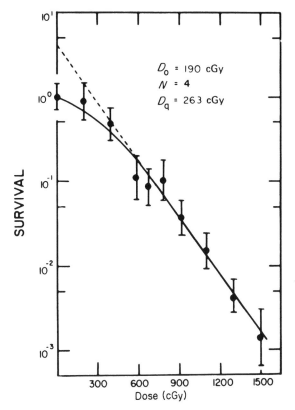

Figure 13.14. Dose–response curve for thyroid cells. (Reproduced from De Mott et al, 1979, by permission of Academic Press, Inc.)

onset may range from 6 months to many years, the interval being related to the dose and overall time of treatment. The severity of lens opacities in mice in relation to dose and time after exposure is illustrated in Figure 13.15.

The anterior epithelial cells differentiate into the fibres of the lens and it is this population that provides the cellular basis for the formation of radiation cataracts. Following irradiation there is a decrease in the mitotic activity of the germinative cells, and abortive attempts to elaborate into normal lens fibres are seen. As a result there is accumulation of abnormal cells and debris, which becomes visible when they reach the posterior pole. With higher doses, all the structures within the capsule may eventually be involved and the lens may become completely opaque in a progressive deterioration that may continue over 10 years or more after irradiation.

Neutrons have been reported to be particularly effective in producing cataracts and very high relative biological effectiveness (RBE) values have been reported from experiments on mice. However, because the murine

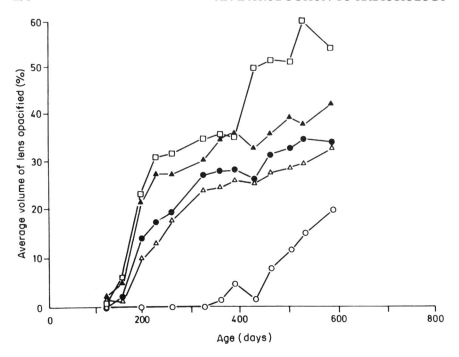

Figure 13.15. The severity of radiation cataracts formed in mice after irradiation with different doses of X-rays: (○) controls; (△), 50 cGy; (●), 100 cGy; (▲), 200 cGy; (□) 400 cGy. (Reproduced from Upton, 1969, by permission of Radiological Society of North America.)

lens is so sensitive to this effect, extremely low doses of radiation have been used and therefore very high RBE values are obtained because of the difference in the shape of the initial slopes of the survival curves of X-rays and neutrons. In humans it seems likely that the RBE for cataract formation may be of the same order as that for other cellular effects.

SUMMARY OF CONCLUSIONS

(1) The faster the growth kinetics of a cell population, the earlier will be its response to radiation. But this *radioresponsiveness* does not depend upon the *radiosensitivity* of the cells.

(2) Clonogenic assays of radiosensitivity are available for skin, intestine and bone-marrow stem cells. These are the stem-cell populations that respond early to radiation. The time of response is constant but the extent is dose dependent (see (4) below).

(3) Vascular tissue responds less quickly to radiation but vascular insufficiency will indirectly damage dependent tissues, in addition to direct effects on the parenchymal cells of such tissues.

(4) The target cells in lung, CNS and kidney, show a 'flexible' response to radiation, leading to an 'avalanche' towards functional insufficiency. The higher the dose, the earlier the avalanche (see (2) above).

(5) Pharmacological agents can be used to reduce the effect.

(6) Radiation appears to have an 'ageing' effect with some tissues such as the kidney and the lens of the eye. These show a low level of damage in the elderly, even without radiation. The higher the radiation dose, the earlier this damage occurs and the higher the level.

(7) The lens of the eye is very sensitive to high linear energy transfer (LET) radiation, and high RBE values have been reported for cataract formation.

REFERENCES

Bergonié, J. and Tribondeau, L., 1906. See English translation by Fletcher G. H., 1959. Interpretation of some results of radiotherapy and an attempt at determining a logical technique of treatment. *Radiation Research*, **11**, 587–588.

Bertalanffy, F. D. and Lau, C., 1962. Cell renewal. *International Review of Cytology*, **13**, 359–366.

Bond, V. P., Fliedner, T. M. and Archambeau, J. O., 1965. *Mammalian Radiation Lethality. A Disturbance in Cellular Kinetics*. Academic Press, New York.

Casarett, A. P., 1968. *Radiation Biology*. Prentice-Hall, New York.

Chapel, H. and Haeney, M., 1988. *Essentials of Clinical Immunology*. Blackwell Scientific Publications, Oxford.

De Mott, R. K., Mullahy, R. T. and Clifton, K. H., 1979. The survival of thyroid cells following irradiation: a directly generated single-dose survival curve. *Radiation Research*, **77**, 395–403.

Denekamp, J., 1973. Changes in the rate of repopulation during multifraction irradiation of mouse skin. *British Journal of Radiology*, **46**, 381–387.

Hopewell, J. W., van den Aardweg, G. J. M. J., Morris, G. M., Rezvani, M., Robbins, M. E. C., Ross, G. A., Whitehouse, E. M., Scott, C. A. and Horrobin, D. F., 1994. Amelioration of both early and late radiation-induced damage to pig skin by essential fatty acids. *International Journal of Radiation Oncology, Biology, Physics*, **30**, 1119–1125.

Lord, B. I., 1995. Haemopoiesis. In *Radiation Toxicology: Bone Marrow and Leukaemia*, edited by J. H. Hendry and B. I. Lord. Taylor and Francis, London.

Millar, W. T. and Hendry, J. H., 1997. Haemopoietic injury after irradiation: analysis of dose responses and repair using a target-cell model. *International Journal of Radiation Biology* (in press).

Morris, G. M., Hopewell, J. W. and Morris, A. D., 1992. The influence of methotrexate on radiation-induced damage to different lengths of the rat spinal cord. *British Journal of Radiology*, **65**, 152–156.

Moulder, J. E., Robbins, M. E. C., Cohen, E. P., Hopewell, J. W. and Ward, W. F., 1997. Pharmacological modification of radiation-induced late normal tissue injury.

In *Radiation Therapy*, edited by B. B. Mittal, J. A. Purdy and L. L. Ang. Kluwer Academic, Dordrecht.

Nias, A. H. W., 1963. Some comparisons of fractioned effects by erythema measurements on human skin. *British Journal of Radiology*, **36**, 183–187.

Nias, A. H. W., 1974. The clinical significance of cell survival curves. In *Biological and Clinical Basis of Radiosensitivity*, edited by M. Friedman. Charles C. Thomas, Springfield, IL, pp. 156–169.

Nias, A. H. W., 1988. *Clinical Radiobiology*, 2nd edn. Churchill Livingstone, Edinburgh.

Upton, A. C., 1969. Radiation cataractogenesis. *Radiology*, **80**, 610–614.

Upton, A. C., Kimball, A. W., Furth, J., Christenberry, K. W. and Benedict, W. H., 1960. Age distribution of death with nephrosclerosis in male mice. *Cancer Res.*, **20** (8/2), 23 (1960).

van den Brenk, H. A. S., 1971. Radiation effects on the pulmonary system. In *Pathology of Radiation*, edited by C. C. Berdjis. Williams and Wilkins, Baltimore, pp. 569–591.

Wheldon, T. E., Michalowski, A. S. and Kirk, J., 1982. The effect of irradiation on function in self-renewing normal tissues with differing proliferative organisation. *British Journal of Radiology*, **55**, 759–766.

Withers, H. R., 1967. The dose–survival relationship for irradiation of epithelial cells of mouse skin. *British Journal of Radiology*, **40**, 187–194.

Withers, H. R. and Elkind, M. M., 1969. The response of intestine to radiation. I Radiosensitivity and fractionation response of crypt cells of mouse jejunum. *Radiation Research*, **38**, 598–601.

Withers, H. R., Mason, K. A. and Thames, H. D., 1986. Late radiation response of kidney assayed by tubule-cell survival. *British Journal of Radiology*, **59**, 587–595.

14 Whole-body Radiation

The energy in a lethal dose of total body irradiation (TBI) is only sufficient to boil a teaspoonful of water. This small amount of energy is nevertheless sufficient, when delivered in the form of ionizing radiation, to have profound effects on cellular systems in the body. The effects will depend on the proportion and/or part of the body exposed to radiation and the dose delivered. A single acute dose of 20 Gy delivered to a 1 cm^2 area of skin will lead to localized moist desquamation but no systemic effects will be observed. Half of this dose delivered to the whole body will lead to death within 2 weeks, after a prostrating illness. Between these extremes, partial body irradiation will produce different results (dose for dose) depending on the particular tissues and organs exposed. In this chapter, these effects will be related to the cellular damage inflicted on various parts of the body and it will be shown that the lethal and other profound effects of acute irradiation can be attributed to damage to specific cell populations. These populations are found in different parts of the body, and they will be discussed first as part of the total body syndrome and then as part of different partial body syndromes.

THE CELLULAR BASIS OF THE TOTAL BODY SYNDROMES

The nature of radiation lethality, the timing of death and whether death occurs at all, or whether recovery ensues, can be shown to depend on the depletion of various cell populations and whether they are able to recover to normal numbers. In fact, the main discussion will be confined to two modes of death: gastrointestinal and haemopoietic. A cellular explanation does not apply to central nervous system (CNS) death because in practice the effects are so acute that there is not time for such a mechanism to become manifest. The CNS syndrome is due to neuronal damage secondary to vascular damage, oedema and increased intra-cranial pressure.

The radiation responses of gut and bone marrow were discussed individually in Chapter 13 with other normal tissues. The kinetics of the two stem-cell populations merit further study, however, in the context of the radiation response of the total body. Figure 14.1 shows a theoretical diagram of the kinetics of these various cellular systems. The diagram follows, over a course of time, the percentage of viable cells after a dose of

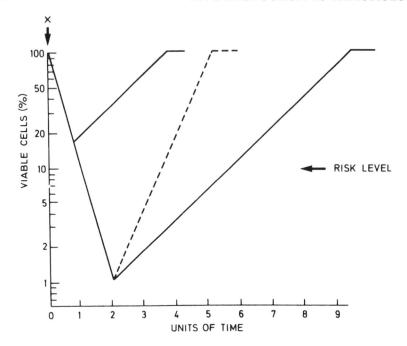

Figure 14.1. Response kinetics to irradiated cells.

X-rays. The larger the dose of X-rays, the smaller the surviving fraction of viable cells. The result of a small or a large dose of radiation is shown in the diagram. The normal rate of recovery is shown by the solid lines, but a faster rate may be possible in the case of bone marrow, as shown by the dashed line. (This might follow the use of a bone-marrow growth factor.)

The time scale can be days, or whatever is appropriate to the particular cell population, depending on the length of the cell cycle. During the first few days, the number of cells falls at a steady rate until the surviving fraction of cells has regenerated sufficiently to begin repopulation, when the curve begins to rise again. This pattern was evident in the peripheral blood count of rats after TBI, which was shown as Figure 13.7 in Chapter 13 (and for a tumour in Chapter 12, Figure 12.7). In that example the dose was 5 Gy, which was a sublethal dose and so the blood counts showed both the initial decline and the subsequent recovery. By contrast, Figure 14.4 shows what happens to the intestinal cell count after a dose of 30 Gy. This is a lethal dose and so no recovery pattern can be seen.

Figure 14.1 also indicates the fraction of viable cells below which the integrity of the tissue and therefore the viability of the whole animal may be at risk. Thus, the size of dose and therefore the extent of cellular depletion and the rate of its recovery may influence the period of time during which the animal is at risk with respect to a damaged cellular system.

CELL RENEWAL SYSTEMS

Figure 14.2 shows a model of a cell renewal system (in fact, myelopoiesis in the dog from bone-marrow stem cells, described in Chapter 13) whose pattern can be applied to any proliferative cell population. It can be assumed that there is a pool of stem cells that have survived a dose of radiation and that this pool can replace itself. After a given time, it will be able to replenish the population of mature cells that is required for the integrity of the tissue and of the animal as a whole. Figure 14.2 shows that a certain time period is necessary before the new cells will become available from the surviving stem cells. During this time the already mature cells will remain viable, dependent on their lifespan. It is the balance between the gradual removal (by death) of the ageing mature cells and the arrival of the new mature cells that will determine whether the tissue remains intact to a

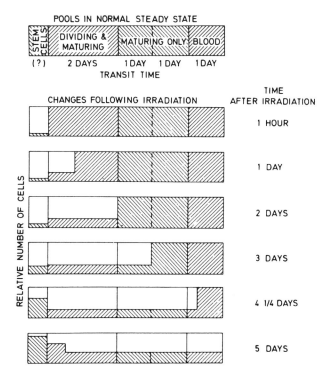

Figure 14.2. Model of cell renewal system. (Reproduced from Bond et al, by permission of Academic Press, Inc.)

sufficient degree to maintain the integrity of that tissue and therefore the health of the animal.

From this specific example, it is possible to generalize to other cellular systems in other animals. It is only the time scale that requires alteration. The kinetics of a depression in cell number followed by recovery will follow the same general shape shown in Figure 14.1. The relationship is illustrated in Figure 14.3, where the transit times of a number of cellular systems are compared. There is a constant relationship between the transit time of non-proliferating maturing cells (the cells that are going to form the functional part of the system) and the period of time after irradiation before the previous mature cells were depressed in number. The earliest cellular system in Figure 14.3 is the intestine; the bone-marrow systems come later, and finally the testis (which will be discussed in Chapter 18).

It is because of these different cellular responses that the various modes of death of the total body syndrome follow the time course already discussed. The reason for gastrointestinal death occurring before haemo-poietic death is the faster depression in the gastrointestinal epithelial cell population. This is due to its shorter transit time, and is illustrated in Figure 14.4, where the mouse intestinal epithelial cell count falls rapidly to a point where diarrhoea ensues. While this shorter transit time explains why the

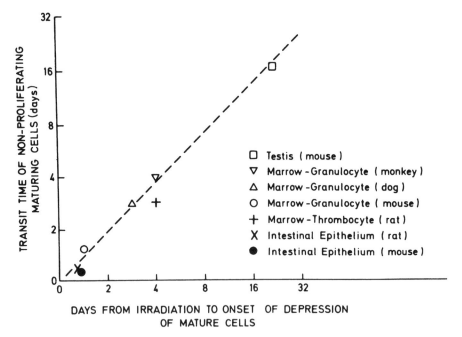

Figure 14.3. Relation of transit time to time of radiation response. (Reproduced from Patt, 1963, by permission of American Roentgen Ray Society.)

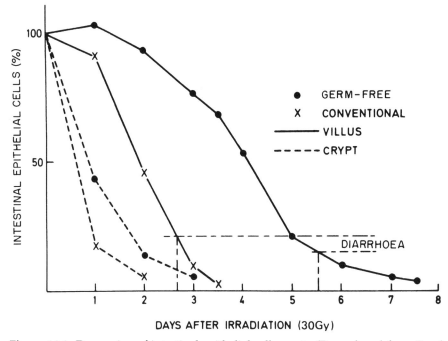

Figure 14.4. Depression of intestinal epithelial cell counts. (Reproduced from Bond et al, 1965, by permission of Academic Press, Inc.)

intestinal syndrome occurs before the haemopoietic syndrome, the reason why survivors of the intestinal syndrome may still suffer haemopoietic death is explained by Table 14.1. This shows that haemopoietic stem cells are much more radiosensitive than intestinal stem cells, with lower values of both D_0 and D_q (see Chapter 13, Figures 13.8 and 13.5).

Another way to consider the probability of a lethal outcome is to measure the minimum number of stem cells that must remain after irradiation in order to ensure survival of the animal. For each critical tissue this will be a 'tissue rescuing unit' (TRU). Hendry and Thames (1986) found that for mouse bone marrow a TRU would be 100 colony-forming cells (CFC-S); for mouse intestine it would be 5×10^5 crypts (or 1.5×10^7 stem cells). These would be the values that apply to a radiation dose spanning the LD_{50}.

Table 14.1. Radiosensitivity and rate of response of mouse stem cell populations

Stem cells	D_0 (cGy)	D_q (cGy)	Transit time (days)
Intestinal	115	430	1
Haemopoietic	90	100	4

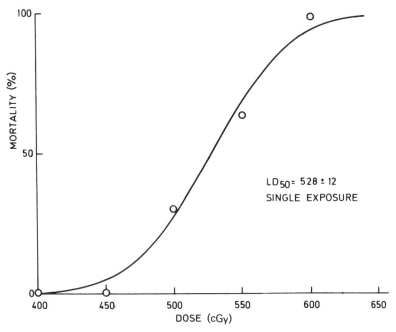

Figure 14.5. Lethality curve for rhesus monkeys. (Reproduced from Paterson, 1954, by permission of Blackwell Science.)

MEAN LETHAL DOSE – LD_{50}

Figure 14.5 illustrates a lethality curve for rhesus monkeys. A dose of 528 cGy is quoted as the (LD_{50}), but it can be appreciated that this is a statistical statement, implying that in a large enough sample of animals 50% would be killed by a dose of 528 cGy of TBI. It is important to note, however, that many animals will survive a dose of 550 cGy, but few will survive 600 cGy, and a few animals may die from a dose as low as 450 cGy. Nevertheless, the dosage range in Figure 14.5 is comparatively narrow, i.e. the survival curve has a broad shoulder of 400 cGy above which there is a rapid rise in the fraction of animals that die. This implies a threshold survival of some critical group(s) of cells, which in this case is the haemopoietic system.

The LD_{50} is a useful statement when comparing different animals or different methods of delivering the total body radiation, or perhaps of treating the animals after this irradiation, but it is still only a guide as far as assessing the prognosis of any individual animal. The expression LD_{50} is thus a convenient way of overcoming the problems of heterogeneous populations, including the results that would be obtained from unduly

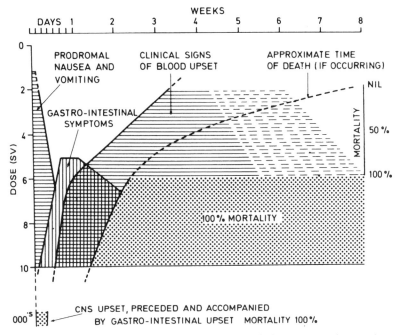

Figure 14.6. Time sequence of the main events of the total body syndrome in humans. (Reproduced from Blakely, 1968, by permission of the author.)

sensitive or unduly resistant subjects. The LD_{50} values are known for a number of animals and vary with body weight; the heavier the animal, the lower the LD_{50}. For hamsters it is at least 10 Gy, while for sheep it can be lower than 2 Gy (Hendry and Yang, 1995). Figure 14.7 shows a figure of 2.6 Gy for the dog. The value for humans has been estimated to be about 4 Gy. This is shown as 4 Sv in Figure 14.6, using the sievert unit of dose equivalence (see Chapter 20).

There is a further definition that must be added to the expression (LD_{50}), however, in order to assess the type of radiation death. Table 14.2

Table 14.2. Dose (cGy) of total body radiation and time of death

Species	$LD_{50/30}$	$LD_{50/8}$	$LD_{50/5}$	$LD_{50/2}$
Mouse	640	–	1260	20 000
Germ-free mouse	705	2000	–	–
Rat	714	–	808	20 000
Monkey	600	1500	–	10 000

Reproduced from Bond et al, 1965, by permission of Academic Press, Inc.

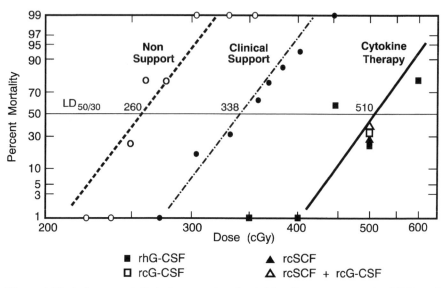

Figure 14.7. Influence of clinical support and cytokine therapy on survival ($LD_{50/30}$) of irradiated dogs. (Reproduced from MacVittie and Farese, 1995, by permission of Taylor & Francis.)

illustrates the dosages that will kill 50% of a sample of different animals; in this table a subscript has been added to the expression LD_{50}. Under these different headings different dosages of TBI are required to kill 50% of the animals. The subscript is the number of days at which the number of deaths is assessed. In the left-hand column, ($LD_{50/30}$), a considerable time (30 days) has elapsed since the TBI and this is usually regarded as sufficient for the final results of the syndrome to be established. This is the most convenient form of the expression (LD_{50}), and when no subscript is used it is usually assumed that this is the expression, although the corresponding time interval for humans is 60 days. (If the TBI is delivered at a lower dose rate, the usual radiobiological mechanisms will apply and so the LD_{50} will be higher; see Chapter 17, Table 17.4). The other columns give the LD_{50} values for shorter time intervals, and for these a higher dosage of radiation is quoted.

Central nervous system death

The right-hand column, ($LD_{50/2}$), is death at 2 days after the dose of radiation and this applies to death from the CNS syndrome, which occurs with very high doses. The choice of 2 days as a time limit reflects the observations that animals dying before 2 days show few, if any, gastrointestinal signs and symptoms, and certainly no haematological changes, unlike those animals dying later than this time, which do. It is probable that deaths attributed to the CNS syndrome on this basis actually include a variety of causes of death that cannot be separated out.

Gut death

The choice of the next time limits of 5 and 8 days reflects the tendency of deaths in the transition zones to group themselves around two sometimes overlapping modes at less than 5 or 8 days, with signs and symptoms of the gastrointestinal syndrome. This is not to say that the bone-marrow syndrome may not already have become evident, but it is the mode of death that is under consideration here. Just as it was CNS death at a much earlier phase, it is now the gastrointestinal syndrome that is causing death in this phase.

Figure 14.4 shows that there is more delay in the fall in intestinal cell number in mice that have been kept germ-free than in conventional mice. Death from the gastrointestinal syndrome would also be delayed for this period in such animals, which is why Table 14.2 quotes the LD_{50} figure for germ-free mice under the $LD_{50/8}$ column rather than the $LD_{50/5}$ column.

The consequences of a large dose of radiation to the intestines were described in the classical paper by Quastler (1956):

> A mammal with a leaky intestinal barrier can survive. If a large segment of the intestinal barrier is missing for some time, however, then death is bound to occur. The problem of the immediate cause of death in acute intestinal radiation death boils down to the question of which one (or ones) of a number of likely mechanisms kills the animal before the others become effective. The timing is important; animals will succumb only if the recuperative activity in the crypts does not become effective before denudation is complete. If it were possible to tide the animal over the fastest dangerous reaction, then it might be possible to avert acute intestinal radiation death altogether.
>
> . . . The loss of the intestinal barrier has three likely consequences: intestinal bacteria and their toxins can enter the submucosa and invade the bloodstream and the peritoneal cavity; proteolytic enzymes in the intestinal lumen can digest submucous tissue and enter into the peritoneal cavity; in the other direction, water and electrolytes will be lost into the intestinal lumen.

This description was applied to the mouse, and much of our radiobiological information depends on the study of that species, for both normal tissues and tumours. This information is much more accurate than that obtainable in human studies, which is necessarily limited for ethical reasons. Intestinal death in humans will be discussed later but the radiobiological principles that lead to it are similar to those described here for the mouse. Only the time scale is different, with the turnover time for human cell populations tending to be longer by a factor of about two. The time of death is likely to be earlier in the mouse, but the mechanism of death is similar.

Regeneration of the small intestine is rapid. There is evidence of mitotic activity 1 day after exposure but many of the new cells are abnormal. By the third day, the rate of mitosis in the crypts is greater than normal, although the villi are covered by only a thin layer of stretched cells. By the end of 1 week, new cells have covered the villi and the intestinal epithelium appears about normal. Removal of cellular debris is slow. Regeneration commonly occurs in the presence of degenerative changes. The initial damage is more severe following large doses, and repopulation of the epithelium may not then occur. The villi appear to be shortened and only partially covered by degenerating cells. Death of the animal usually occurs between the third and fifth day, in the absence of regeneration of the epithelium of the small intestine.

Bone-marrow death

Death of animals from the bone-marrow syndrome occurs commonly at 12–14 days. This time interval is well outside the 8-day period for gut death but, because there is not a fourth mode of death from acute radiation to follow that of the bone-marrow syndrome, the interval of 30 days has been accepted as a convenient experimental period after which animals may be considered to be survivors from acute radiation. Subsequent deaths can reasonably be excluded from an acute radiation cause.

It should now be obvious why Table 14.2 is set out in this form. Central nervous system death is an acute manifestation because of immediate vascular effects ($LD_{50/2}$). The middle columns deal predominantly with the gastrointestinal syndrome, which occurs before 5–8 days because of the time course of depletion of the gastrointestinal epithelium below a risk level (Figure 14.1). If death from this syndrome is to occur, it will occur in this period of time, otherwise the epithelial system will already be regenerating and the animal will recover as far as this system is concerned. However, it has been shown that the haemopoietic system, as far as its functional peripheral compartment is concerned, has still to reach its time of greatest risk, which may occur between days 10 and 20. For this reason, the first column in Table 14.2 is expressed as $LD_{50/30}$ days in order to allow for death to occur during this 30-day period.

The $LD_{50/30}$ value can be increased if a support regime is used to replace or substitute for the function of those mature cells depleted as a consequence of lethal radiation exposure to haemopoietic stem and progenitor cells. Antibiotics, blood transfusion and parenteral fluids are used. Figure 14.7 shows how the $LD_{50/30}$ value for dogs was increased from 260 to 338 cGy by such a clinical support regime. An even larger increase to 510 cGy was obtained by the use of cytokines such as recombinant human G-CSF or canine SCF, and G-CSF (see Chapter 13).

HUMAN SYNDROMES

The three expressions ($LD_{50/2}$), ($LD_{50/5}$) or 8 and ($LD_{50/30}$) are statistically convenient, but deaths from acute radiation cannot always be divided into separate categories. The three syndromes may often co-exist. Nevertheless, the three modes of death can be applied to the response in humans. The precise value of a lethal dose of TBI has not been determined, for obvious reasons, but there is evidence from various industrial radiation accidents, such as that at Chernobyl in 1986, from the atomic bombs at Hiroshima and Nagasaki in 1945 and from various groups of cancer patients receiving TBI (discussed later). All the accidental evidence is confused by the difficulty of obtaining dosimetry in the individuals exposed, but the best estimate of the median lethal dose (LD_{50}) for humans is 4 Gy TBI, received as a single acute dose. The actual value depends on the quality and distribution of the radiation. This does not mean that humans can tolerate this amount of radiation, because all individuals exposed to it would have serious symptoms, and 50% would die. It must be stressed that exposure to 2 Gy of acute TBI may sometimes cause death but all the fatalities from the Chernobyl accident had received doses higher than 6 Gy to their bone marrow.

That accident in 1986 provided, sadly, some useful examples of the doses that lead to the various degrees of TBI syndrome in humans. Biological dosimetry was based upon chromosome aberrations in peripheral blood lymphocytes (see Chapter 5) in samples taken within a few hours of the accident. The most severely affected personnel received doses ranging from 6 to 16 Gy, and 17 out of the 20 in this category died at between 10 and 50 days. These 'fourth-degree' victims suffered a rise in temperature within half an hour, with vomiting and headaches. There was almost total disappearance of lymphocytes from the blood within 3 days. Within a week there were severe intestinal symptoms, a decline in the other white cells in the blood and general intoxication leading to death.

There were 23 'third-degree' victims who received doses of 4–6 Gy; seven of these died 2–7 weeks after the accident. Their headaches and vomiting did not start until 30 min after irradiation and they then developed fever, infections and bleeding. Fifty-three people received 2–4 Gy ('second-degree' victims) and others received lower doses, none of which were fatal. These examples of whole-body irradiation at Chernobyl confirmed the patterns of response depicted in Figure 14.6.

General clinical picture

All the syndromes overlap to a certain extent, depending on the dose delivered to the whole body. Prodromal nausea and vomiting will be found, even after doses that do not prove lethal, but will last longer after higher doses. Any CNS symptoms will also occur in the initial period after irradiation, but these indicate a very high and lethal dose. Gastrointestinal symptoms will usually also indicate a fatal outcome, but the time scale is dose dependent, as is the time of onset of haematological changes. These are not necessarily fatal over the lower dose range. The time scale extends from hours to weeks. The longer an irradiated individual survives after the first 2–3 weeks, the better the prognosis. This will also be much better if a support regime has been employed (e.g. cytokines).

Central nervous system syndrome

After a single dose of several thousand centigrays to the whole body, particularly the head, the clinical onset is prompt and death may occur in minutes to hours. After the initial phase of radiation sickness, there is swift progression from listlessness, drowsiness and languor to severe apathy, prostration and lethargy. The development of vasculitis or encephalitis gives rise to cerebral oedema. After more than 50 Gy, there are seizures ranging from generalized muscle tremor to epileptoid convulsions similar to grand mal. This convulsive phase lasts a few hours and is followed by ataxia. Total body radiation causing the CNS syndrome is fatal.

Gastrointestinal syndrome

Gastrointestinal syndrome predominates with lower doses received by the whole body, particularly the abdomen (5–20 Gy). The prodromal nausea and vomiting begin promptly and do not subside. For some people these symptoms develop within 0.5 h after exposure; in others, these symptoms do not occur for several hours. Gastrointestinal symptoms may continue (anorexia, nausea, vomiting and diarrhoea). Sometimes the symptoms disappear after 2–3 days and recur by about the fifth day (just when the patient's condition seemed to have improved) owing to injury of intestinal epithelium, which by then is denuded of cells leaving few and even bare villi. Rather abruptly, malaise, anorexia, nausea and vomiting prevent normal food and fluid intake, leading to serious electrolyte imbalance. Simultaneously, high fever and persistent diarrhoea – rapidly progressing from loose to watery, bloody stools – appear. The abdomen is distended and peristalsis is absent. Rapid deterioration leads to severe paralytic ileus. Exhaustion, fever and perhaps delirium follow, dehydration and haemo-concentration develop, the circulation fails and the patient becomes comatose and dies 1 or 2 weeks after exposure.

After doses where regeneration of the gastrointestinal epithelium is possible, antibiotics, fluid replacement and other supportive therapy may keep the patient alive. The epithelium regenerates and vomiting and diarrhoea subside. Unfortunately, this will only be a temporary respite because of the onset of the haemopoietic syndrome, when evidence of bone-marrow aplasia and pancytopenia appears within 2–3 weeks, as shown in Figure 14.6. After doses that cause this severe intestinal damage, bone-marrow regeneration is unlikely, so that even if there is spontaneous recovery or successful treatment, individuals will inevitably suffer the severe effects of the haemopoietic syndrome that follows such doses.

Haemopoietic syndrome

After lower doses of irradiation, i.e. less than 5 Gy, the symptoms and signs are due to different causes and appear in two successive phases. Leucopenia, thrombocytopenia and haemostatic abnormalities are a direct consequence of lesions of the haemopoietic organs. Symptoms such as haemorrhage and anaemia may be secondary to the visceral lesions and associated with oedema or thrombosis in capillaries and ulceration of mucous membranes. Anorexia, apathy, nausea and vomiting and some diarrhoea are maximum 6–12 h after exposure. The symptoms may subside so that by 24–36 h individuals feel well, but their bone marrow, spleen and lymph nodes are atrophying. The patient enjoys apparently normal health until about the third week. Then chills, malaise, fever, headache, fatigue, anorexia and dyspnoea on exertion develop, and at this time partial or complete loss of hair is likely.

Within a few days the general condition worsens and the patient then develops a sore throat and pharyngitis, with a tendency to bruise easily. This is followed by bleeding from gums and ulcerations in gingiva and tonsils. Similar ulceration in the intestines causes a renewal of diarrhoea. The patient has a high fever with complete anorexia. During weeks 5–6, agranulocytosis, anaemia and infection become critical. The increased susceptibility to infection is caused by the dose-dependent decrease in circulating granulocytes and lymphocytes, impairment of antibody production, impairment of granulocyte and reticuloendothelial functions and haemorrhagic ulceration permitting entrance of bacteria through the gastrointestinal tract. Thereafter, if the patient recovers, fever subsides, ulcerations heal and convalescence begins at about the end of the second month after exposure.

Prognosis

A knowledge of these symptoms and signs allows a prognosis to be determined in those cases of accidental TBI where biological dosimetry has not been possible, so that there is considerable uncertainty as to the dose received by the patient. Individuals showing the CNS syndrome will die, as in general will those with intractable nausea, vomiting and diarrhoea. Those in whom nausea and vomiting is brief, i.e. for 1–2 days followed by well-being, have a good chance of survival.

After initial symptoms, the effects of haemopoietic damage predominate. The lymphocyte count is valuable as an early criterion for judging radiation injury. In normal individuals, a fall in lymphocyte number is seen within the first 24–48 h. If, at 48 h, the lymphocyte count is 1200/mm³ or above, it is unlikely that the individual has received a fatal exposure; if the lymphocyte count is in the 300–1200 range, a dose in the lethal range may be suspected; counts below 300 indicate an extremely serious exposure.

The total white cell count is of particular value for following the patient throughout the course of sickness. In general, the drop in neutrophils will reflect the degree of exposure; a fall in white counts beginning within the first week denotes a rather high exposure, whereas late falls indicate a less serious exposure. Because of this time course of the total blood count and its various elements, a consideration of death from the total body syndrome must include a discussion of the time intervals involved. The relationship between time span and radiosensitivity is shown in Figure 14.8. The upper part shows that when mice are given more than 10 Gy of TBI they die

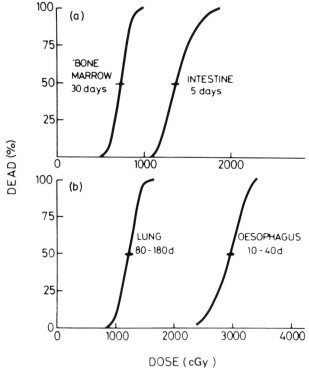

Figure 14.8. Dose–response curves for mouse lethality after (a) total body and (b) thoracic irradiation. (Reproduced from Denekamp, 1986, by permission of *Int. J. Radiat. Biol.*, Taylor & Francis.)

within 4–7 days from the gastrointestinal syndrome. After a lower dose of TBI the intestinal epithelium regenerates sufficiently rapidly to avoid gastrointestinal syndrome, but the mice succumb from the bone-marrow syndrome between 12 and 30 days. Bone-marrow stem cells are more radiosensitive than intestinal stem cells but have a slower transit time (Table 14.1).

PARTIAL BODY IRRADIATION

The cellular basis of TBI can also be applied to partial body irradiation. If it is known which part of the body has been irradiated, one can consider which cell population may be at risk. Table 14.3 compares the $LD_{50/30}$ values of rats treated through either the upper or lower body. There is considerable difference between the two doses and both are higher than that shown for the $LD_{50/30}$ of the total body in Table 14.2. This is because much less tissue is at risk, but the particular tissue at risk still influences the lethal effects. With the lower body, it is predominantly the gastrointestinal tract that is affected and death occurs at an average of 5 days, as is usual with the gastrointestinal syndrome, although a higher dose is tolerated because of the smaller amount of tissue involved.

When only the upper part of the body is irradiated, an even higher dose is tolerated and the mean survival time rises to 11 days, which is more typical of the haemopoietic syndrome. This is related to the incidence of the radiation on the bone marrow present in the upper body. But much bone marrow is still spared, so the LD_{50} value is considerably higher than that for the whole body. Other cell populations are involved, of course, and the lower part of Figure 14.8 shows how the relationship between radio-sensitivity and the time span of radiation response applies to thoracic irradiation. With a dose of about 30 Gy the mice die after 10–40 days from oesophageal damage. After a lower dose they may die of pulmonary damage, but not until much later.

CLINICAL TBI

Clinical TBI is now used for bone-marrow transplantation (Parker and Tait, 1995). The object of the exercise is to eradicate the malignant bone-marrow cells, e.g. leukaemic cells, and then transplant healthy bone-marrow cells from a suitable donor. Great care has to be taken to prevent infection. Patients also have to have their lungs shielded in order to maintain their lung dose below 8 Gy. A fractionation regime will assist because of the different radiosensitivity of lung parenchymal cells and bone-marrow stem cells (see Chapter 8, Figure 8.7).

Table 14.3. Dose of partial body radiation and time of death

Rat	$LD_{50/30}$ (Gy)	Mean survival time (days)
Upper body	18	11
Lower body (abdomen)	10	5

Reproduced from Bond et al, 1965, by permission of Academic Press, Inc.

DOSES AND TIMES

This chapter has covered those circumstances in which a large proportion of the body is exposed to an acute dose of radiation. Death will occur within hours if the CNS syndrome is caused by a very high dose. If the whole of the gastrointestinal tract is given 10 Gy, the outcome will be fatal within days. If the haemopoietic system is given 6 Gy this will also be lethal, but after a longer interval of time. Individuals exposed to lower doses may survive after radiation sickness of varying severity. Survival is more probable if the radiation dose is more protracted (as may occur with fall-out) and if only part of the body is exposed (as may occur in a built-up area). The effect of protracted radiation is discussed in Chapter 17, where the effect of reduced dose rate on $LD_{50/30}$ is shown in Figure 17.4.

This is the only chapter of this book where the biological effect of radiation has had to be described in general terms without a very precise dose response. The reason for this is simply that physical dosimetry is rarely available in these circumstances and even biological dosimetry may be imprecise. The general principles of the radiosensitivity and rate of response of the relevant normal-cell populations have been applied, however. The rate of response of tumour cell populations is the subject of the next chapter, where the radiation doses *will* have been precisely measured.

SUMMARY OF CONCLUSIONS

(1) When a very large volume of tissue is irradiated, damage will be evident after a relatively low dose; 4 Gy to the whole human body will kill half of a group of people (LD_{50}).

(2) Death occurs because of depletion of haemopoietic stem cells below a critical number, leading to haematological insufficiency and the 'bone-marrow syndrome'. Cytokines can be used to stimulate the recovery of bone marrow.

(3) After a higher dose of total body irradiation the gastrointestinal system will be lethally damaged. The gut syndrome will occur earlier than

haematological insufficiency because of the faster kinetics of intestinal stem cells.

(4) Lower doses of TBI (2 Gy) are more likely to cause radiation sickness than death, from which survival and recovery is possible provided that the sufferer can be kept free of infection.

(5) When dosimetry is not possible after a radiation accident to a person, the likely outcome can be predicted from the type and severity of the clinical syndromes.

(6) When only half of the body is irradiated, a larger dose can be tolerated than by the whole body but the bone-marrow syndrome (upper body) or the gut syndrome (lower body) will still occur after the same time intervals.

(7) Protracted radiation is less lethal than acute radiation for the usual radiobiological reasons.

REFERENCES

Blakely, J., 1968. *The Care of Radiation Casualties*. Heinemann, London.

Bond, V. P., Fliedner, T. M. and Archambeau, J. O., 1965. *Mammalian Radiation Lethality. A Disturbance in Cellular Kinetics*. Academic Press, New York.

Denekamp, J., 1986. Cell kinetics and radiation biology. *International Journal of Radiation Biology*, **49**, 357–380.

Hendry, J. H. and Thames, H. D., 1986. The tissue-rescuing unit. *British Journal of Radiology*, **59**, 628–630.

Hendry, J. H. and Yang, F.-T., 1995. Response of bone marrow to low LET radiation. In *Radiation Toxicology: Bone Marrow and Leukaemia*, edited by J. H. Hendry and B. I. Lord. Taylor and Francis, London.

MacVittie, T. J. and Farese, A. M., 1995. Experimental approaches for therapeutic treatment of radiation-induced haemopoietic injury. In *Radiation Toxicology: Bone Marrow and Leukaemia*, edited by J. H. Hendry and B. I. Lord. Taylor and Francis, London.

Parker, C. C. and Tait, D. M., 1995. Total body irradiation. In *Treatment of Cancer*, 3rd edn, edited by P. Price and K. Sikora. Chapman and Hall, London.

Paterson, E., 1954. Factors influencing recovery after whole-body radiation. *Journal of the Faculty of Radiologists*, **5**, 189–199.

Patt, H. M., 1963. Quantitative aspects of radiation effects at the tissue and tumour level. *American Journal of Roentgenology*, **90**, 928–937.

Quastler, H., 1956. The nature of intestinal radiation death. *Radiation Research*, **4**, 303–320.

15 Proliferation Kinetics after Radiation

The methods used to analyse the growth of unirradiated cell populations were described in Chapter 3. This chapter will apply those methods to show how radiation affects the proliferation kinetics of tumour cell populations. This is of special interest to radiotherapists who treat cancer patients and need to know how best to stop the growth of tumours and cure patients of their disease.

Throughout this book emphasis has been placed upon the cellular basis of radiobiology. Tumours consist of tissues, well or poorly differentiated, with a stroma of connective and vascular tissue. When it comes to improving the therapeutic ratio between tumour and normal-tissue response, however, it is the total tumour cell mass that is the critical target, limited by the reaction of the essential normal-cell populations and tissues. Figure 15.1 follows the peripheral blood count of a patient with chronic myeloid leukaemia who received radiotherapy to the spleen on five occasions between 1962 and 1964. On each occasion there was an immediate fall in the white cell count followed by a gradual rise to the starting level, when treatment had to be repeated (until busulphan therapy was instituted

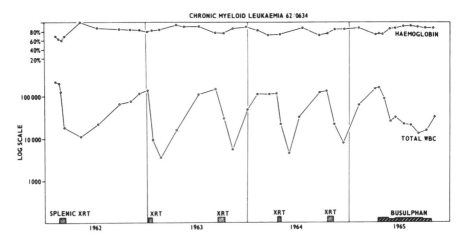

Figure 15.1. Blood count after irradiation for chronic myeloid leukaemia. (Reproduced from Nias, 1988, by permission of Churchill Livingstone.)

in 1965). This illustrates the concept of the 'total cell mass' in a very obvious way that is not often possible to record with solid tumours. A question arises as to why some tumours respond in this almost predictable way and some do not. Studies on the kinetics of animal tumours will lead to the conclusion that carcinomas have a higher cell-loss factor than sarcomas and that radiotherapy accentuates this. For the C_3H carcinoma the cell-loss factor starts at 70% and rises to 76%; for the RIB5 sarcoma there is no cell loss at all before irradiation but a factor of 64% can be measured afterwards. The old data in Table 15.1 showed how these principles apply to human tumours where the response of squamous-cell carcinomas to radiotherapy also lies in the high cell-loss factor of such a histological type. This also serves to explain the radiation responsiveness of reticuloses and embryonal tumours. Table 15.1 shows why adenocarcinomas and sarcomas may be less responsive because of their lower values of cell-loss factor.

The consequences of rapid shrinkage, due to cell loss, on tumour reoxygenation will be discussed in Chapter 16. This shrinkage of an irradiated tumour may be due to any one of the three processes of apoptosis, autolysis and phagoctyosis. Apoptosis was discussed in Chapter 6 and just means the shedding of cells, i.e. cell loss. The process of autolysis depends on a good blood supply for diffusion; if the blood supply is poor then 'coagulative necrosis' will occur. Finally, phagocytosis requires a new growth of capillaries and connective tissue, leading to 'organization' in the irradiated tumour volume. The effect of radiation on cell loss will be described later in this chapter.

TUMOUR MODELS

In this book the emphasis has been chosen to be upon scientific laboratory observations of the response of experimental animal tumours to radiation, as distinct from clinical observations, which are usually less well defined

Table 15.1. Kinetics of human tumours

Histological type	Number of tumours	Doubling time (days)	Growth fraction (%)	Cell loss (%)
Embryonal	6	27	90	94
Reticulosis	15	29	90	94
Sarcoma	32	41	11	68
Squamous cell carcinoma	68	58	25	90
Adenocarcinoma	121	83	6	71

Reprinted from *Eur. J. Cancer*, **9**, 305–312 from Malaise et al, 1973. The relationship between growth, labelling index, and histological type of human solid tumours, with kind permission from Elsevier Science Ltd, The Boulevard, Langford Lane, Kidlington OX5 1GB, UK.

and relatively imprecise. Nevertheless, it is useful that the examples of experimental radiotherapy should be performed on those animal tumours that are reasonable models of human cancers. The histological classification of human tumours into carcinomas, sarcomas, lymphomas, etc. can be related to animal models (although most experimental animal tumours grow much faster than human tumours). The growth characteristics of some of these human tumour cell populations were discussed in Chapter 3 and examples of the kinetic parameters were given using the growth-fraction model (Figure 3.10). In this model, tumour cell populations were shown to have four compartments: cells in cycle with a measurable cycle time; resting cells (or the non-growth fraction), which may still have the capacity to grow; sterile cells, which are still alive but have lost the capacity to reproduce; and dead cells, which eventually will be 'lost' from the population.

Table 15.1 lists five histological types of human tumour with the average values for their growth fraction and volume doubling time, as well as their cell-loss factor discussed already. Although Table 15.1 comprises observations from 242 human tumours, some of the histological types are poorly represented. Nevertheless, the parameters provide some basis for comparison with the animal tumours that have been used for radio-biological studies. For convenience, the tumours are listed in increasing order of volume doubling time, but there are variations in the values for cell-loss factor and particularly for growth fraction. These account for the fact that the cells in such tumours are often cycling at a very much faster rate than the volume doubling time would suggest. Thus, for squamous-cell carcinoma, labelling studies indicate a cycle time of about 6 days. The volume doubling time is very much longer at 58 days because only 25% of the tumour cells are in the growth 'compartment' and 90% of their surplus progeny are 'lost'.

Table 15.2 lists four of the many animal tumour systems used in radiobiology that have been described in this book. They serve to illustrate the problem of finding a suitable 'model' tumour. The L1210 leukaemia was described in Chapter 8. This system has been widely used for the screening

Table 15.2. Kinetics of animal tumours

Animal	Code	Histological type	Doubling time (h)	Growth fraction (%)	Cell loss (%)
Mouse	L1210	Leukaemia	10	95	5
Rat	RIB5	Fibrosarcoma	24	45	0
Rat	R1	Rhabdomyosarcoma	66	29	62
Mouse	C$_3$H	Mammary carcinoma	110	30	70

Reproduced from Nias, 1988, by permission of Churchill Livingstone.

of cancer chemotherapy compounds, but until it is irradiated (Figure 15.2) it normally has a very low cell-loss factor and this shows it to be quite unlike any of the human tumours. The same criticism can be applied to the RIB5 fibrosarcoma. Some of the radiobiological findings with these tumours will nevertheless be quoted in this chapter because they illustrate some important general principles. The more 'relevant' tumours are the R1 rhabdomyosarcoma and the C_3H mammary carcinoma (whose kinetics were described in Chapter 3). These two are examples of tumours that can have as high a cell-loss factor (60–70%) and as low a growth fraction (30%) as some of the more common human tumours.

They are all examples of 'model' tumours that may be grown and transplanted in small animals. (Small animals are used for the convenience of laboratory space.) Furthermore, strictly controlled breeding of strains of mice and rats enables the radiobiologist to perform studies on large numbers of similar tumours under constant and reproducible conditions to a high scientific standard. Tumours can be transplanted into groups of animals that are identical genetically (isologous), so that the only variable in the experiment will be the radiobiological factor to be tested. There remains one important difference between mice and humans, however: the growth

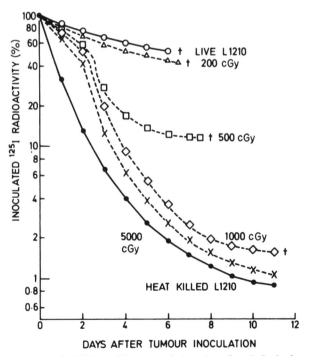

Figure 15.2. Death of L1210 cells treated *in vitro* for 2 h before inoculation. (Reproduced from Hofer, 1970, by permission of Academic Press, Inc.)

rate of the tumours. Many of the murine tumours can have a volume doubling time of only 2–3 days, whereas many human tumours have a volume doubling time of around 70 days. This large discrepancy might be accounted for by comparing the normal lifespan of mice and humans: 2–3 years and 70 years, respectively.

Unfortunately the growth kinetics of the limiting normal tissues of the two species do not show anything like that discrepancy (see Chapter 13). Furthermore, many experimental mouse tumours are allowed to grow to a relatively very large size. A 1 g tumour in a mouse would be equivalent in proportion to a 3 kg tumour in a human, which would be enormous by any standards. With such large tumours the mice often develop anaemia, with the haemoglobin level falling below 10%. This is associated with an increase in the fraction of hypoxic cells to 21%, but this fraction can be reduced back to the usual 10% by a transfusion of packed red cells.

The only solution to this problem of comparison is to study tumours of a small size (say 5 mm diameter, 0.2 g in mice). Each experiment should preferably be carried out on a range of animal tumours, chosen to cover a range of variables, that show similarity to the human situation in at least one respect, because no exact matching can be achieved. As long as the animal tumours are used as models for the purpose of examining specific effects and responses, then the tremendous advantage of obtaining statistically significant results will outweigh the disadvantages of the differences in the biological characterization of tumours in mice and humans.

CELL LOSS

The first example of the effect of irradiation on a tumour cell population is provided by a study of cell loss from L1210 tumour cells. A direct measure of cell loss is possible if the tumour cells can be pre-labelled with a DNA precursor, which will be completely removed when the cells die. In this respect [125]IUdR is the labelling precursor of choice because, following cell death, it is re-utilized to a lesser extent than [3H]-thymidine. Figure 15.2 illustrates the method for L1210 leukaemia cells, which were labelled *in vitro* with [125]IUdR and then exposed to various treatments, including increasing doses of radiation and heat inactivation, before being inoculated into mice. The whole-body ^{125}I radioactivity of the mice was then monitored at daily intervals by placing the mice in a scintillation counter. Figure 15.2 shows the rapid fall in radioactivity for the mice that received killed cells, a slow fall with untreated cells (until the animals died of leukaemia at the point indicated) and progressively more rapid rates of fall after increasing doses of radiation. The rates of fall in ^{125}I radioactivity indicate the actual disintegration of labelled tumour cells, rather than radiation-induced loss of reproductive integrity, and cell loss can be calculated directly.

Chapter 3 described how cell loss can be calculated from the discrepancy between the rate of production of new cells, t_{pot}, and the observed growth rate in the tumour, t_D. There are clearly a number of assumptions built into such a calculation but it is still a useful parameter because cell loss is often the major factor in determining the slow growth rate of primary tumours. Cells can be lost in a number of ways. In addition to loss to other parts of the body by the usual processes of metastasis from a primary tumour, cells are lost by death from damaged mitotic mechanisms, death from immunological attack, apoptosis and loss from exfoliation (as in normal skin and gut) and death from inadequate nutrition (as in a tumour). This last mode of death, from chronic hypoxia in necrotic areas, reflects the latent inability of the vascular system to keep up with the rate of cell production in a tumour, and this explains the shape of many tumour growth curves (see Figure 3.1).

GROWTH DELAY

Growth delay is one of the objectives of palliative radiotherapy and it can be studied with an animal tumour that shows a poor response to radiation. The second tumour model in Table 15.2 is the RIB5 fibrosarcoma, which can be transplanted into Wistar rats and the growth of the transplants can be measured in terms of the diameter of the tumour, as shown in curve A of Figure 15.3. The vertical axis in Figure 15.3 is a linear scale of mean diameter. In other graphs of tumour growth the scale may be logarithmic, with volume as the measurement. An estimate of volume may be derived from diameter, and the volume doubling time calculated in this way is the parameter used in Tables 15.1 and 15.2. Most tumours do not show an exponential growth curve during their whole lifespan. A semi-logarithmic plot for the R1 rhabdomyosarcoma in rat is shown in Figure 15.5, and this is bending towards the time axis, indicating a slowing in volume doubling time throughout the whole series of measurements. This is probably due to deteriorating nutritional status as the distance between blood vessels increases and widespread local necrosis results. Kinetic values were given for mouse tumours in Chapter 12, Table 12.2, which show that there is a decreasing gradient in proliferation between cells near blood vessels and those near necrotic areas in tumours. This slower proliferation applies to larger tumours in general.

It is important always to study tumour growth rate data with care. Are they mean values for the whole tumour? How was this volume measured: indirectly by weighing, or by calculation from records of the diameter of one or more of the three dimensions of a tumour? A well-documented

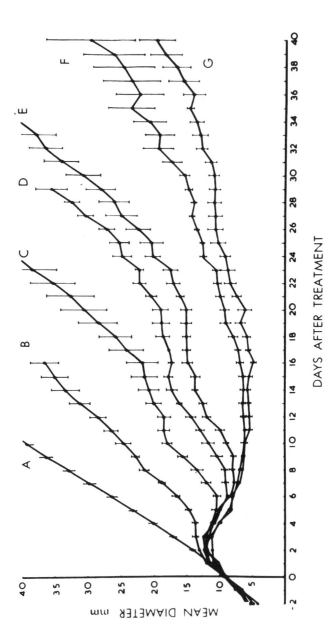

Figure 15.3. Growth curves of rat fibrosarcoma. (Reproduced from Thomlinson, 1961, by permission of *Brookhaven Symp. Biol.*)

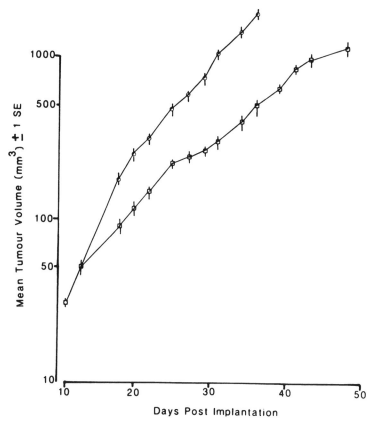

Figure 15.4. Growth curve for RIF-1 tumours implanted into unirradiated beds (circles) or irradiated (20 Gy) beds (squares). (Reproduced from Penhaligon et al, 1987, by permission of *Int. J. Radiat. Biol.*, Taylor & Francis.)

clinical case history should contain a series of measurements of tumour diameter. Most of these must necessarily follow treatment but the sort of patterns illustrated for the rat fibrosarcoma in Figure 15.3 and rhabdomyosarcoma in Figure 15.5 are typical. For ethical reasons those parts of the two figures that show tumour growth before or without treatment will usually remain absent from clinical records. But these can be derived by extrapolation, on the assumption that these animal models apply to human tumours.

Figure 15.3 shows (on a linear scale of diameter) how increasing single doses of radiation leads to growth restraint for increasing periods of time (A–G correspond to 0, 10, 20, 30, 40, 50 and 60 Gy). If the surrounding tissues could only tolerate an even larger dose then this period of growth restraint would become so long that 'cure' would have been achieved. More

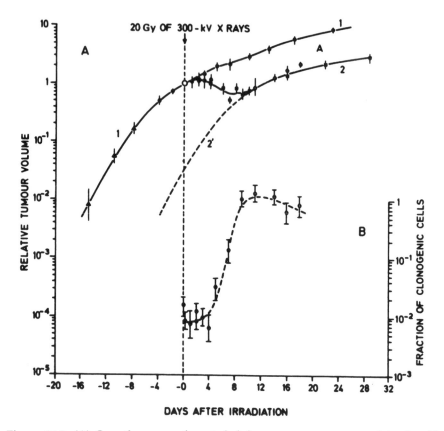

Figure 15.5. (A) Growth curves of a rat rhabdomyosarcoma, measured *in vivo*: (1) without treatment; (2) after 20 Gy. (B) Survival of the irradiated tumour cells, assayed *in vitro*. (Reprinted from *Euro. J. Cancer*, **5**, 173–189, from Hermens and Barendsen, 1969. Changes of cell proliferation characteristics in a rat rhabdomyo-sarcoma before and after X-irradiation, with kind permission from Elsevier Science Ltd, The Boulevard, Langford Lane, Kidlington OX5 1GB, UK.)

commonly, residual cells grow and the tumour then regenerates at a rate that may be similar to the rate before treatment. On the linear plot in Figure 15.3, however, the post-treatment curves are not parallel to that of the untreated tumour and show a dose-dependent slowing in growth.

TUMOUR BED EFFECT

The explanation for the above-mentioned slowing in growth is that irradiation damages the vascular stroma in which the tumour cells are growing and this leads to defective angiogenesis in the tumour cells. The damaged stroma is less able to support the needs of the growing tumour. Figure 15.4 shows that if tumour cells are implanted into an unirradiated bed they will grow at the normal rate. By contrast, if such unirradiated cells are implanted in an irradiated bed they grow more slowly.

IN VIVO/IN VITRO ASSAY

Many of the tumours studied in animals as transplantable tissues can also be examined in tissue culture. The third tumour model in Table 15.2 is the R1 rhabdomyosarcoma, which was one of the first animal tumour models to be investigated in this way. Figure 15.5 was described in Chapter 12 (Figure 12.9) and compares the growth pattern *in vivo* (A) with a clonogenic assay *in vitro* (B) after a dose of 20 Gy. There is an apparent contradiction in that the fraction of clonogenic cells assayed from the tumour fell to 10^{-2} before returning to unity, whereas the maximum volume change in the tumour was only about 25%. A major factor was that cells that had lost the capacity for indefinitely continued division remained *in situ* and, in many cases, continued with a limited number of divisions while repopulation was proceeding from surviving tumour stem cells. Certainly, the growth of a mixed-cell population such as this tumour is complex even without perturbation by a dose of radiation. Thus, the volume doubling time of the tumour is 4 days but when the tumour cells are cultured *in vitro*, their population doubling time is as short as 20 h (Barendsen et al, 1977).

In such cultures there will be very little cell loss, and the growth fraction is maximal so that the cell cycle time will be very similar to the population doubling time. For the tumours growing *in vivo*, however, cell loss is as high as 62% and the growth fraction is only 29% (Table 15.2) before irradiation. This is enough to explain why a tumour may take 4 days to double in volume despite the fact that its tumour cell cycle time is less than 1 day.

FRACTIONATION STUDIES

The R1 tumour has been used to provide a further illustration of the difference between the radiosensitivity of tumour cells and the radio-responsiveness of the whole tumour. Figure 15.6 shows how the rhabdomyosarcoma responds to five treatments per week of 4, 3 or 2 Gy per treatment. The larger the fraction dose and the more weeks of treatment, the longer the period of growth restraint and the greater the chance of cure. However, the rate of tumour shrinkage is the same whatever the regime, and when the tumour recurs it also regrows at the same rate. This illustrates the fact that the time scale of shrinkage of a tumour and its possible recurrence depends upon the kinetics of the particular cell

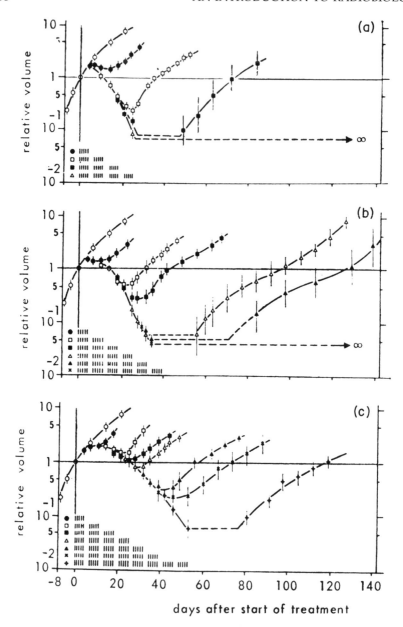

Figure 15.6. Growth curves for a rat rhabdomyosarcoma irradiated five times a week for different numbers of weeks with (a) 400 cGy, (b) 300 cGy and (c) 200 cGy fractions of X-rays. (Reprinted from *Eur. J. Cancer*, **6**, 89–109, from Barendsen and Broerse, 1970. Experimental radiotherapy of a rat rhabdomyosarcoma with 15 MeV neutrons and 300 kV X-rays, with kind permission from Elsevier Science Ltd., The Boulevard, Langford Lane, Kidlington OX5 1GB, UK.)

population. This is the *radioresponsiveness* of the tumour, but it does not give a direct indication of its *radiosensitivity*.

The sensitivity of a cell population can be measured only by the number of cells that survive or do not survive a radiation dosage. The extent of this cell killing will determine whether the tumour can be cured. Figure 15.6 shows that a total of 80 Gy from the regime of 4 Gy fractions per day given over 4 weeks (a) and 90 Gy given as 3 Gy daily fractions over 6 weeks (b) produced sufficient 'cell kill' to cure the tumour. This depended upon the radiosensitivity of the cell population, which is more easily measured from a cell survival curve (see Figure 12.10).

PATTERN OF RESPONSE

The fourth tumour model in Table 15.2 is the C_3H mouse mammary carcinoma. The results of a study of the effects of radiation on the growth of that tumour were mentioned in Chapter 12 and are shown again in Figure 15.7. On this occasion the tumours were given single doses of irradiation at

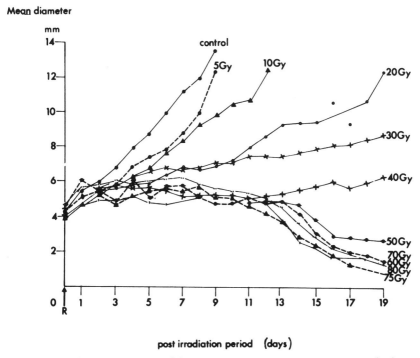

Figure 15.7. Radiation response of C_3H mouse mammary tumours to single doses of X-rays (R = day of irradiation). (Reproduced from Abdelaal and Nias, 1979, by permission of Royal Society of Medicine.)

an earlier stage in the growth curve when they were only 4–5 mm in diameter and the doubling time was just over 1 day. Figure 15.7 shows the gross response of this tumour to increasing doses of X-irradiation: from 5 to 80 Gy. Just as with the fractionated regime used in Figure 15.6, the higher the total dose, the more the effect on tumour growth. Single doses of 50 Gy or more produce actual regression of the tumour and the highest dose of 80 Gy will effect a complete cure in every case. In between those dosage levels the temporary regression shown in Figure 15.7 is followed by regrowth in a proportion of cases (the lower the dose, the more likely the regrowth and the earlier this occurs).

In Figure 15.7 a 20 Gy dose was enough to halt tumour growth for 1 week. When a stathmokinetic analysis was done on such irradiated tumour cells (using the same technique that was described in Chapter 3, Figure 3.12, for an unirradiated cell population), the rate of cell production was shown to be unchanged after 20 Gy. This was because regression and growth delay following irradiation was mainly due to increased cell loss from the tumour. Figure 15.8 shows how the proportion of pyknotic cells (i.e. those showing severe damage) rose to a peak 2 days after irradiation and then fell

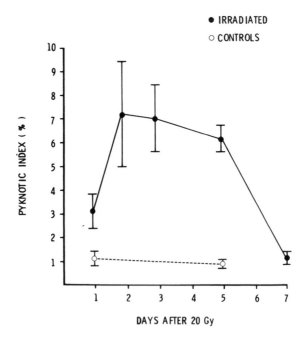

Figure 15.8. Changes in pyknotic index with time after irradiation of C_3H mouse mammary tumours. (Reproduced from Jones and Camplejohn, 1982, by permission of Springer-Verlag GmbH & Co. KG.)

to a normal level after 7 days. During this period the tumour repopulated itself with viable cells while the dead cells were cleared away by macrophages. The tumour then began to grow again (as happened with the R1 tumour in Figure 15.5) when cell loss returned to the normal level. This sort of time pattern will be shown to be important in the next chapter when reoxygenation is discussed as one of the mechanisms involved in fractionated radiotherapy.

PROGNOSIS

The question arises as to whether the proliferation kinetics of a tumour will affect the response of such a tumour to irradiation and the likelihood of it being cured. This was discussed in Chapter 12, where Table 12.3 showed that the longer the doubling time of a tumour, the slower it grows and the longer a patient will survive. Those were data based upon lung metastases from a variety of types of human tumour.

Figure 15.9 shows a similar relationship between the response of squamous cell carcinomas of the oral cavity that had been given two doses of 850 cGy. The labelling index was measured before irradiation and

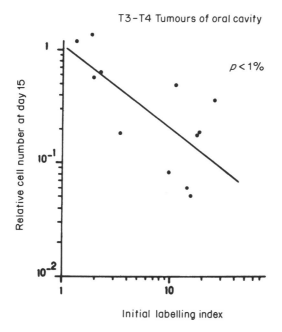

T3–T4 Tumours of oral cavity

$p < 1\%$

Relative cell number at day 15

10^{-1}

10^{-2}

Initial labelling index

Figure 15.9. Relationship between the labelling index of squamous cell carcinomas before treatment and the relative cell number in the tumour 15 days after irradiation. (Reproduced from Malaise et al, 1978, by permission of S. Karger AG. Basel.)

the number of cells per unit of surface was compared before and 15 days after the radiation. The higher the initial labelling index, the more the tumour cell depletion at 15 days.

These two examples only refer to the *rate* of response of tumours to radiation. The extent of the response (i.e. whether or not the tumours are cured) depends upon the radiosensitivity of the tumour cells and the size of the radiation dose that has been used. This is an important distinction. It means that estimates of the cell proliferation kinetics of tumours cannot be used to predict the final outcome of radiotherapy, only the immediate response. Most kinetic studies of human tumours depend upon an estimate of the potential doubling time, t_{pot}, derived from the labelling index (by autoradiography) or the S-phase fraction – or BUdR uptake – of the tumour cells by flow cytometry (see Chapter 3). These data depend upon the provision of suitable biopsy specimens from the patient. The trouble with such biopsies is that, at best, they can only represent a sample of the whole tumour. Many tumours are heterogeneous in structure and so a single sample may give a misleading picture. Because the derivation of t_{pot} values is also based upon some mathematical assumptions (see Chapter 3), the data can be only of limited value. They may only provide a basis for comparison between different tumours, but this may be of prognostic values. The t_{pot} is likely to vary during fractionated radiotherapy, however, because even if the tumour cell cycle time does not change, the growth fraction certainly will. It is difficult to verify this because repeated tumour samples cannot usually be obtained from the same patient during treatment, for ethical reasons; even if they were, the measurements would be confounded by the presence of dying cells.

Where a knowledge of tumour cell kinetics *may* be useful is in the choice of time interval between fractions of radiotherapy. It may be beneficial to a patient to leave only a short time interval if the tumour is growing very quickly. This will be discussed in the next chapter. But the problem will remain that although the t_{pot} may be known, it is *the cell cycle time* (t_C) of the tumour cells that really needs to be determined for this purpose.

SUMMARY OF CONCLUSIONS

(1) To cure a cancer the total tumour cell mass must be eradicated.
(2) To achieve this it will be necessary for irradiation to increase the rate of cell loss above the usual level for the histological type of tumour.
(3) L1210, R1B5, R1 and C_3H tumours are useful animal models for certain radiobiological studies.
(4) The rate of regrowth of a tumour after irradiation can be used as an alternative endpoint to tumour cure.

(5) Irradiation of the tumour bed will generally slow down the growth of a tumour.

(6) The *in vivo* response of a tumour can be assayed *in vitro* in terms of the clonogenic survival of the tumour cells.

(7) The *rate* of response to irradiation depends less on the dose than on the growth kinetics of the tumour. The *amount* of regrowth delay (or the probability of cure) depends upon the total dose of radiation and the radiosensitivity of the tumour cells.

(8) The growth kinetics of a tumour (measured as t_C or t_{pot}) will also determine the likely time of any recurrence.

REFERENCES

Abdelaal, A. S. and Nias, A. H. W., 1979. Regression recurrence and cure in an irradiated mouse tumour. *Journal of the Royal Society of Medicine*, **72**, 100–105.

Barendsen, G. W. and Broerse, J. J., 1970. Experimental radiotherapy of a rat rhabdomyosarcoma with 15 MeV neutrons and 300 kV X-rays: II. Effects of fractionated treatments applied 5 times a week for several weeks. *European Journal of Cancer*, **6**, 89–109.

Barendsen, G. W., Janse, H. C., Deys, B. F. and Hollander, C. F., 1977. Comparison of growth characteristics of experimental tumours and derived cell cultures. *Cell and Tissue Kinetics*, **10**, 469–475.

Hermens, A. F. and Barendsen, G. W., 1969. Changes of cell proliferation characteristics in a rat rhabdomyosarcoma before and after X-irradiation. *European Journal of Cancer*, **5**, 173–189.

Hofer, K. G., 1970. Radiation effects on death and migration of tumour cells in mice. *Radiation Research*, **43**, 663–678.

Jones, B. and Camplejohn, R. S., 1982. Cell kinetic response of an experimental tumour to irradiation. Use of the stathmokinetic method. *Virchows Archiv B*, **40**, 405–410.

Malaise, E. P., Chavaudra, N. and Tubiana, M., 1973. The relationship between growth, labelling index and histological type of human solid tumours. *European Journal of Cancer*, **9**, 305–312.

Malaise, E. P., Chavaudra, N., Guichard, M., Courdi, A. and Vazquez, T., 1978. The influence of tumor growth kinetics on the response to radiation therapy and drug therapy in man. *Fundamentals in Cancer Chemotherapy*, **23**, 181–190.

Nias, A. H. W., 1988. *Clinical Radiobiology*, 2nd edn. Churchill Livingstone, Edinburgh.

Penhaligon, M., Courtenay, V. D. and Camplejohn, R. S., 1987. Tumour bed effect: hypoxic fraction of tumours growing in pre-irradiated beds. *International Journal of Radiation Biology*, **52**, 635–641.

Thomlinson, R. H., 1961. The oxygen effect in mammals. In *Fundamental Aspects of Radiosensitivity. Brookhaven Symposia in Biology*, **14**, 204–216.

16 Fractionated Radiotherapy

Although the purpose of this book is to describe the damaging effect of ionizing radiation upon mammalian cell populations, there are three applications that are intended to be beneficial to mankind. X-rays are used to diagnose disease (Chapter 18) and nuclear reactors generate energy (Chapter 19). In both these cases, the radiation doses to the public are kept as low as is reasonably achievable (ALARA; Chapter 20). This chapter deals with the third application: radiotherapy. In this case the radiation doses are deliberately chosen to be as high as the body can tolerate in order that a cancer may be cured.

Radiotherapy is most commonly administered every day during the working week. This used to be 6 days at the time when Strandqvist (1944) published the first iso-effect curve for dose fractionation (see Figure 16.11) but is now 5 days a week, Monday to Friday. Five treatments a week for 3–6 weeks has been shown to be a clinically acceptable regime but it is based more upon expediency than upon radiobiological principles. A single regime of fractionation cannot possibly be optimal for every type of tumour and normal tissue.

The practice of giving multiple small daily fractions of radiation was first introduced in an attempt to irradiate as many tumour cells as possible during mitosis, because this was recognized as the most sensitive phase of the cell cycle (Chapter 8). Pioneer radiotherapists found that fractionation of the total dose of radiation had a relatively favourable effect on normal tissues while still having a lethal effect on tumours. The object of fractionation in radiotherapy is to kill all tumour cells without producing serious damage to the surrounding normal tissues, which necessarily must be included in the volume of high-dose irradiation.

This chapter will explain how radiobiological principles may guide radiotherapists in their choice of alternative fractionation regimes, which may increase tumour response without increasing damage to normal tissues.

BIOLOGICAL FACTORS

The effects of fractionated radiation are influenced primarily by the four 'Rs' of radiobiology:

(1) *Recovery* of mammalian cells from radiation damage.
(2) *Repopulation* of the tumour and normal tissues between fractions.

(3) *Reoxygenation* of the tumour during the course of treatment.
(4) *Redistribution* of normal and tumour cells in the cell cycle.

Another factor that may influence the clinical response to radiotherapy is the intrinsic radiosensitivity of the cells measured by the parameters D_0, $\overline{D}$ or SF2 (Chapter 8), although there is no consistent difference between normal tissues and tumours (Chapter 12). Indeed, there is often a close similarity between the mean lethal dose of tumours and the normal tissues from which they arise. When it comes to the other biological factors, however, there are some differences between tumours and normal tissues that will influence their response to fractionated therapy. These will be discussed now, and then later in relation to iso-effect curves and fractionation formulae.

RECOVERY FROM SUBLETHAL DAMAGE

Data from *in vitro* experimental results do not demonstrate any consistent difference in the repair capacity of tumour cells and normal tissue under aerated conditions, when measured by the shape of the shoulder of their survival curves. The quasi-threshold dose, D_q, was formally used for this purpose and a wide range of D_q values from 100 cGy to 550 cGy was recorded in a large series of mouse experiments, some of the results of which were given in Chapter 7, Table 7.1. This showed the differences in the ability of normal cells to repair sublethal damage. Haemopoietic stem cells show little repair capacity, while the epithelial cells of the skin and gastrointestinal tract have a large capacity to repair sublethal damage.

The short and long repair half-lives for several tissues were shown in Chapter 7, Table 7.2, and they illustrated the biphasic pattern of repair (Canney and Millar, 1997). It is estimated that 66% of the total damage will be repairable by the shorter phase, which takes a matter of minutes (as distinct to the hours of the remaining 33% of the longer phase of repair).

Many tumours are known to be hypoxic and diminished capacity to repair sublethal radiation damage has been reported in mammalian cells that are deficient in oxygen. If this is generally true, then the accumulated damage of fractionated irradiation might be somewhat greater in tumours than in the surrounding normal tissues that are well oxygenated. Furthermore, some tumour cells, such as those found in malignant lymphoma, have little or no capacity to repair sublethal damage and this may also explain how effectively they may be managed by radiotherapy.

During fractionated radiotherapy both recovery and repopulation will tend to reduce the effectiveness of the total radiation dosage, but repopulation is a less important factor than recovery. This was shown by some experimental studies in which pigs were irradiated with one single dose or with five fractions either in 4 days or 28 days. The doses required to

Table 16.1. The doses required to produce the same skin reaction

Fractionation	Total dose (cGy)	Dose increment (cGy)
One fraction	2000	–
Five fractions in 4 days	3600	1600
Five fractions in 28 days	4200	600

Reproduced from Fowler et al, 1963, by permission of BJR.

produce the same skin reaction are shown in Table 16.1. These observations lead to the conclusion that even fractionation over the shortest period necessitated 1600 cGy extra to produce the same effect. This is mainly attributable to recovery because repopulation would be minimal over that 4-day period. It does occur over the 28-day period but the dose increment for the same number of fractions amounts to only another 600 cGy. The recovery phenomenon is obviously more important than repopulation in such a situation. However, when large numbers of small fraction doses are given, so that recovery is quite small after each dose, repopulation may then be comparable to, or even greater than, recovery. This would apply to a regime of 30 fractions given over 6 weeks.

Recovery from radiation damage is thus the first of the four 'Rs' of radiobiology. Cells may recover from sublethal damage and from potentially lethal damage. Both of these phenomena influence the dose–response relationship of mammalian cells to fractionated radiotherapy. Recovery is also a factor in an extreme form of fractionation, namely protracted irradiation from radium and similar sources used for implantation and intracavitary treatment at a relatively low dose rate (see Chapter 17).

POTENTIALLY LETHAL DAMAGE

It has been established that mammalian cells in the stationary phase (G_0) of the cell cycle when cultured at 37 °C may recover from what would otherwise have been lethal damage following irradiation. This effect, which is called potentially lethal damage, is dose dependent, is distinct from sublethal radiation damage and occurs predominantly in *non*-cycling cells (see Chapter 7). Cells that are not in cycle at the time of irradiation are capable of shedding this particular type of injury and are in effect a more radioresistant population of cells than those in the cell cycle. They could be the origin of recurrent cancer after fractionated radiotherapy if their number accounted for a high proportion of the tumour during the course of treatment. However, this effect is dose dependent and, although of real importance after high-dose fractions, it is likely to contribute little to the biological damage that follows the relatively low doses of radiation usually given in a conventional fractionation regime.

REPOPULATION

In the ideal clinical situation one would hope that normal tissues would be completely repopulated, while the tumour showed no growth between fractions of the X-ray treatment. If that were so, the tumour would be progressively depopulated while the surrounding normal tissue was maintained in a steady state. While it is true that there is no general difference in cell cycle times between cycling cells in tumours and normal tissues, the effective volume doubling times of tumours and of normal tissues may show considerable differences owing to the effects of cell loss and other factors influencing the cell population kinetics (see Chapters 3 and 15).

In some normal tissues following the initial radiation injury there may be a surprisingly large increase in the proliferation rate until the normal tissue is fully reconstituted. The effect may be seen in haemopoietic stem cells, where the response is immediate and the growth fraction increases together with a reduction in maturation rate. The pool of precursor cells is renewed quickly and there may even be an over-production of leucocytes, for example, for a time after X-ray treatment to a large volume of bone marrow. The epithelium of the gastrointestinal tract is capable of rapid repopulation after an initial radiation injury while daily dose fractions continue to be given.

Skin can also show considerable repopulation during the latter half of a fractionated course of radiotherapy. This was mentioned in Chapter 13, where Figure 13.2 showed how extra dosage is needed after 2 weeks to counteract the proliferation of skin in the mouse. A similar phenomenon occurs with human tumours but Figure 16.1 shows that, in this case, extra dosage is not needed until after 4 weeks of treatment has been given.

The fact that both normal and tumour cells have a similar radiosensitivity raises the question of how radiotherapy can ever succeed. Figure 16.2 provides a possible answer to this question. The diagram makes use of the idea that clonogenic cells may form only a very small proportion of a tumour cell mass and that the rate of proliferation of some normal-cell populations can exceed that of the tumour after fractionated radiotherapy.

The diagram therefore starts with a lower number of tumour cells, which are proliferating, and a higher number of normal cells, which are not (because they are in the steady state of an adult cell population). After the first treatment there is a similar reduction in both cell populations but now the normal cells will begin to proliferate, and do so at a faster rate than the tumour cells. If the optimum time interval is allowed between treatments

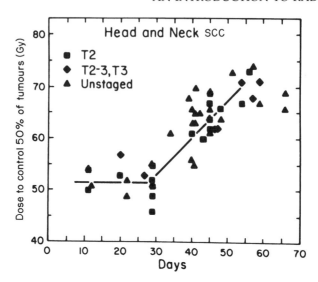

Figure 16.1. The increase in dose required to control human tumours when fractionated radiotherapy is prolonged beyond 4 weeks. (Reproduced from Withers et al, 1988, by permission of Scandinavian University Press.)

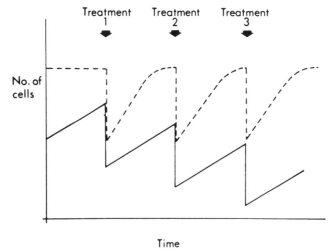

Figure 16.2. Effect of fractionated radiotherapy on normal (- - -) and tumour (—) cell populations. (Reproduced from Priestman, 1980, by permission of Farmitalia Carlo Erba.)

then the normal population is restored to its original level, whereas the tumour cell population will progressively decrease. Given enough fractions, the number of clonogenic tumour cells might then be reduced to the level required for cure.

Table 16.2. Proliferation parameters of human tumours

Tumour type	LI	T_s (h)	T_{pot} (days)
Head and neck	4.9	9.9	6.4
Lung	8.0	15.1	7.3
Oesophagus	7.8	12.4	5.2
Cervix	11.6	15.8	4.5
Melanoma	4.2	10.7	7.2
Colorectal	9.0	13.1	3.9

Reproduced from Wilson, 1993, by permission of Springer-Verlag GmbH & Co. KG.

Potential doubling times t_{pot} of human tumours have been estimated by the BUdR technique described in Chapter 3. Table 16.2 shows mean values for the parameter, together with the labelling index (LI) and DNA synthesis time (t_s) for six tumour types. The t_{pot} times were quite short for these tumours, averaging 6 h. Earlier estimates for other tumour types using *in vitro* labelling with tritiated thymidine (Trott and Kummermehr, 1985) showed much longer times for tumours of the breast (12 h), kidney (30 h) and prostate (60 h). When the t_{pot} is less than 5 days there may be an advantage in shortening the overall treatment time. (Accelerated fractionation is discussed at the end of this chapter.)

REOXYGENATION

The proportion of hypoxic cells in a tumour will influence its response to irradiation. Most tumours are thought to contain some hypoxic cells, but with small doses the response to irradiation will be determined almost exclusively by the well-oxygenated cells. Only when relatively high radiation doses are employed will cell survival be influenced by hypoxia. However, as fractionated radiotherapy proceeds, a hypoxic cell population would become increasingly important unless the oxygenation of these cells improved. Reoxygenation does take place in most tumours, but at different rates and to different extents. The processes involved in reoxygenation have been illustrated by Thomlinson (1968) in Figure 16.3:

When a tumour is very small there are not likely to be any anoxic cells (A), and in some tumours they may never occur. In other tumours anoxic cells appear as the tumour grows (B) but the proportion becomes limited to a level (C) which is characteristic of the type of tumour and dependent on its growth rate, degree of differentiation and site. When a dose of radiation (R_1) is given the proportion of anoxic cells amongst the surviving clonogens is likely to rise (D) to 100% and remain at this proportion (E) until the other effects of radiation begin to develop. As injury leads to cell death the

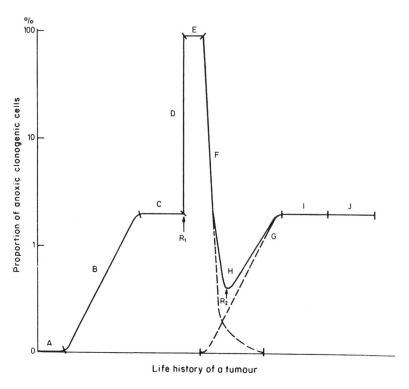

Figure 16.3. Schematic representation of the proportion of viable anoxic cells in a tumour during its growth and following irradiation. (Reproduced from Thomlinson, 1968, by permission of S. Karger AG. Basel.)

proportion of anoxic cells will fall (F) because of increased availability of oxygen to hypoxic cells following reduced consumption by damaged cells, and improved circulation following shrinkage of the tumour. Then surviving cells regrow the tumour (G) at a rate dependent on the post-irradiation environment. As a result of these two processes, the proportion of anoxic cells reaches a minimum (H) at a time which is dependent on the type of humour and its growth rate. This is the time which will be optimal for the second dose of radiation (R_2) to be given. Otherwise, the characteristic level (I) will be restored. Late radiation ischaemia is not likely to alter the proportion of anoxic cells (J) unless it was previously zero.

In this example the proportion of hypoxic cells is not much more than 1% but for many solid tumours the proportion is 15–20% (Moulder and Rockwell, 1984). The temporal pattern of reoxygenation also varies from one tumour to another. After irradiation the proportion of hypoxic cells falls to a minimum at 1 day for the rat fibrosarcoma, 3 days for the mouse carcinoma and 5 days (or later) for the mouse sarcoma.

The fact that 3 days was an optimum time interval for the mouse carcinoma was shown in Chapter 15 (Figure 15.8). Figure 16.4 now shows the results of treating this tumour in C_3H mice with five fractions of (caesium) γ-rays. The time interval between fractions was either zero (i.e. the total dose was given as a single treatment) or 1, 2, 3 or 5 days. The total doses were chosen so that the median tissue culture dose (TCD_{50}) could be determined, and this was done 120 days after treatment. The tumours were hypoxic (i.e. clamped), aerated or hyperbaric (with the mouse in a hyperbaric oxygen chamber) at the time of irradiation. The curve for hypoxic tumours shows a rapid increase in TCD_{50} when the fractionation interval becomes 1 day, and this is mainly due to recovery from radiation damage. The slower increase with longer fractionation intervals is due to repopulation. No effect of reoxygenation will be shown in these clamped tumours.

Reoxygenation does apply, however, to the aerated tumours and this explains the reduced rate and extent of recovery for fractionation intervals up to 3 days. Thereafter, repopulation leads to the same rate of increase in TCD_{50} as in the hypoxic tumours. The addition of hyperbaric oxygen at the time of irradiation produces a further improvement in tumour oxygenation,

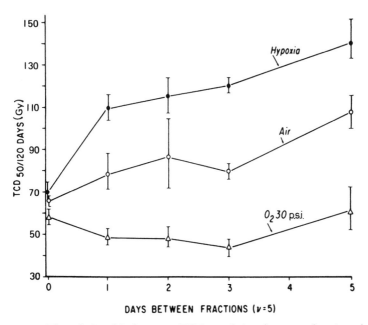

Figure 16.4. The relationship between TCD_{50} and time between fractions for various conditions of oxygenation at the time of irradiation of C_3H mouse mammary tumours. (Reproduced from Howes and Suit, 1974, by permission of Academic Press, Inc.)

sufficient to overcome completely any effects of recovery and repopulation with intervals up to 3 days. Thereafter, the TCD_{50} does rise at the same rate as that for hypoxic and aerated tumours, presumably because of an increased number of hypoxic cells resulting from rapid repopulation.

It is obvious that the optimum fractionation interval for this tumour is 3 days, which is due to the fact that reoxygenation cancels out the radiobiological effects of recovery and repopulation during that time interval, to a large extent in air and completely with hyperbaric oxygen. Sadly, little is known about the time course of such events in humans, but the same sort of variation is also likely to occur between different types of tumour. This may be influenced further by the size and spacing of fractionated doses of radiotherapy. Certainly, there is no radiobiological basis for the same fractionation regime to be used for all different types of human tumour, as far as reoxygenation is concerned.

REDISTRIBUTION OF CELLS IN THE CYCLE

The radiosensitivity of mammalian cells varies throughout the cell cycle (Chapter 8). The effect of redistribution of cells throughout the phases of the cell cycle will be complex. Following a radiation dose the cells in the most sensitive phases will be killed preferentially. The remainder of the population will be in the more resistant phases, such as late-S phase. The proliferating cells will therefore be synchronized to some extent. As these cells progress, they will be more radiosensitive for a time.

The importance of redistribution in fractionated radiotherapy depends primarily on the proportion of cells in the tumour or tissue that are in cycle. In human tumours, the proportion of cells in the growth fraction is normally low and redistribution is unlikely to contribute greatly to the beneficial effects of fractionation. Also, acutely responding normal tissues are no less influenced by this factor than tumours.

When there is a significant differential radiosensitivity in the phases of the cell cycle, fractionated radiotherapy will lead to partial synchronization by means of a selective depopulation of the most sensitive cells, leaving an increasing proportion of relatively resistant cells. The partially synchronized cell population will progress through the cycle to a more or less resistant phase when the next X-ray treatment is given. This was shown in Figure 8.12 by the considerable variation in the radiosensitivity of mouse intestinal stem cells following synchronization by hydroxyurea (which causes an accumulation of cells at the beginning of the S phase). The clinical effect will therefore depend not only on the level of dose delivered at each fraction but also on the interval between treatment fractions if synchronization occurs.

Unless some phase-specific drug (Chapter 2) is being combined with a fractionated radiotherapy regime, it is unlikely that even partial synchronization of the relevant cell population will be produced. It follows that it is unlikely that any significant differential effect of this kind will be obtained that will increase the depopulation of the tumour compared to normal tissues.

DIVISION DELAY

All cells will be delayed by irradiation to some extent in proceeding to division, and this block in the cell cycle is influenced by the size of the radiation dose and also by the age of the cell at the time of irradiation (see Chapter 7). Mammalian cells will accumulate in the phase of the cycle just before mitosis, G_2, which is a period of increasing radiosensitivity. The delay amounts to approximately one cell cycle time for every 10–15 Gy. When one considers the size of dose fractions normally given in radiotherapy, it can be appreciated that this effect is probably of little importance in determining the clinical end result.

PHYSICAL FACTORS

The clinical response to fractionated radiotherapy is also determined by a number of physical factors that influence the relative importance of the biological effects that have been described.

RADIATION QUALITY

The biological effect is determined by the quality of the beam of radiation. Quality of orthovoltage X-ray beams is usually defined by specifying the peak generating voltage and the half-value thickness of the effective treatment radiation. With megavoltage radiation only the peak generating energy is given, as half-value thickness is too crude an index with such penetrating radiations (Chapter 4). The absorption of radiation beams in tissues may be regarded as taking place in discrete events and the biological effect is thought to depend on one, or at most a few, of these events. The rate at which secondary charged particles deposit energy in the tissues in unit distance is known as the linear energy transfer (LET), expressed as keV/μm. The relative biological effectiveness (RBE) of radiation was correlated with the estimates of LET values in Chapter 9.

As the LET increases above 10 keV/μm the shape of the cell survival curve becomes significantly different in the shoulder region compared with the curve for low-LET radiation, and the RBE depends on the level of biological effect produced. The greater the effect or the larger the radiation dose, the smaller the RBE, and vice versa. The RBE value of fast neutrons measured by large single-dose exposures is usually about 2, but this significantly underestimates their relative effectiveness when multiple small fractions of dose are given and the RBE rises to 3 or 4. This is the explanation of the 'fractionation trap', which led to many patients in the first neutron therapy trial having severe high-dose effects.

The radiosensitivity of the cell depends on its position in the cell cycle but this effect is smaller with high-LET than with low-LET radiations, particularly when low doses of radiation are employed. The possibilities of differences in repopulation in tumours and normal tissues have also been examined after high-LET radiations, but in the small number of experiments reported no differences have been found in the rates of repopulation after high-LET or low-LET radiations.

Radiation dose rate

Study of cell survival curves will show that as the dose rate is decreased below that normally used for external beam therapy, the killing effect is reduced on well-oxygenated cells and the extrapolation number tends to unity. At low rates of X- and γ-radiation much of the accumulated damage is repaired during irradiation. A difference in response is evident down to about 10 cGy/h, when all repairable damage is shed during irradiation with X- or gamma rays. Under hypoxic conditions, however, the dose rate dependence is much reduced – probably because of greatly reduced recovery from sublethal damage during prolonged hypoxia. All this will be discussed in Chapter 17.

Volume factor

The clinical response to irradiation is influenced by the volume of tumour and normal tissues contained in the treatment zone. Dose–effect curves like those in Figure 16.5 illustrate the constant dilemma that faces radio-therapists. As the volume of cancer enlarges due to an increase in the number of clonogenic cancer cells, so the dose of radiation required for a certain probability of local cure of the tumour is increased. However, as the volume of related normal tissues will also have to be increased, the dose of radiation that can be tolerated without unacceptable morbidity may have to be reduced. The cure rate that may reasonably be achieved with radiation therapy is always determined by the level of morbidity that is acceptable. In Chapter 13, Figure 13.12 showed how the longer the length of spinal cord that is irradiated, the lower the radiation dose that will lead to paralysis.

The dose–effect curves in Figure 16.5 are sigmoid in shape, with a large threshold range of dose before the effect begins to be observed. These curves are similar in shape to those obtained from total body exposure of

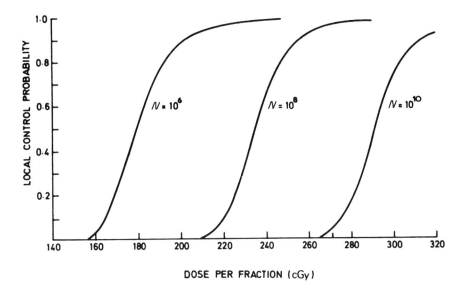

Figure 16.5. Calculated dose–effect curves for different numbers of cells in a tumour. (Reproduced from Nias, 1988, by permission of Churchill Livingstone.)

animals (Chapter 14, Figure 14.5) whose death is simply a reflection of the depletion of stem cells below a critical level in essential tissues such as the bone marrow or gastrointestinal tract. At the lower dose region of the dose–effect curve relatively small increases in dose will produce a large increase in the probability of tumour control. Figure 16.5 shows that in a tumour of 10^8 clonogenic cells an increase in dose per fraction from 225 cGy to 240 cGy, i.e. an additional 15 cGy per fraction, may increase the control probability from about 20% to 65%. The number of clonogenic cells that determine the clinical results in a tumour or normal tissue will not be constant, because one must expect some repopulation during radiotherapy.

Figure 16.5 also shows dose–effect curves for tumours with different numbers of clonogenic cells. Other curves will apply to cells with different radiation sensitivities. If the sensitivity of a group of tumours is not uniform, the dose–effect curve will be less steep. This is observed when there is a significant hypoxic cell fraction in a cancer. The clinical data in Figure 16.6 show the difference between the dose–effect curves of smaller and larger skin cancers. The single-dose irradiation required for 50% local control increases from about 18 Gy for small tumours to 22 Gy for larger tumours. For the smaller tumours it is possible to increase the dose so as to achieve a 90% probability of local control without risk of skin necrosis; but the 50% control dose for the larger tumours already leads to some skin

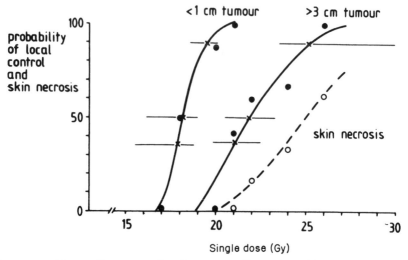

Figure 16.6. Dose–effect curves for skin cancer. (Reproduced from Trott et al, 1984, by permission of Elsevier Science Ireland Ltd, Bay 15K, Shannon Industrial Estate, Co. Clare, Ireland.)

necrosis, so no increase in dose can be acceptable and 90% control cannot be attempted.

Therapeutic ratio

In clinical practice the response curve of normal tissues must always lie to the right of the tumour response curve in order to obtain a favourable therapeutic ratio. This is shown diagrammatically in Figure 16.7, where the two dose–effect curves are sufficiently far apart for tumour cure to begin at much lower doses than those causing normal-tissue damage. The normal response curve begins to rise at a dose level where the tumour control curve had already risen to 60%. The diagram shows that if 10% damage is acceptable, then 90% tumour control can be achieved.

It was seen in Figure 16.5 that the dose–response curves for larger tumours are moved to the right, indicating that a larger radiation dose is necessary to maintain the same probability of local control. As the size of the tumour increases, so the mean lethal dose increases. At the same time, the curve representing the incidence of late-tissue effects will approach the tumour response curve as the volume of tissue irradiated increases. Accordingly, the margin of safety is much reduced and in these circumstances it will be found that the therapeutic ratio becomes so low that curative or radical radiotherapy may no longer be feasible. This was nearly the case for the larger tumours in Figure 16.6.

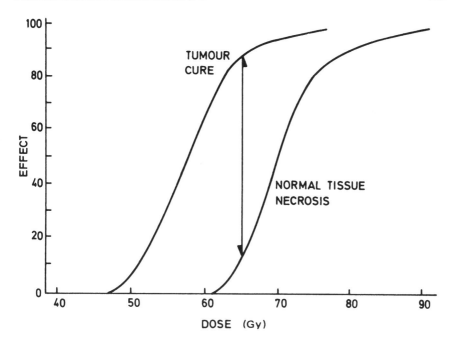

Figure 16.7. Schematic diagram of dose–effect curves for tumour cure and normal-tissue damage. (Reproduced from Nias, 1988, by permission of Churchill Livingstone.)

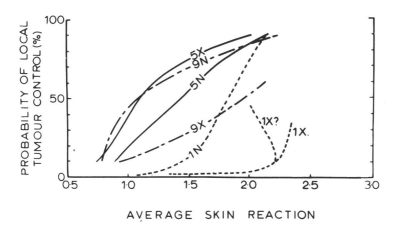

Figure 16.8. Relationship of tumour cure to skin reaction in the treatment of the mouse mammary carcinoma by X-rays and fast neutrons using one, five or nine fractions. (Reproduced from Fowler et al, 1972, by permission of BJR.)

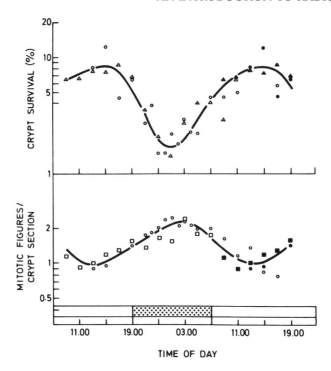

Figure 16.9. Curves showing whole-crypt survival after a 1300 cGy single exposure and the mean mitotic figure per crypt section. (Reproduced from Hendry, 1975, by permission of BJR.)

It may be possible, by using other methods, to increase the therapeutic ratio and enhance the effectiveness of radiotherapy. Figure 16.8 illustrates the use of fast neutrons instead of X-rays in the treatment of transplanted C_3H mouse mammary tumours. The therapeutic ratio between tumour control and skin reaction was least favourable with single doses of X-rays. Single doses of neutrons and nine fractions of X-rays provided a better ratio, and five fractions of neutrons was even better, but the best ratio was obtained with either five fractions of X-rays or nine fractions of neutrons. The equivalent radiobiological data necessary to design rational and optimum treatment regimes in patients are not yet available.

CHRONOBIOLOGICAL EFFECTS

The timing of fractionation schedules may prove inappropriate if circadian rhythms are ignored. Figure 16.9 illustrates the consequence of this so-called chronobiological effect on the radiosensitivity of mouse intestine. The upper part of the figure shows the considerable variation in crypt survival (assayed by the technique described in Chapter 8, Figure 8.13) if the mice receive the single dose of 1300 cGy of γ-irradiation at different times of the day. The lower part of the figure shows that the mitotic index is maximal during the night, which is when the intestine is most radiosensitive in such nocturnal animals. There is evidence of a similar variation in the radiation response of bone marrow.

Because circadian rhythms are a feature of most biological systems, it follows that it may prove to be more beneficial not to treat human tumours at the time of peak mitotic activity of limiting normal tissues such as gut and bone marrow. This would mean avoiding radiotherapy during the hours of the day when it is normally administered, but only if the circadian rhythm of the tumour cell population is shown to be significantly different from that of the normal tissues, as was shown in Chapter 2, Figure 2.9. Only then would the reduction in gut and bone-marrow damage justify such a change in the practice of radiotherapy.

ISO-EFFECT CURVES AND FRACTIONATION FORMULAE

Much clinical information has been collected about dose–time relationships and to a lesser extent about dose–fraction number relationships. More accurate data are now available for animal tissues and tumours and they clearly indicate the essential importance of fraction size (for a given total dose), rather than the number of fractions, in obtaining a favourable therapeutic ratio.

The classical study of dose–time relationships was reported by Strandqvist in 1944. He described certain levels of skin damage that could be tolerated in patients treated for skin cancer with a range of radiation doses given in different overall treatment times. He showed that the dose-dependent responses gave a straight line when plotted on a log–log graph of dose against time in days, and that the slope of these lines for all degrees of skin damage and for the cure of skin cancer was the same (Figure 16.10). The slope of such an iso-effect curve was 0.22 but Cohen's (1952) data for breast cancer fitted a slope of 0.34 when plotted against the number of fractions.

Ellis (1965) proposed an iso-effect formula for normal-tissue tolerance that related the total dose (D) given in a prescribed overall time (T) in days, in a specific number of fractions (N), to what he called the nominal standard dose or NSD. The NSD unit of 'iso-effective' dose has been called the ret (rad equivalent therapy):

$$D = NSD \cdot T^{0.11} \cdot N^{0.24}$$

When combined, these functions are consistent with the slope of Cohen's curve, but they separate the effects of time and the number of fractions. This

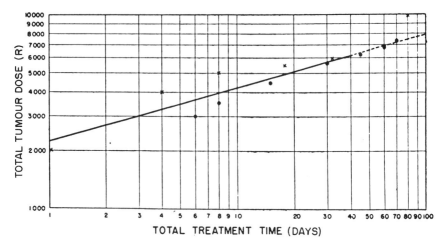

Figure 16.10. Iso-effect curves relating the total dose and overall treatment time for skin tolerance. (Reproduced from Strandqvist, 1944, *Acta Radiol.*, by permission of the author.)

important distinction was shown by the results of experiments on pig skin described earlier (Table 16.1). Ellis found that such data were consistent with the clinical data that he had collected and analysed. The time function 'T' is related to the rate of repopulation of normal tissues, and the 'N' function is related to the capacity of normal-tissue cells to recover from sublethal radiation damage.

The dotted line in Figure 16.11 shows how N can be plotted as a straight line on a log–log graph of total dose against number of fractions and has a constant slope of 0.24. If T was taken into account, the slope would rise to 0.35. The use of the Ellis formula provided a means for radiotherapists to compare the tolerance levels of doses delivered by different treatment regimes in respect of this effect on early-reacting tissues such as skin. It does not represent the isobiological effect of late-reacting tissues, however, and was never intended to apply to tumours. Ellis pointed out that it should not be used for less than five or more than thirty fractions, and the term $T^{0.11}$ does not apply beyond 100 days.

In order to simplify the system and make it more generally applicable, Orton and Ellis (1973)) introduced factors that relate time, dose and fraction size (TDF) and are proportional to partial tolerance. These TDF factors provide a simple and more reliable way of comparing and equating all regimes of radiotherapy. However, this formalism is subject to the same limitations as the Ellis formula.

The two curved solid lines in Figure 16.11 show alternative plots of iso-effective dose calculated on the basis of the linear-quadratic (LQ) relationship for the dose response of early- and late-reacting tissues. Cell

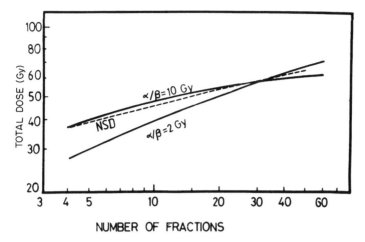

Figure 16.11. Increase of iso-effective dose with number of fractions, based upon dose–response curves using either the NSD formula or linear-quadratic ratios of 10 Gy or 2 Gy. (Reproduced from Fowler, 1984, by permission of *Int. J. Radiat. Biol.*, Taylor & Francis.)

survival curves can also be fitted by the LQ model and the data fit reasonably well in the low-dose region, which is of greatest interest in fractionated radiotherapy. On the other hand, this model gives a continuously bending curve and at high doses this may not be accurate for most cell survival curves, which have a truly exponential final slope (Chapter 8, Figure 8.3).

The LQ model is described by the equation:

$$\text{Surviving fraction} = e^{-(\alpha D + \beta D^2)}$$

The α/β ratio is defined as the dose at which killing by single-hit activation (α component) and multi-hit activation (β component) are equal (Figure 16.12a). Cell types with high α/β ratios have more slowly bending survival curves, while cells with low α/β ratios have sharply bending survival curves. The α/β terms can be derived from the intercept and the slope of the iso-effective dose plot (Figure 16.12b).

These plots show that slowly dividing (and therefore late-reacting) tissues have low α/β ratios, while acutely responding tissues have high ratios. The α/β ratio is about 10 Gy for early-reacting tissues such as skin and gut (Figure 16.11). Such α/β plots only take into account the number of fractions because there is not normally any dimension for time in LQ equations. It is for that reason that the usual LQ model overestimates the effect on normal tissues of most radiotherapy protocols. These may use up to four treatment fields and the time interval between each field will permit

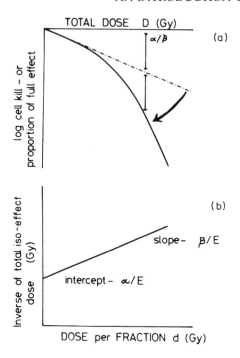

Figure 16.12. Diagram to show the significance of α and β in terms of a cell survival curve (a) and the way these are derived from an iso-effect plot (b). (Reproduced from Denekamp, 1986, by permission of *Int. J. Radiat. Biol.*, Taylor & Francis.)

cellular repair and result in a reduction of the biological effect (Canney and Millar, 1997).

The plot for early-reacting tissues in Figure 16.11 is not dissimilar to that for the NSD, except that it is curved and not straight. The other plot is quite different and fits an α/β ratio of 2 Gy; this is the one for late-reacting tissues such as spinal cord and lung (Figures 16.13 and 16.14). The curves in Figure 16.11 cross over at the 32-fraction point, which would apply to an 'orthodox' radiotherapy regime using 2 Gy fractions. If the regime is changed to use fewer fractions with a larger dose per fraction over the same length of time, there is an increasing divergence of the early (10 Gy) and late (2 Gy) curves. This means that a total dose that would be within the tolerance level of a tissue such as skin would exceed the tolerance level of a tissue such as spinal cord and lung.

Modifications of the NSD formula were suggested by Cohen and Creditor (1983) to take account of this sort of variation in the time–dose factors of different tissues. Thus, for spinal cord, the N exponent would be increased to 0.42 and the T exponent decreased to 0.06. The total slope of 0.48 is similar to that shown for radiation myelitis in Figure 16.13. For lung

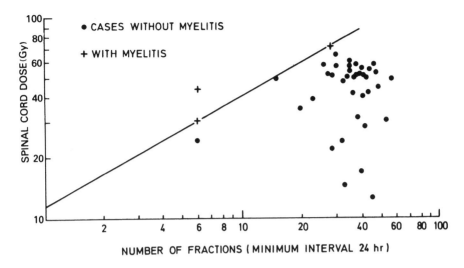

Figure 16.13. Dose–response curve for fractionated irradiation producing myelitis of the spinal cord in the thoracic region. The line shows the lowest doses with myelitis. (Reproduced from Phillips and Buschke, 1969, by permission of American Roentgen Ray Society.)

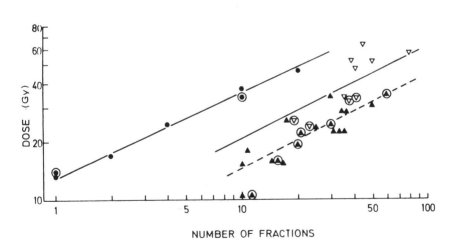

Figure 16.14. Dose–response curves for fractionated irradiation producing pneumonitis in the mouse (closed circles) and human subjects (triangles). The mouse data were measured by the $LD_{50/160}$. The open triangles indicate cases of pneumonitis and the closed triangles indicate cases without pneumonitis. The circles show the additional effect of actinomycin D, which reduces lung tolerance in patients. (Reproduced from Phillips and Margolis, 1972, by permission of S. Karger AG. Basel.)

damage the N exponent is increased to 0.38 and the T exponent again is decreased to 0.06. Figure 16.14 shows iso-effect curves for radiation pneumonitis in both mice and humans. The slopes of these curves are about 0.45. The lower time exponents take into account the slower kinetics that apply to such late-reacting tissues.

Radiotherapists in different centres in England use a wide variety of fractionation regimes, ranging from 30 fractions 5 days a week for 6 weeks, to 6 fractions twice a week for 3 weeks. The largest centre uses 16 fractions 5 days a week for 3 weeks. In each centre the regime has been found to be tolerated by normal tissues and to be effective in tumour control. In theory all the regimes should be iso-effective, but it has yet to be proved that any of them is optimal with respect to the highest local tumour control rates and the lowest radiation morbidity.

For fast-growing tumours it may even be worth giving radiation doses more than once a day, and this is then called 'hyperfractionation'. If the usual number of fractions is given, then the regime will amount to 'accelerated' fractionation because the overall time will be much shorter than usual. One example is the CHART regime (continuous hyperfractionated accelerated radiation treatment) which consists of 36 fractions given three times each day with 6-h intervals for 12 consecutive days, including the weekend. A trial with patients suffering from lung cancer has shown some advantage over a conventional regime of fractionated radiotherapy, but no advantage with head and neck cancer (Saunders et al, 1996). Flow cytometry after BUdR labelling is being used to answer the question of whether it is the faster growing tumours that benefit from such a fractionation regime. However, while the regime may overcome repopulation, the time interval may be too short to allow reoxygenation between fractions, and the slower phase of a biphasic repair process will also have less opportunity for completion.

SUMMARY OF CONCLUSIONS

(1) Radiotherapy is intended to eradicate tumour tissue without causing too much damage to normal tissue.
(2) This is best achieved by giving the total dose of radiation in a number of fraction doses over a period of time.
(3) The effects of such fractionated radiotherapy are influenced by radiobiological factors: recovery, repopulation and reoxygenation (described in earlier chapters).
(4) The quality and the dose rate of the radiation will influence the killing of tumour cells.

(5) The larger the tumour volume, the lower the radiation dose that can safely be given without exceeding the tolerance of the associated normal tissue.

(6) A therapeutic ratio between the effects of radiation upon tumour and normal tissue determines how successful a treatment can be.

(7) Various formulae have been devised to calculate the doses of radiation that can safely be given in different numbers of fractions over different periods of time.

(8) The late effects of radiation determine such tolerance dosage, e.g. damage to lung, kidney or spinal cord.

REFERENCES

Canney, P. A. and Millar, W. T., 1997. Biphasic cellular repair and implications for multiple field radiotherapy treatments. *British Journal of Radiology*, **70**, 817–822.

Cohen, L., 1952. Radiotherapy in breast cancer – the dose–time relationship; theoretical considerations. *British Journal of Radiology*, **25**, 636–642.

Cohen, L. and Creditor, M., 1983. Iso-effect tables for tolerance of irradiated normal human tissues. *International Journal of Radiation Oncology, Biology, Physics*, **9**, 233–241.

Denekamp, J., 1986. Cell kinetics and radiation biology. *International Journal of Radiation Biology*, **49**, 357–380.

Ellis, F., 1965. The relationship of biological effect to dose–time fractionation factors in radiotherapy. *Current Topics in Radiation Research*, **4**, 357–397.

Fowler, J. F., 1984. Review: total doses in fractionated radiotherapy – implications of new radiobiological data. *International Journal of Radiation Biology*, **46**, 103–120.

Fowler, J. F., Morgan, R. L., Silvester, J. A., Bewley, D. K. and Turner, B. A., 1963. Experiments with practical X-ray treatment of the skin of pigs. *British Journal of Radiology*, **36**, 188–196.

Fowler, J. F., Denekamp, J., Page, A. L., Begg, A. C., Field, S. B. and Butler, R. S., 1972. Fractionation with X-rays and neutrons in mice: response of skin and C$_3$H mammary tumours. *British Journal of Radiology*, **45**, 237–249.

Hendry, J. H., 1975. Diurnal variations in radio-sensitivity of mouse intestines. *British Journal of Radiology*, **48**, 312–314.

Howes, A. E. and Suit, H. D., 1974. The effect of time between fractions on the response of tumors to irradiation. *Radiation Research*, **57**, 342–348.

Moulder, J. E. and Rockwell, S., 1984. Hypoxic fractions of solid tumours: experimental techniques, methods of analysis and a survey of existing data. *International Journal of Radiation Oncology, Biology, Physics*, **10**, 695–712.

Nias, A. H. W., 1988. *Clinical Radiobiology*, 2nd edn. Churchill Livingstone, Edinburgh.

Orton, C. G. and Ellis, F., 1973. A simplification of the use of the NSD concept in practical radiotherapy. *British Journal of Radiology*, **46**, 529–537.

Phillips, T. K. and Buschke, F., 1969. Radiation tolerance of the thoracic spinal cord. *American Journal of Roentgenology*, **105**, 659–664.

Phillips, T. K. and Margolis, L. W., 1972. Radiation pathology and clinical response of lung and oesophagus. *Frontiers of Radiation Therapy and Oncology*, **6**, 254–273.

Priestman, T. J., 1980. *Cancer Chemotherapy – An Introduction*. Farmitalia Carlo Erba, Barnet, Herts, p. 71.

Saunders, M. I., Dische, S., Barrett, A., Parmar, M. K. B., Harvey, A. and Gibson, D., 1996. Randomised multicentre trials of CHART vs conventional radiotherapy in head and neck and non-small-cell lung cancer: an interim report. *British Journal of Cancer*, **73**, 1455–1462.

Strandqvist, M., 1944. Studien uber die kumulative Wirkung der Rontgenstrahlen bei Fraktionierung. *Acta Radiologica*, **55** (Suppl.), 1–293.

Thomlinson, R. H., 1968. Changes of oxygenation in tumours in relation to irradiation. *Frontiers of Radiation Therapy and Oncology*, **3**, 109–121.

Trott, K. R. and Kummermehr, J., 1985. What is known about tumour proliferation rates to choose between accelerated fractionation or hyperfraction? *Radiotherapy and Oncology*, **3**, 1–9.

Trott, K. R., Maciejewski, B., Preuss-Bayer, G. and Skolyszewski, J., 1984. Dose–response curve and split-dose recovery in human skin cancer. *Radiotherapy and Oncology*, **2**, 123–129.

Wilson, G. D., 1993. Limitations of the bromodeoxyuridine technique for measurement of tumour proliferation. In *Current Topics in Clinical Radiobiology of Tumours*, edited by H.-P. Beck-Bornholdt. Springer-Verlag, Berlin.

Withers, H. R., Taylor, J. M. F. and Maciejewski, B., 1988. The hazard of accelerated tumor clonogen repopulation during radiotherapy. *Acta Oncologica*, **27**, 131–146.

17 Protracted Radiation

When cells and tissues are given a short dose of radiation they show a dose response that is uncomplicated by other radiobiological phenomena. Most of the survival curves used for this book have been obtained with single doses of 'acute' radiation given at a rate of about 100 cGy/min. This dose rate is convenient for the radiotherapy of cancer patients and for studies by radiobiologists because the dose is delivered in just a few minutes. There is no time for any recovery from sublethal damage (Chapter 7) or repopulation by the surviving cells and tissues to take place before the completion of such an acute dose of radiation.

If radiation is delivered more slowly, however, then recovery may occur during the irradiation with the result that the cells and tissues show less damage. Track structure considerations (Goodhead, 1992) suggest that, at

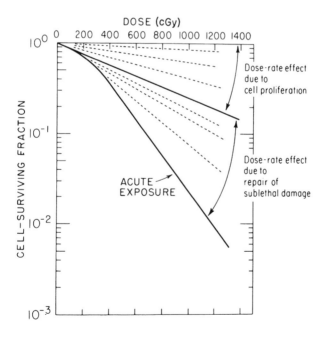

Figure 17.1. The effect of (a) repair of sublethal damage and (b) cell proliferation on a cell survival curve when the radiation dose rate is reduced. (Reproduced from Hall, 1978, by permission of Lippincott-Raven.)

sufficiently low dose rates, multiple-track effects will become negligible because the tracks become effectively independent in time. The dose response thus will be solely from single tracks and should be simply linear with dose. It will extend down to zero dose with no threshold.

If the dose rate is very slow then the cells that survive the radiation and recover from sublethal damage will also have time to proliferate during the irradiation. As a result of these processes the radiation may appear to have little or no effect at all. This will depend upon the rate of the irradiation, the rate of recovery from sublethal damage and the rate of cell proliferation. The effect of these three mechanisms on cell survival is illustrated in Figure 17.1.

As the dose rate is reduced, the survival curve becomes less and less steep as more and more sublethal damage is repaired. The D_0 becomes larger and the extrapolation number becomes smaller. If the dose is delivered within a few hours, then recovery can be completed but repopulation will still be minimal. The pattern may be further complicated by an 'inverse dose rate effect' if growth is stopped in the G_2 phase (described later). An even more protracted period of irradiation will give time for proliferation also to occur while the dose is being delivered. The 'survival' curve will then become even less steep. It is because of these processes that the very low dose rate of background radiation from the environment (Chapter 19) cannot be shown to have any effect in terms of such survival curves.

IN VITRO STUDIES

Frozen cells

Mammalian cells can be frozen to liquid nitrogen temperature (-196 °C) as long as this is done very slowly and a cryo-protective agent is added, such as dimethyl sulphoxide (DMSO). In this way they can be stored for a long period and when they are thawed (quickly, this time) they are still viable and can be plated out for the usual assay of survival of colony-forming ability. If they are irradiated at that very low temperature, cells should neither proliferate nor shed sublethal damage. Because of this, there should then be absolutely no dose rate effect at all.

Figure 17.2 shows some of the results of this sort of study. The lowest curve shows the standard dose–response curve for HeLa cells with a D_0 value of 150 cGy (see Chapter 8). Because the cryo-protective agent DMSO is also a radiation-protecting agent, the second curve is less steep with a D_0 of 275 cGy. The third curve shows the effect of cooling aerated cells to liquid nitrogen temperature and the survival curve is even less steep ($D_0 = 625$ cGy). The last curve is for hypoxic cells, and this shows that there is still a small oxygen effect even at liquid nitrogen temperature: the D_0 value is 960 cGy and the oxygen enhancement ratio (OER) is 1.5.

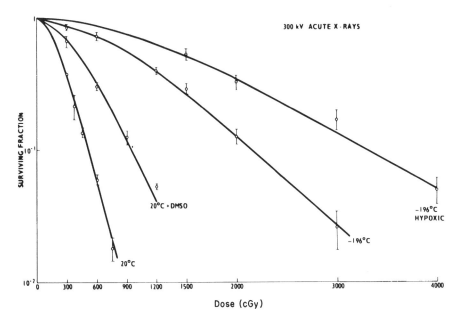

Figure 17.2. HeLa cell survival curves for four conditions of acute radiation. (Reproduced from Nias and Ebert, 1969, by permission of *Int. J. Radiat. Biol.*, Taylor & Francis.)

These data were all obtained with acute irradiation at a dose rate of 100 cGy/min. When the frozen cells were irradiated at the much lower dose rate of 100 cGy/day the survival data were unchanged for both aerated and hypoxic cells. Furthermore, split-dose experiments showed no recovery from sublethal damage so there was indeed no dose rate effect with radiation at that very low temperature.

Cells at room temperature

Another way of studying such low dose rates is to reduce the temperature of a cell culture from 37 °C to 20 °C. This also halts cell proliferation but recovery from sublethal damage does occur. The top part of Figure 17.3 shows how the growth of a CHO cell population ceased for the 72-h period at 20 °C and then resumed at the normal rate when the temperature was raised back to 37 °C. The bottom part of the figure shows that the DNA labelling index fell rapidly to zero during that period and then rose, but only to the starting level, indicating that the cells had remained in an asynchronous cycle phase distribution during this period at 20 °C. Neither had they lost their viability, because the plating efficiency remained unchanged. Furthermore, the acute radiosensitivity of these cells was the same at the end of this period of 72 h without proliferation as it was at the

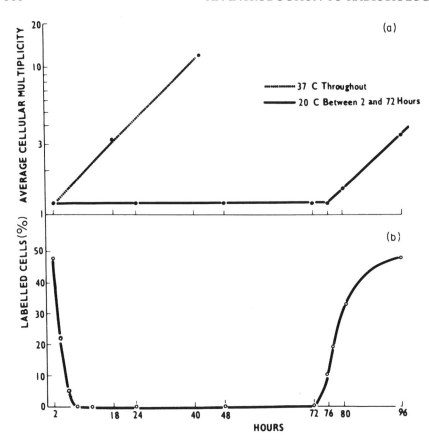

Figure 17.3. The effect of reducing the temperature of CHO cells from 37 °C to 20 °C on (a) growth rate and (b) DNA labelling.

beginning. The lower curve in Figure 17.4 shows the dose response that was found in both cases.

Table 17.1 shows the other half of the evidence: namely, that the relative survival after a split-dose experiment was just as high when the cells were maintained at 20 °C between the doses as it was when they were maintained at 37 °C, i.e. recovery from sublethal damage was unchanged during this cold period (Chapter 7).

This technique was used to obtain the data shown in Figure 17.4, where the cells were either given acute doses of radiation at 100 cGy/min or were continuously irradiated at 25 cGy/h during this 72-h period when the cells did not proliferate (Figure 17.3) but did recover from sublethal damage (Table 17.1). The D_0 value increased from a value of 200 cGy for cells given acute radiation to 625 cGy for the cells given protracted radiation; the

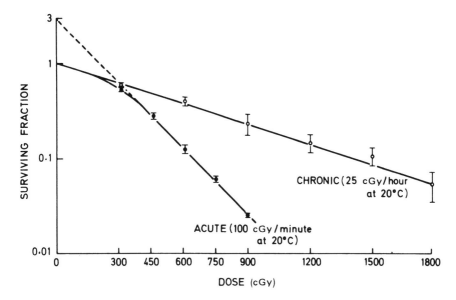

Figure 17.4. CHO cell survival curves after irradiation at 100 cGy/min or 25 cGy/h at 20 °C. (Reproduced from Fox and Nias, 1970, by permission of Elsevier Science-NL, Sara Burgerhartstraat 25, 1055 KV Amsterdam, The Netherlands.)

extrapolation number fell from 3 to 1. The protracted dose rate was so low that there was ample time for the cells to recover from sublethal damage. Because the half-time for the repair of such sublethal damage is about 1 h, the damage would be shed as fast as it was delivered. Thus, the upper survival curve in Figure 17.4 applies only to the lethal damage in such a cell population that has not been able to proliferate during the irradiation (as predicted in Figure 17.1).

Table 17.1. Relative survival (divided dose/single dose)[a] of CHO cells maintained at 37 °C or 20 °C between divided doses

Time between doses (h)	Relative survival when maintained at:	
	37 °C	20 °C
1	2.25 + 0.05	1.75 + 0.40
2	2.25 + 0.65	2.15 + 0.10
4	1.9 + 0.50	2.26 + 0.56
6	2.3 + 0.30	2.41 + 0.54

[a]Relative survival is expressed as mean + standard error of mean; 800 cGy single dose, ca. 6% survival; 400 + 400 cGy divided dose.
Reproduced from Fox and Nias, 1970, by permission of Elsevier Science-NL, Sara Burgerhartstraat 25, 1055 KV Amsterdam, The Netherlands.

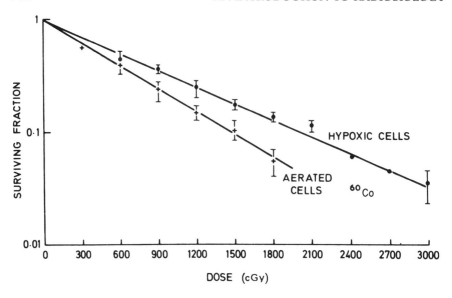

Figure 17.5. CHO cell survival curves after protracted irradiation at 100 cGy/h in air or under hypoxic conditions. (Reproduced from Nias, 1988, by permission of Churchill Livingstone.)

If these CHO cells had been able to proliferate, they would have doubled in number every 12 h. In that case, the upper part of Figure 17.1 would have been applicable. After 12 h of irradiation at that low dose rate when the cells would have received a dose of 300 cGy, Figure 17.4 shows that the surviving fraction would still only have been reduced to 80%, even without proliferation during that time. With proliferation it is obvious that just one population doubling would more than keep pace with this small amount of lethal damage, which is why the end result of both of the processes shown in Figure 17.1 would be a surviving fraction of 100% and the irradiation would have had no apparent effect.

A similar technique was used to obtain the survival curves shown in Figure 17.5, but this time the dose rate was 100 cGy/h. This faster dose rate was used because a comparison was being made with the effect of protracted radiation upon hypoxic cells, and mammalian cells begin to die if they are kept hypoxic for very long periods of time. Figure 17.5 shows that the OER under these conditions of protracted radiation has a value of only 1.4, which is very much lower than the usual value of 2.5 found when cells are given acute radiation (Chapter 10). The explanation for this reduction in OER is that while the aerated cells can recover from sublethal damage during the irradiation, hypoxic cells cannot. Radiotherapists use three dose rates of protracted radiation when they insert ^{137}Cs sources into various tumour tissues. The effectiveness of this sort of treatment may well be because of the advantage of this reduced OER over that obtained with acute X-ray treatments.

Continuous irradiation at very low dose rates

Figure 17.6 shows a family of growth curves for CHO cells that were continuously irradiated by means of incorporating tritiated water into the culture medium. This provides a continuous beta irradiation of the cells, and the effect of various dose rates are shown. The higher the dose rate, the earlier the growth curve begins to slow down and then plateau off. This occurred at 300 cGy/day after 5 days, when the cell population had grown to more than 10^5. Figure 17.7 shows a similar family of growth curves, but this time for HeLa cells. Again, the higher the dose rate, the earlier the

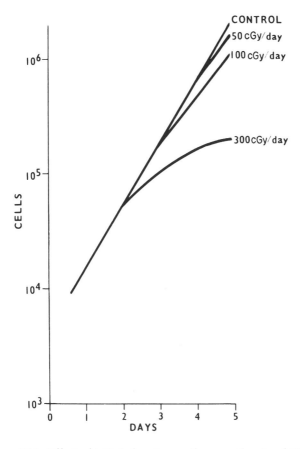

Figure 17.6. Effect of tritiated water on the growth rate of CHO cells.

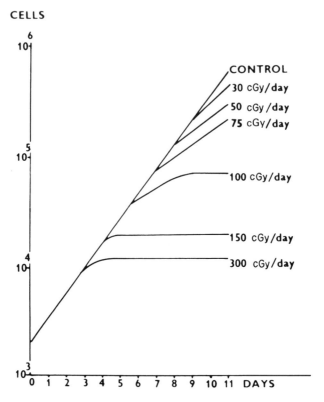

Figure 17.7. Effect of tritiated water on the growth rate of HeLa cells. (Reprinted from Nias and Lajtha, 1964, with permission of *Nature*, Macmillan Magazines Limited.)

growth curve departs from the control and flattens, but these effects occur at lower dose rates. Thus, 300 cGy/day led to the HeLa cell growth curve levelling off after only 3 days, when the cell population had only grown to 10^4.

Comparison of Figures 17.6 and 17.7 shows that the minimum dose rate to slow the growth of CHO cells is 50 cGy/day, but only 30 cGy/day is needed to slow the growth of HeLa cells. In both cases the effect is only noticeable towards the end of the growth curve, i.e. 5 days with CHO cells and 10 days with HeLa cells, when the cell populations reach approximately 10^6 in number. At this stage a monolayer culture becomes crowded and subculture with trypsinization is required.

The subsequent growth curves show a different pattern, with an inflection after a few days of growth and then resumption of the normal growth rate. This is the result of the accumulated radiation damage that is revealed by the trypsinization step. Figure 17.8 shows that this occurs with

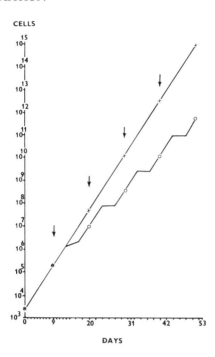

Figure 17.8. Effect of trypsinization on the growth rate of HeLa cells continuously irradiated with tritiated water at 30 cGy/day: (→) time of trypsinization; (x) control; (○) irradiated cells. (Reprinted from Nias and Lajtha, 1964, with permission of *Nature*, Macmillan Magazines Limited.)

every subculture and so the overall effect is a slowing of the population doubling time. This also occurs with suspension cultures, but because subculture does not need trypsinization the growth curves do not show an inflection. Table 17.2 shows how the cell cycle time of suspension cultures of P388F lymphoma cells is elongated in proportion to the dose rate of continuous irradiation and that this is due to division delay in the G_2 phase.

Such lymphoma cells normally have a cell cycle time of only 12 h, which is the same as that of the CHO cells used for Figure 17.6. During 5 days of culture, therefore, the cells will have completed 10 cell divisions. By contrast, the HeLa cells used in Figures 17.7 and 17.8 divide only once every 25 h, which is why they can be grown for 10 days before subculture is needed.

A comparison of Figures 17.6 and 17.7 might seem to indicate that CHO cells are only half as radiosensitive as HeLa cells. This anomaly is explained by Table 17.3. The top line shows that CHO cells had to be irradiated at twice the dose rate (100 cGy) per day to produce the same level of damage as in HeLa cells irradiated at 48 cGy per day. However, when allowance is made for the twofold difference in the population doubling times of these

Table 17.2. G_2 lengthening induced in P388F lymphoma by 15 days of continuous irradiation with tritiated water at various dose rates

Dose rate (cGy/day)	G_2 lengthening (h)	Cell cycle (h)
Control	–	12.0
60	0.5	12.5
90	1.3	13.3
120	2.1	14.1
150	2.25	14.25

Reproduced from Fox and Gilbert, 1966, by permission of *Int. J. Radiat. Biol.*, Taylor & Francis.

two cell lines, the dose rate becomes identical at 50 cGy per doubling time. There is still a difference in surviving fraction (derived by backward extrapolation from the inflected growth curves), but this is accounted for by the fact that HeLa cells are more sensitive to acute radiation ($D_0 = 150$ cGy) than are CHO cells ($D_0 = 200$ cGy). When allowance is made for this, the effect of such a similar dose rate of continuous irradiation is to produce a similar level of damage in terms of equivalent acute doses.

This similarity can be shown to apply over a wide range of dose rate of continuous irradiation as long as the dosage is expressed in relation to the doubling time of the cell populations. The dose–response curves in Figure 17.9 were derived from a large number of growth curves of CHO and HeLa cells irradiated by different concentrations of tritiated water in the growth medium. Because of small variations in the doubling times of the cells, horizontal error bars have to be used for the dose rate data and vertical error bars for the survival data. The two curves differ in slope by a factor of 1.36 (for HeLa, $D_0 = 260$ cGy per doubling time; for CHO, $D_0 = 340$ cGy per doubling time) but this is similar to the ratio of the acute D_0 values.

The concept of cGy per cell cycle time is obviously more biologically relevant than cGy per physical unit of time. The HeLa/CHO cell comparisons show that, as a general rule, a given dose rate of continuous irradiation will be more effective in the cells with a longer cell cycle. When

Table 17.3. Continuous irradiation in a monolayer

	HeLa cells	CHO cells
Dose rate (cGy/day)	48	100
Population doubling time (h)	25	12
cGy/doubling time	50	50
Survival (%)	16	27
Equivalent acute dose (cGy)	440	460

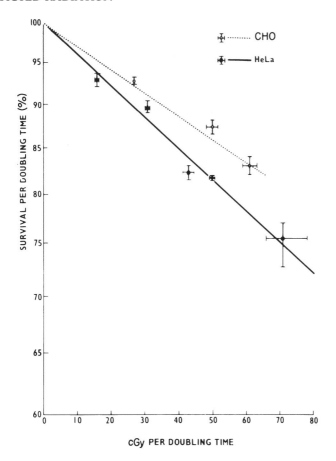

Figure 17.9. Dose–response of CHO and HeLa cells to continuous irradiation. Survival was estimated by backwards extrapolation from a series of growth curves at each dose rate. (Reproduced from Fox and Nias, 1970, by permission of Elsevier Science-NL, Sara Burgerhartstraat 25, 1055 KV Amsterdam, The Netherlands.)

the dose rate is very low, however, there will be no apparent accumulation of damage in the cell population at all.

The maximum dose rates that can be tolerated by mammalian cell systems *in vitro* appear to be of the order of 50–100 cGy per cell cycle. This is shown in Figure 17.10 in terms of the survival of HeLa cells from a dose rate of 2 cGy/h. Every 5 days, samples of the cell population were plated out to measure survival while the remaining population was continuously irradiated with tritiated water. Initially the survival fell, but after 20 days a plateau was reached and this shows that a 'steady state' had been reached between cell death and cell proliferation. Clearly, the processes of recovery and repopulation were both evident at this dose rate, which was roughly

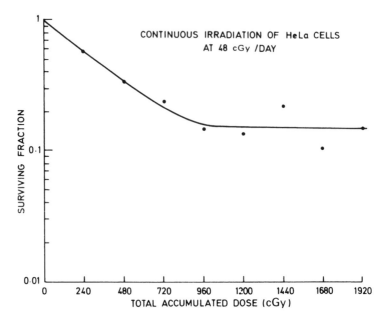

Figure 17.10. HeLa cell survival curve after protracted irradiation in air. (Reproduced from Nias, 1988, by permission of Churchill Livingstone.)

50 cGy per doubling time. Figure 17.11 shows more examples of steady states, but this time for P388F cells, which divide twice as quickly as HeLa cells. The comparable level of cell survival was reached with a dose rate of 120 cGy/day but this is equivalent to 60 cGy per doubling time, which is not very different from the HeLa cell dose rate.

Dose rate to stop growth

Figures 17.10 and 17.11 showed that a given dose rate of radiation will eventually stop the growth of a cell population but that this is related to the doubling time of the cells. Figure 17.12 shows that this relationship also applies to division delay (Chapter 7). There is an inverse relationship between these two phenomena. Cells that require a higher dose rate to stop growth show less division delay and, conversely, the longer the division delay, the lower the dose rate required to stop the growth of a cell population. This is not surprising, because a cell that stops cycling during continuous irradiation will accumulate more radiation dose during that cycle. Such division delay was shown for P388F cells in Table 17.2. With some cells this may lead to the so-called 'inverse dose rate effect' (Hall, 1994). If cells are blocked in the G_2 phase, when they are more radiosensitive, the survival curve in Figure 17.1 would become steeper until a further lowering

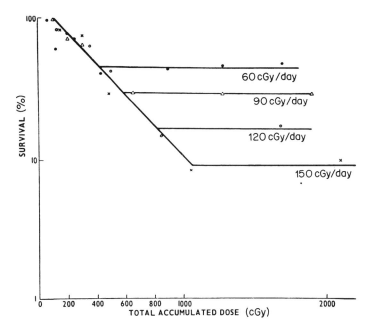

Figure 17.11. P388F cell survival curves after protracted irradiation at various dose rates. (Reproduced from Fox and Nias, 1970, by permission of Elsevier Science-NL, Sara Burgerhartstraat 25, 1055 KV Amsterdam, The Netherlands.)

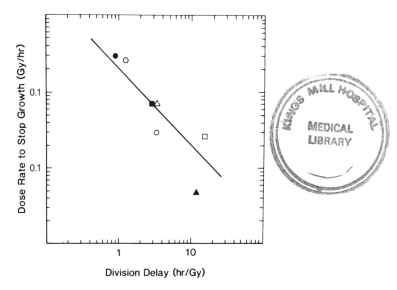

Figure 17.12. Relationship between dose rate to stop growth and division delay after continuous irradiation of different cell lines. (Reproduced from Mitchell et al, 1979, by permission of Academic Press, Inc.)

of the dose rate allowed cells to escape the G_2 block, and then the effect of proliferation leads to an ever shallower survival curve.

CONTINUOUS IRRADIATION *IN VIVO*

All the examples given in this chapter so far have been from cells cultured *in vitro*, but the same phenomena occur *in vivo*. Figure 17.13 shows dose–response curves of mouse intestinal crypt cells using the assay technique described in Chapter 8. Figure 8.13 in that chapter showed a survival curve for acute doses of radiation that is similar to the 274 cGy/min curve. As the dose rate is progressively reduced down to 0.54 cGy/min the curves become progressively less steep in slope.

The 'steady state' phenomenon has also been shown to apply *in vivo*. Figure 17.14 shows what happened when rats were exposed to continuous irradiation at a dose rate of 415 cGy/day. The response of the small intestine was a fall in the number of cells per crypt during the first 2 days and then a 'steady state' was established for the next 3 days. This is such a

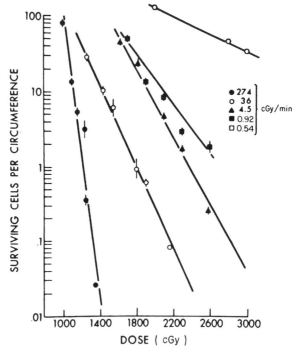

Figure 17.13. Dose–response of mouse jejunal crypt cells irradiated at different dose rates. (Reproduced from Fu et al, 1975, by permission of Radiological Society of North America.)

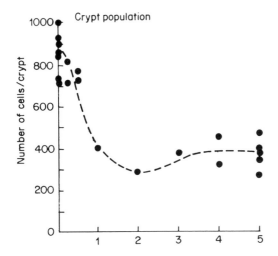

Figure 17.14. The response of small intestinal crypt cells in rats irradiated at 415 cGy/day. (Reproduced from Lamerton and Lord, 1964, by permission of Oxford University Press.)

high dose rate that the animals die from the haemopoietic syndrome after about 10 days. If the dose rate is reduced to 176 cGy/day then they will survive for 16 days and the steady state of intestinal crypt cells will be at a higher level. Because the cell cycle time of these intestinal epithelial cells is less than 12 h, the effective dose rates per cell cycle will be less than half those rates per day.

The cell cycle time of cells in the rat bone marrow is very much longer: 57 h for early normoblasts and myelocytes. In terms of dose rate per population doubling time, therefore, these bone-marrow cells can only maintain a steady state with a much lower dose rate per day that can be tolerated by intestinal cells. A dose of 84 cGy/day can be tolerated for 50 days, but only 50 cGy/day for longer periods of continuous irradiation (Lord, 1964).

WHOLE-BODY RADIATION

The effects of an acute dose of radiation to the whole body were described in Chapter 14 with three lethal syndromes: central nervous system (CNS), intestinal and haemopoietic. The median lethal dose is usually taken to be the dose that can be tolerated by the haemopoietic system within 30 days (LD$_{50/30}$), because intestinal and CNS deaths occur much earlier and after much higher doses.

Table 17.4. Variation of mortality with dose rate

Dose rate (cGy/min)	$LD_{50/30}$ (cGy)
68	850
7.7	950
4.4	1030
2.4	1100

Reproduced from Neal, 1960, by permission of *Int. J. Radiat. Biol.*, Taylor & Francis.

Table 17.4 shows that the median lethal dose to CBA mice rises progressively as the dose rate falls. So, once again, the effect of reducing the dose rate is to reduce the biological effect of the radiation. At even lower dose rates, the radiation would not be lethal because the effects of recovery from sublethal damage and repopulation in the haemopoietic system would compensate for the radiation damage – as has been shown in the other examples in this chapter.

At even lower dose rates, all the same phenomena will occur but the cell population will now show a negligible fall below the normal level even when the population has been exposed to an accumulated dose of many hundreds of centigrays. This effect of very low dose rates is mentioned because it applies to background irradiation from the environment (Chapter 19). Low doses of acute radiation are used in diagnostic radiology (Chapter 18), and cells will shed sublethal damage and repopulate after such doses in the same way as they do after the continuous doses described in this chapter. Until there is good evidence for a 'safe' lower limit of radiation dosage, it must be assumed that any dose delivered at any dose rate will be associated with the sort of cell damage that has been demonstrated here, even though such damage may be very difficult to observe at the time. In addition to these effects on cell survival, however, there are genetic and carcinogenic effects that must also be assumed to have occurred, even though they will also be difficult to observe after such low doses and dose rates. These will be discussed in Chapters 18 and 19.

SUMMARY OF CONCLUSIONS

(1) When the radiation dose rate is lowered from 100 to 1 cGy/min there will be more and more time for recovery from sublethal damage to be completed during the radiation exposure. As a result, the cell survival curve will be much less steep because only lethal damage will be expressed.

(2) If the dose rate is lowered still further there will also be time for proliferation of undamaged cells. As a result, the cell survival curve may show no apparent damage at all.

(3) In order to take account of differences in cell proliferation, it is best to express the radiation dose rate in terms of cGy per population doubling time, rather than cGy per day.

(4) At intermediate dose rates a cell population may only fall to a survival level that amounts to a 'steady-state' between the effects of continuous radiation damage on the one hand and recovery plus repopulation on the other.

(5) This is presumed to occur in people who are exposed to continuous background radiation, even though the dose rate is much too low to cause any detectable damage.

REFERENCES

Fox, M. and Gilbert, C. W., 1966. Continuous irradiation of a murine lymphoma line P388F *in vitro*. *International Journal of Radiation Biology*, **11**, 339–347.

Fox, M. and Nias, A. H. W., 1970. The influence of recovery from sub-lethal damage on the response of cells to protracted irradiation at low dose rate. *Current Topics in Radiation Research*, **7**, 71–103.

Fu, K. K., Phillips, T. L., Kane, L. J. and Smith, V., 1975. Tumor and normal tissue response to irradiation *in vivo*: variation with decreasing dose rates. *Radiology*, **114**, 709–716.

Goodhead, D., 1992. Track structure considerations in low dose and low dose rate effects of ionizing radiation. *Advances in Radiation Biology*, **16**, 7–44.

Hall, E. J., 1978. *Radiobiology for the Radiologist*, 2nd edn. Harper and Row, New York.

Hall, E. J., 1994. *Radiobiology for the Radiologist*, 4th edn. Lippincott, New York.

Lamerton, L. F. and Lord, B. I., 1964. Studies of cell proliferation under continuous irradiation. *National Cancer Institute Monograph*, **14**, 185–198.

Lord, B. I., 1964. The effects of continuous irradiation on cell proliferation in rat bone marrow. *British Journal of Haematology*, **10**, 496–507.

Mitchell, J. B., Bedford, J. S. and Bailey, S. M., 1979. Dose-rate effects in mammalian cells in culture. III. Comparison of cell killing and cell proliferation during continuous irradiation for six different cell lines. *Radiation Research*, **79**, 537–551.

Neal, F. E., 1960. Variation of acute mortality with dose rate in mice exposed to single large doses of whole body X-radiation. *International Journal of Radiation Biology*, **2**, 295–300.

Nias, A. H. W., 1988. *Clinical Radiobiology*, 2nd edn. Churchill Livingstone, Edinburgh.

Nias, A. H. W. and Ebert, M., 1969. Effects of single and continuous irradiation of HeLa cells at $-196\,^{\circ}C$. *International Journal of Radiation Biology*, **16**, 31–41.

Nias, A. H. W. and Lajtha, L. G., 1964. Continuous irradiation with tritiated water of mammalian cells in a monolayer. *Nature*, **202**, 613–614.

18 Diagnostic Radiology

Over 85% of the nuclear radiation received by humans comes from natural sources and we are all exposed to it whether we like it or not (Chapter 19). The remainder comes from artificial sources, however, and nearly all of this comes from medical procedures such as diagnostic radiology and nuclear medicine. In most cases the radiation doses are very low, but these doses are delivered to quite a lot of people. The annual frequency of X-ray examinations varies from about 300 to 900 per 1000 inhabitants in developed countries. The frequency is much lower for nuclear medicine procedures: 10–40 per 1000 inhabitants.

In some cases the diagnosis can be reached without using radiation. Imaging can be done using ultrasound or magnetic resonance. Many body cavities can be examined using fibre-optic endoscopy. If there is no alternative to using radiation, then the doses used are kept to low levels according to the following principles:

(1) No radiological practice shall be adopted unless its introduction produces a positive net benefit.
(2) All doses shall be kept as low as is reasonably achievable (ALARA).
(3) The effective dose to individuals must not exceed limits recommended by the International Commission on Radiological Protection.

These dose limits will be discussed in Chapter 20. In this chapter, the doses delivered by the commoner radiological procedures will be described and the genetic effects of radiation will be considered, together with effects on the developing embryo. Because the doses are so much lower than those considered in earlier chapters, it will be convenient to make most of the comparisons of absorbed doses in terms of mGy (1 cGy = 10 mGy) and effective doses (defined later) in terms of mSv.

RADIATION DOSE PER EXAMINATION

The dose received will vary widely throughout the body, the maximum being to the skin in the primary beam of radiation. This incident skin dose gives an indication of the maximum dose received by any cell population in the body, and ranges from less than 0.1 mGy for a large-film examination of the chest to as high as 1 Gy for cardiac catheterization.

Table 18.1. Typical bone-marrow doses during diagnostic X-ray examinations

Examination	Median dose (mGy)	
	Male	Female
Barium meal	5.1	8.0
Mass survey chest	0.6	1.0
Lumbar spine	2.7	2.7
Abdomen	1.2	1.3
Descending urography	5.8	4.5
Retrograde urography	4.4	3.3
Dental	0.02	0.02

Reproduced from UK Committee on Radiological Hazards to Patients, 1966. Crown copyright is reproduced with the permission of the Controller of HMSO.

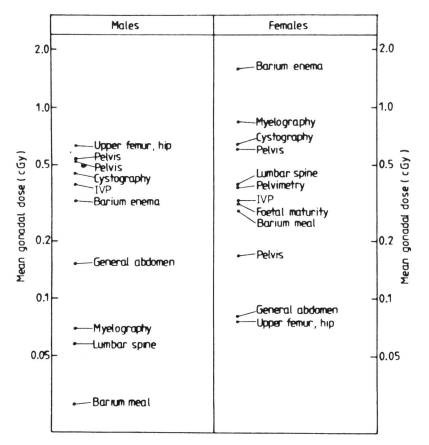

Figure 18.1. Mean gonad doses from diagnostic X-ray examinations. (Reproduced from Mould, 1985, by permission of Adam Hilger.)

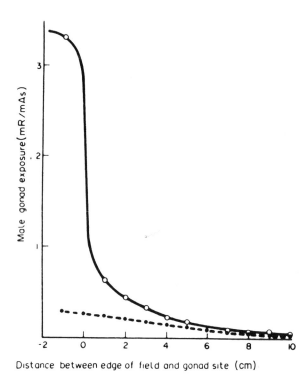

Distance between edge of field and gonad site (cm)

Figure 18.2. Male gonad exposure as a function of distance between the edge of the X-ray field and the location of the gonads. -o-, no shielding; --●--, contact shielding. (Reproduced from ICRP, 1982, by permission of ICRP.)

The two tissues that are most important in this respect are the bone marrow, because of the possibility of leukaemogenesis (Chapter 19), and the gonads, because of genetic effects. Table 18.1 shows some typical doses to bone marrow, which is localized in both the sternum and pelvis. These doses range from 0.02 mGy from dental examinations to 8 mGy from a barium meal in a woman.

The effects of radiation on the gonads will be described later but gonad doses will be less than 0.1 mGy from X-ray examinations of the heart, chest and extremities. By contrast, in examinations of the lower trunk the gonads are irradiated directly, so the dose is usually greater than 5 mGy and may be as high as 20 mGy. Figure 18.1 shows the gonad doses (in cGy) measured during various X-ray examinations of men and women. It shows that the doses from many types of examination tend to be higher in females than males.

On the other hand, the gonads can be avoided in many cases by carefully centring and adjusting the field to irradiate only the field of interest. The testes can be shielded and this may reduce the dose considerably. Figure 18.2 shows that even without contact shielding, the gonad dose will be much lower if the edge of the field can be placed some centimetres away from the testis. (This old report expressed the dose in milliroentgens, with a given milliamp current setting per second of exposure from the X-ray machine.) Lead shielding can also be used in other sites. In dental radiography, for example, the patient can be protected by wearing a rubber apron containing the equivalent of 0.25 mm of lead. Such aprons can also be worn by radiological staff, but they can also take advantage of such simple precautions as distance (due to the inverse square law, the intensity of the X-ray beam falls by the square of the distance) and they can obviously avoid standing in the path of the X-ray beam.

Doses to patients can also be reduced by using rare earth screens, quicker-acting film and slot radiography. This is important with children, especially when repeated X-rays are needed (e.g. to control the development of pelvic abnormalities). The benefit of these technical advances has been cancelled out, however, by the increasing use of computed tomography (CT) scanning. Table 18.5 will show how much larger the doses are and this explains why, although CT scans account for less than 1% of all diagnostic imaging procedures, they contribute nearly 3% of the 'effective dose'.

EFFECTIVE DOSE OF RADIOLOGICAL EXAMINATIONS

The sievert unit is used when doses of absorbed radiation in gray units are converted to units of *equivalent dose*. This is done by multiplying the absorbed doses by the appropriate quality factor (see Chapter 9, Table 9.1) to take into account the relative biological effectiveness (RBE) of different types of radiation. One sievert of any such radiation will have the same radiobiological effect on a tissue but some tissues are more sensitive than others, and this has to be taken into account by using the '*effective dose*'. This is obtained by using weighting factors (Table 18.2) that account for the varying susceptibility of different organs or tissues to the stochastic effects

Table 18.2. Tissue weighting factors

Weight	0.01	0.05	0.12	0.20
Organs	Bone Skin	Bladder Breast Liver Oesophagus Thyroid Remainder	Colon Lung Red bone marrow Stomach	Gonads
Total	0.02	0.30	0.48	0.20

Reproduced from Clarke, 1991, by permission of NRPB/SO.

of fatal and non-fatal cancer and severe hereditary effects, i.e. a method of risk assessment (Mountford, 1997). The effective dose is simple to calculate in the case of a uniform total body exposure (e.g. from natural background radiation) using a factor of 1. The calculation is more complicated when only certain parts of the body are exposed for diagnosis. For most diagnostic procedures, mSv units are used.

Nuclear medicine

In nuclear medicine, the radiation is delivered internally from radioactive isotopes administered to the patient by injection or by mouth. Some of the isotopes are chosen for their property of localizing in the different tissues of the body for which diagnostic information is required (e.g. iodine in the thyroid). Other isotopes have a more general distribution but are useful because of their imaging properties (e.g. technetium, Tc).

The dose absorbed by an organ is calculated from the dose rate and duration of exposure. The dose rate depends on the fraction of the administered dose reaching the organ and the size and shape of that organ. The duration depends on the biological half-life of the isotope. Variation in excretion due to disease can influence the radiation dose: for example, if a patient has impaired renal function, radioactive isotopes that are normally rapidly excreted by the kidneys can cause a much higher exposure. Most investigations use ^{99m}Tc because it is a γ-emitter with a short radioactive half-life of 6 h, which limits the radiation dose. If the compound is excreted in the urine, prompt emptying of the bladder will significantly reduce the duration of exposure.

Table 18.3 shows how the equivalent dose, effective dose and the associated uterine dose are related for a few examples of common nuclear medicine procedures. For thyroid, lung and kidney the doses are fairly low, but higher doses are delivered with bone, heart and brain scans. For studies of brain metabolism the PET (positron emission tomography) technique uses ^{18}F in the form of FDG (2-fluoro-2-deoxy-d-glucose); with this isotope technique the effective dose is 7 mSv and the uterine dose is 5 mGy.

Table 18.3. Typical doses from nuclear medicine procedures with ^{99m}Tc

Site	Vehicle	Equivalent dose (mSv)	Effective dose (mSv)	Uterine dose (mGy)
Bone	Phosphate	4.8	3.7	4
Heart	Red cells	7	5	4
Thyroid	Pertechnate	1	1	0.6
Lung	Albumin	1.2	1.2	0.3
Kidney	DMSA	1.3	0.7	0.4
Brain	Pertechnate	7	7	6

Based on NRPB, 1993, by permission of NRPB/SO.

Diagnostic X-rays

Table 18.4 shows how the effective doses for some of the commoner X-ray examinations have been reduced between 1984 and 1995. The table also shows the mean entrance surface doses (ESD) for these procedures. These values are per radiograph but the number of films taken for each examination has not changed during this period, so modern techniques have led to a reduction in dose in conventional radiography. By contrast, the doses delivered in CT examinations are much higher; this is shown by the comparisons in Table 18.5. Other high-dose examinations include cardiac catheterization, but this is an X-ray examination used for direct diagnosis of a known disease.

In other cases, the examination may be part of a screening procedure when the patient has no symptoms. The question of cost–benefit then arises. The problem is best illustrated by breast cancer screening, where it is estimated that for women under the age of 50 years more cancer deaths may be induced by exposure to radiation than are prevented by early diagnosis.

On the other hand, chest X-rays are the most common of all radiological procedures, with an average dose of only 0.04 mSv. To put this into context,

Table 18.4. Reduction in effective dose for common radiographs

Radiograph	Mean ESD per radiograph (mGy)		Effective dose per radiograph (mSv)	
	1984	1995	1984	1995
Lumbar spine	23.2	16.0	0.46	0.29
Chest	0.23	0.16	0.024	0.017
Abdomen	8.2	5.6	1.1	0.7
Pelvis	6.5	4.4	1.05	0.66
Skull	2.6	1.5	0.02	0.01
Thoracic spine	14.0	13.0	0.34	0.29

Reproduced from Hart et al, 1996, by permission of NRPB/SO.

Table 18.5. Effective dose for conventional and CT X-ray examinations

Examination site	Conventional dose (mSv)	CT dose (mSv)
Skull	0.10	1.8
Chest	0.04	8.3
Thoracic spine	1.1	5.8
Abdomen	1.4	7.2
Pelvis	1.0	7.3

Reproduced from NRPB, 1993, by permission of NRPB/SO.

over half of the routine examinations have effective doses that are less than the annual dose of 2.6 mSv from background radiation in the UK. The recommended dose limit for the general public is now 1 mSv per year, and for occupational exposure it is 20 mSv per year (see Chapter 20).

GENETIC EFFECTS OF RADIATION

The radiation doses resulting from diagnostic radiology have been described with particular emphasis on the doses received by the gonads and by bone marrow. At these levels, the most detrimental effect upon bone marrow will be leukaemogenesis, which will be discussed in Chapter 19. As far as the gonads are concerned, the risk from low doses is genetic. Before such risks are discussed, however, the effects of higher doses of radiation will be described.

Testis

In the testes of adult males, all germ-cell stages are present in the seminiferous tubules: stem-cell spermatogonia, differentiating spermatogonia, spermatocytes, spermatids and spermatozoa. In men, the duration of spermatogenesis is about 74 days, with a further 16 days added for stem-cell division. In between the seminiferous tubules is the interstitial tissue, consisting of clumps of Leydig cells that secrete testosterone, which is part of the complex hormonal mechanism that regulates fertility. The seminiferous tubules contain not only the germ cells but also Sertoli cells, which support and nourish them. The germ cells are an example of a stem-cell population (cf. bone marrow, Chapter 13).

Some types of spermatogonia are sensitive and are killed after exposure of the testes to relatively low doses of radiation: they die in early prophase or later metaphase. As the supply of germ cells derived from spermatogonia becomes exhausted, the testes are progressively depleted of these cells until, at 2–4 weeks after exposure, mature sperm cells have disappeared. If the dose has not been excessive, regeneration begins from type A spermatogonia spared from radiation death. The time course of this phenomenon over a 5-year period has been described for a man who had received an accidental dose of 390 cGy of soft X-rays to the whole body (Figure 18.3). The sperm count reached its lowest level 6 months after irradiation and then recovered to a normal level at 2–3 years. In contrast, the Leydig and Sertoli cells of the interstitial tissues are relatively radioresistant; for this reason, testes that are atrophied because of radiation damage appear to contain more interstitial cells than germ cells.

Histological examination of mouse testes after irradiation shows that regeneration of spermatogenic epithelium occurs in discrete foci. On this basis, a single-dose 'cell' survival curve has been derived and this has a D_0

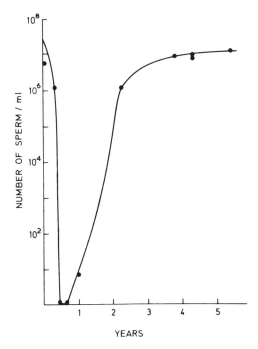

Figure 18.3. Changes in human sperm count for 5 years after total body irradiation. (Reproduced from Oakes and Lushbaugh, 1952, by permission of Radiological Society of North America.)

value of 180 cGy. Fractionation studies show that recovery from sublethal damage also occurs in this tissue and the value of $D_2 - D_1$ is 270 cGy after an interval of 4 h (Withers et al, 1974).

In the human male a dose of 0.15 Sv to the testis is likely to produce temporary sterility for about 12 months and a dose of 3.5 Sv will produce permanent sterility (BEIR, 1990). In most men, however, their libido and potency are normally retained because the interstitial cells, the main source of male hormone production, would not have lost their functional integrity.

Ovaries

Unlike the testis, the ovary does not contain a renewable stem-cell population of germinal cells. By puberty a woman may have 10^5 oocytes, but only 400 will finally ovulate. As time goes on, fewer of the oocytes will be left owing to continuous depletion by ovulation and/or degeneration. As a result, the older ovary appears to be more sensitive to radiation, which is why the dose needed to produce sterilization is smaller in older women.

Early in this century it was recognized that the ovaries atrophy after irradiation and that temporary or permanent sterility may result. In order to evaluate studies of irradiated ovaries, stress must be laid upon the fact that no other organ presents such large differences in response after irradiation between species or between individuals within a species. In the developing foetus, oogonia are relatively radioresistant, but oocytes in primordial follicles are extremely radiosensitive ($D_0 = 91$ cGy, $N = 2$–3). Sensitivity diminishes as the follicles mature, and is low before ovulation.

As in the male, female germ cells are most sensitive during the last pre-meiotic prophase and the development into mature gametes. However, the 'fertile–sterile–fertile' pattern often found in the ovaries after irradiation is not a result of regeneration from a stem-cell pool, as it is in males, but of the higher sensitivity of the intermediate follicular stages compared with that of the primitive and mature stages. Granulosa cells in the developing follicles are damaged even earlier than the oocytes, but in the mature follicles and the corpus luteum they appear more resistant.

Relatively low doses of radiation given during the second and third week after birth have drastic effects on the fertility of the female mouse. This effect can be traced to depletion of the oocyte pool by radiation-induced cell killing. Because the mouse cannot replenish losses from the oocyte pool established during embryonic life, sterility ensues when the supply of oocytes surviving radiation is exhausted.

The effect of age on the radiosensitivity of the ovary is illustrated by the doses of fractionated radiation needed to induce an artificial menopause: 12–15 Gy is needed in young women but only 4–7 Gy in older women (Ash, 1980). Permanent sterility occurs in 60% of young women given 8 Gy of fractionated radiation. On the other hand, occasional pregnancies can occur after doses of up to 5–8 Gy and the children are apparently normal at birth. The question arises of whether these children may be carrying severe genetic lesions.

Genetic effects

The biochemical changes related to chromosome damage and methods for the analysis of lethal aberrations were described in Chapter 5. Structural changes in the chromosomes occur spontaneously and irradiation merely increases the probability of changes of the same type being produced. The expression of non-lethal chromosome aberrations is in gene mutation, whereby some feature of a cell's form or function is changed and that change is handed down in the progeny. The mutations that follow irradiation are identical to those that occur spontaneously, but their frequency after irradiation will be increased by several orders of magnitude, depending on the dose of radiation.

Chromosome mutations are the result of either an increase or decrease in the number of genes in the nucleus. Changes in gene structure may involve quite small alterations in the DNA molecules; these result in *point mutations* and imply no change in the number of genes. Point mutations occur in simple proportion to dose and are independent of dose rate over a very wide range. These changes are also independent of any fractionation effect and the quality of the radiation. A question arises as to whether chromosome aberrations lead to a viable cell population that is so altered in genetic information as to be detrimental to the human subject. These will be mutations that may result in malignant disease (Chapter 19) and other changes that may have long-term consequences for future generations.

The *genetic risks* are extremely difficult to evaluate and few data are available on the genetic effects of radiation in humans. Since 1977 the genetic committee of UNSCEAR (United Nations Scientific Committee on the Effects of Atomic Radiation) have recommended that 1 Gy should be considered the *mutation doubling dose*. This is the amount of radiation required to produce as many mutations as those occurring spontaneously in a generation, i.e. the dose of radiation that would double the natural incidence. The International Commission on Radiological Protection (ICRP, 1991) confirmed this doubling dose but recent studies (including data from Hiroshima and Nagasaki) suggest that 1 Gy is a conservative figure, i.e. it overestimates the risk, and that the doubling dose may be as high as 4 Gy (Sankaranarayanan, 1996). The genetic detriment will be manifest in a number of ways: in the form of autosomal and sex-linked gene characters, chromosomal aberrations, abortions and what are called genetic deaths. Genetic death implies the loss of a particular cell line either as a result of premature death or impaired fertility.

Genetically significant dose (GSD)

For the purposes of expressing genetic risk, the most suitable quantity is the *genetically significant dose* (GSD). This is the equivalent dose to the gonads weighted for age and sex distribution in those members of the exposed population expected to have offspring. The GSD is an index of the presumed genetic impact of radiation on the whole population. Because only part of the population receives radiation from medical radiography, colour TV or cosmic rays from flying at high altitudes, the calculation of GSD attempts to average the genetic effects over the whole population. The GSD is therefore the dose that, if given to every member of the population, should produce the same hereditary damage as the actual doses received by the gonads of the particular individuals who receive radiation, and takes into account the child-bearing potential of those receiving the dose.

In 1982 the GSD in Great Britain was estimated to be 0.12 mGy, compared with 0.2 mGy in the USA, 0.3 mGy in Italy and 0.46 mGy in Sweden (Wall, 1982). These figures were obtained from the sort of data in Figure 18.1, which showed the gonad doses likely to be received by patients undergoing diagnostic X-ray examinations. In both sexes the doses rose to around

10 mGy but, of course, these doses were received only by a small number of individuals and the GSD averages this out. But even 10 mGy is well below the mutation doubling dose of 1 Gy.

The genetic effects will be most pronounced in the first generation after irradiation, but the total number of deleterious effects of genetic mutation following irradiation will be much greater in all subsequent generations. Nevertheless, such genetic effects of small doses of radiation are extremely rare compared to the natural mutation rate; indeed, other environmental pollutants and cytotoxic drugs are responsible for much greater genetic damage than radiation.

EFFECTS ON THE EMBRYO AND FOETUS

Many physical, chemical and infective agents are known to carry high risks of producing damaging effects on the embryo and foetus, and great care is taken to minimize such hazards. Severe effects will commonly follow irradiation of the developing offspring. Russell and Russell (1954) have

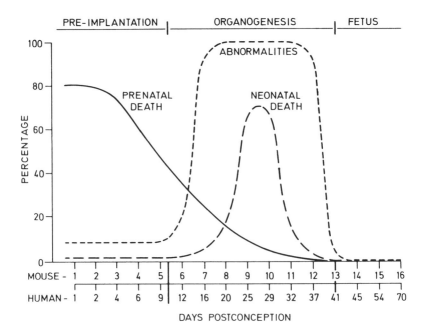

Figure 18.4. Incidence of radiation-induced death and abnormalities in mice related to the period at which irradiation (200 cGy) takes place. A comparative scale of human development is given. (Reprinted from Russell and Russell, 1954, by permission of Wiley–Liss, Inc., a subsidiary of John Wiley & Sons, Inc.)

Table 18.6. Some events in early human development

Day	Event
1	Fertilization
2	Two cells
3	Four cells; rapid division to 16 cells; enter uterus
4	Inner cell mass (embryo proper) forms
5	Blastocyst
6	Implantation begins
8	Establishment of exoderm germ layers
11	Primitive placental circulation
14	Prochordal plate formed; major organogenesis begins
	FIRST MISSED MENSTRUAL PERIOD
18	Neural plate
20	Primitive brain
21	Primordial germ cells visible in yolk-sac wall near allantois
22	Heart begins to beat
27	Arm and leg buds
30	Lens vesicles, optical cups forming
36	Oral and nasal cavities confluent
42	Major organogenesis completed

Reproduced from Moore, 1993, by permission of Saunders.

shown that the important stages of growth in this respect are pre-implantation, organogenesis and foetal development. Figure 18.4 shows this for mice given a dose of 200 cGy at different times during pregnancy (with a comparable time scale for humans).

During the period of pre-implantation (0–9 days in humans) the organism is particularly sensitive to radiation, the $LD_{50/30}$ in mice being one-third that of the mature animal. Irradiation at this stage usually results in death (i.e. abortion) and those organisms that survive may show little abnormality, except those having sex-chromosome aberrations.

It is during the period of active organogenesis (9–42 days) that irradiation will produce severe anatomical malformations. During this phase of development, in which major changes occur quickly in the organization of the embryo, the time of irradiation very much determines the nature and severity of the malformation (Table 18.6). Thus, irradiation at this stage will normally result in severe structural abnormalities, but high doses (in the range of LD_{50} to the mother) will prove lethal to most of the embryos. During the succeeding weeks of foetal development the incidence of anatomical defects after irradiation decreases, except in the brain, eye and gonads, which differentiate relatively late.

Information on the effects of intrauterine exposure of the embryo and foetus has been obtained from studies of the atomic bomb survivors at

Hiroshima and Nagasaki. These investigations over the past 40 years remain the one and only group of studies of the genetic effects of radiation on humans (Neel and Schull, 1991). The principal finding is that there are no statistically significant differences in any of the eight measures used between the 'irradiated' and 'control' groups. The exposed survivors may have sustained an increased germinal mutation rate, but this is too small to be detected.

AVOIDANCE OF IRRADIATION OF EMBRYO

Because of the risks related to irradiation of the embryo and foetus, doctors try to make certain that a pregnant woman is not referred for abdominal X-ray examination. They especially have to consider whether a patient may be in the early stages of pregnancy. In the old days a '10-day' rule was operated. This rule recommended that, unless medical indication required it, X-ray examination of the lower abdomen should be carried out in the first 10 days following the first day of the menstrual cycle. In this way the possibility of irradiating the gravid uterus, even with a low dose, was excluded. However, there is no evidence that irradiation during the first 2 weeks of a pregnancy is any more dangerous than irradiation of the ovum in the weeks before fertilization. The *resting* ovum is relatively resistant to radiation (like other non-dividing cells) but when division begins to occur during the 6–7 weeks before ovulation then radiosensitivity increases. Indeed, it has been calculated that the risk of radiation injury could be greater in the 7 weeks before the mother becomes pregnant than in the first 2 weeks of pregnancy (Russell, 1986).

For this reason the ICRP withdrew support for the 10-day rule in 1984. They said:

> During the first ten days following the onset of a menstrual period, there can be no risk to any conceptus, since no conception will have occurred. The risk to a child who had previously been irradiated *in utero* during the remainder of a four week period following the onset of menstruation is likely to be so small that there need be no special limitation on exposure required within these four weeks.

By the end of that period most women will know if they are pregnant and *then* is the time to avoid unnecessary radiology of the pelvis, when organogenesis is beginning.

If the human embryo is irradiated, the question of therapeutic abortion should be considered. In fact, no hazard has been demonstrated to organogenesis from X-rays at normal diagnostic dose levels in humans, so there is no radiological indication for a termination of pregnancy in a woman accidentally exposed to a uterine dose of less than 5 cGy. Above

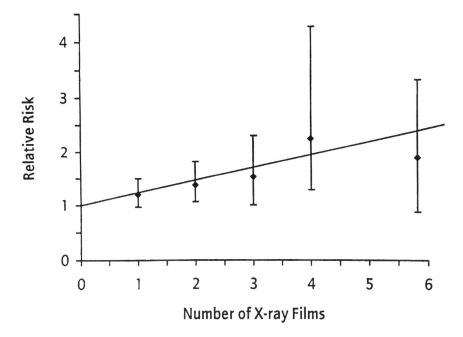

Figure 18.5. The relative risk of childhood cancer after radiation exposure during pregnancy. (Reproduced from Doll and Wakeford, 1997, by permission of BJR.)

that dose level there is increasing risk of congenital abnormality if the radiation was delivered during the period of organogenesis.

Diagnostic radiography during the last 3 months of pregnancy has been shown to increase the risk of childhood cancer. Figure 18.5 shows that the relative risk depends on the number of X-ray films that were taken. The fitted line suggests that there is no threshold dose below which no excess risk arises, but it is concluded that the risk increases with doses of the order of 10 mGy received by the foetus *in utero*.

BENEFIT AND DETRIMENT

Most doses of radiation used in medical diagnosis are at such a low level that it is difficult to find evidence of harm. Many of the effective doses are below the level received from background radiation anyway. That is not to say that the radiation is 'safe', only that the benefit will normally outweigh the detriment. Where that is not so, the question arises of whether that diagnostic procedure is really justifiable and whether some alternative to radiation might be used.

SUMMARY OF CONCLUSIONS

(1) Most 'man-made' ionizing radiation is produced for medical purposes and most of this is for diagnostic examinations using X-rays and radioactive isotopes.
(2) Diagnostic radiation is intended to be beneficial to the patient but doses must still be kept as low as is reasonably achievable (ALARA) so as to reduce harmful effects to a minimum.
(3) Particular care is taken to reduce doses to bone marrow and the gonads. These tissues are given a higher weighting factor when calculating the effective dose delivered by an X-ray examination.
(4) For a chest X-ray the *effective dose* may only be 0.04 mSv, which compares favourably with the 2.6 mSv from background radiation.
(5) With more complicated X-ray examinations and CT scanning the doses will be higher, e.g. 8.3 mSv with a CT chest scan.
(6) Irradiation of the gonads may have genetic effects. The *genetically significant dose* is used to indicate the level of hereditary damage that will follow such gonad doses.
(7) An embryo is most sensitive to radiation during the period of pregnancy from 9 to 42 days, when organogenesis occurs.
(8) Radiation during the last 3 months of pregnancy may increase the risk of childhood cancer.

REFERENCES

Ash, P., 1980. The influence of radiation on fertility in man. *British Journal of Radiology*, **53**, 271–278.
BEIR Committee, 1990. *Health Effects of Exposure to Low Levels of Ionizing Radiation. BEIR V.* Committee on the Biological Effects of Ionizing Radiations of the National Research Council. National Academy Press, Washington, DC.
Clarke, R. H., 1991. 1990 recommendations of ICRP. *Supplement to the Radiological Protection Bulletin*, No. 119, National Radiological Protection Board, Chilton, Oxon.
Doll, R. and Wakeford, R., 1997. Risk of cancer from fetal irradiation. *British Journal of Radiology*, **70**, 130–139.
Hart, D., Hillier, M. C., Wall, B. F., Shrimpton, P. C. and Bungay, D., 1996. Doses to patients from medical X-ray examinations in the UK – 1995 review. *NRPB-R289*. National Radiological Protection Board, HMSO, London.
ICRP, 1982. Protection of the patient in diagnostic radiology. ICRP Publication 34. *Annals of the ICRP*, **9**, 26.
ICRP, 1991. 1990 recommendations of the ICRP. ICRP Publication 60. *Annals of the ICRP*, **21**, 46.
Moore, K. L., 1993. *The Developing Human.* Saunders, Philadelphia.
Mould, R. F., 1985. *Radiation Protection in Hospitals.* Adam Hilger, Bristol.
Mountford, P. J., 1997. Risk assessment of the nuclear medicine patient. *British Journal of Radiology*, **70**, 671–684.
Neel, J. V. and Schull, W. J., 1991. *The Children of Atomic Bomb Survivors, a Genetic Study.* US National Academy, Washington.

NRPB, 1993. Occupational, public and medical exposure. *Documents of the NRPB*, **4** (No. 2). National Radiological Protection Board, HMSO, London.

Oakes, W. R. and Lushbaugh, C. C., 1952. Course of testicular injury following accidental exposure to nuclear radiations. *Radiology*, **59**, 737–743.

Russell, L. B. and Russell, W. L., 1954. An analysis of the changing radiation response of the developing mouse embryo. *Journal of Cellular and Comparative Physiology*, **43** (Suppl. 1), 103–149.

Sankaranarayanan, K., 1996. Radiation mutagenesis in animals and humans and the estimation of genetic risk. In *Health Effects of Exposure to Low-level Ionizing Radiation*, edited by C. W. R. Hendee and F. M. Edwards. IOP Publishing, Bristol.

UK Committee on Radiological Hazards to Patients, 1966. Final report of the Committee, HMSO, London.

UNSCEAR, 1977. *Sources and Effects of Ionizing Radiation*. United Nations, New York.

Wall, B. F., Rae, S., Darby, S. C. and Kendall, G. M., 1982. The NRPB Survey; methods and results. In *Dosimetry in Diagnostic Radiology*, edited by M. Fitzgerald. Hospital Physicists' Association, London.

Withers, H. R., Hunter, N., Barkley, H. T. and Reid, B. O., 1974. Radiation survival and regeneration characteristics of spermatogenic stem cells of mouse testis. *Radiation Research*, **57**, 88–103.

19 Environmental Radiation

Humankind has always been exposed to radiation from the Sun and outer space, and naturally radioactive materials are present in the earth, in the buildings we inhabit and in the food and water we consume. There are radioactive gases in the air we breathe and our bodies are radioactive, but the dose level is relatively low. The average Briton receives an annual dose of 2.6 mSv from these natural sources, amounting to 85.5% of the total annual dose. The rest comes from artificial sources, mostly in medical applications.

Figure 19.1 shows the relative contribution of these various sources to the dose received on average by each person. The largest amounts come from natural radioactivity in the air and from isotopes of radon. These isotopes are the product of the small amounts of uranium and thorium in the ground and in buildings. The main contribution is from radon (i.e. ^{222}Rn), with an average annual dose of about 1.3 mSv. The significance of background radiation from radon will receive more detailed discussion in the next section.

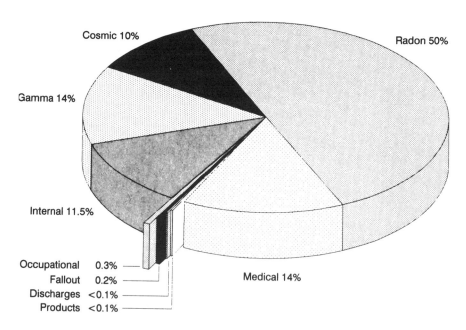

Figure 19.1. Relative contribution of sources of radiation to the population. (Reproduced from Hughes and O'Riordan, 1993, by permission of NRPB/SO.)

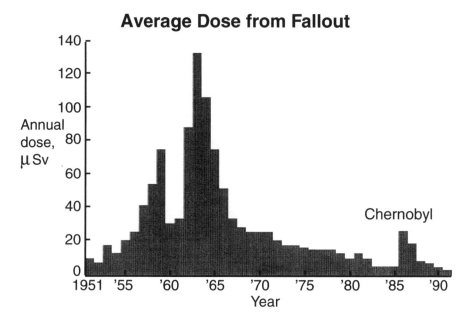

Figure 19.2. Average annual dose from radioactive fallout. (Reproduced from NRPB, 1994, by permission of NRPB/SO.)

Gamma radiation contributes an average of 0.35 mSv/year and arises mainly from long-lived isotopes such as potassium-40 (^{40}K) in rocks and soil. Some of this is incorporated into buildings. Internal exposures come from the ingestion of isotopes such as ^{40}K in food and drink, and the average dose is 0.3 mSv/year. Cosmic radiation from outer space amounts to 0.26 mSv/year on average, but people living at higher altitudes will receive a higher dose because there is less atmosphere to absorb the cosmic radiation, which may rise to three times the dose at about 3000 m.

Apart from the 14% for medical uses (Chapter 18), 'man-made' sources of radiation add up to only a small proportion of the average dose to the public. The fallout from nuclear weapons testing now only produces about 0.005 mSv/year (Figure 19.2), although high rainfall in some parts of the UK raises the fallout dose to 0.015 mSv/year. The Chernobyl accident added an extra 0.037 mSv in 1986 but then the level of radiation rapidly declined. (The same dose would be received during a return flight across the Atlantic! But frequent air travellers receive an annual dose of 3 mSv from cosmic rays and the dose for some couriers may be as high as 8 mSv.) A small proportion of the average involves the exposure of people whose use radiation in their work (0.007 mSv) and an even smaller proportion comes from the nuclear power industry, which amounts to less than 0.001 mSv/year.

This chapter describes the various sources of radiation in the environment that are likely to affect members of the general public and the likely consequences of such radiation. The doses from some sources can be reduced by taking suitable precautions. This applies to radon decay products in the home, ultraviolet radiation in the air and food that has become radioactive from nuclear emissions. The regulatory authorities are supposed to give guidance on these matters to protect the public. Workers in the nuclear industry and industrial radiographers are supposed to take their precautions according to Health and Safety regulations (see Chapter 20). There is an irreducible minimum level of radiation from the natural background and this should only be exceeded for good reason, using the ALARA (as low as is reasonably achievable) principle. The main consequence of unnecessary radiation will be an increase in carcinogenesis, which will be discussed at the end of this chapter.

RADON

Radon-222 is an inert gas that is a decay product of radium-226 (^{226}Ra), the fifth daughter product of uranium-238 (^{238}U). These are present in most soils and rocks from which radon enters the surroundings. As a result, radon is found both indoors and outdoors. It contaminates many underground mines and the miners are found to have an increased risk of lung cancer, especially in smokers. The reason for the lung cancer risk is that radon decays to polonium. This emits alpha particles, which cause 'hot spots' of radiation damage within the lung if the polonium is inhaled with particles of dust or smoke.

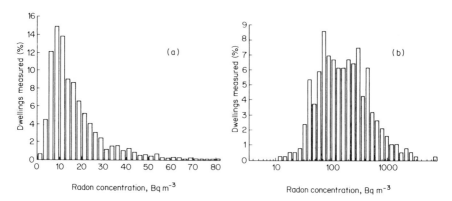

Figure 19.3. Radon concentration in British dwellings: (a) distribution in the United Kingdom; (b) distribution in SW England. (Reproduced from Wrixon et al, 1988, by permission of NRPB/SO.)

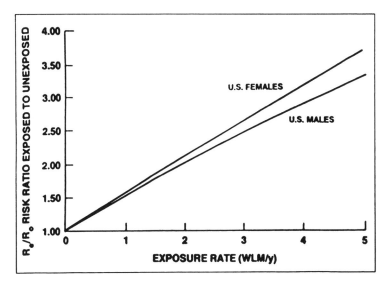

Figure 19.4. Relative risk of mortality from lung cancer after lifetime exposure to radon decay products at constant annual rates. (Reproduced from BEIR Committee, 1988, by permission of National Academy of Sciences.)

Figure 19.1 showed that radon contributes 50% of sources of radiation to the population of the UK. The average concentration of radon in British homes is 20 Bq/m³ (annual dose=1 mSv) but there are areas, such as SW England, where some houses have 20 times that level (Figure 19.3). The average person in Cornwall receives a dose of 7.8 mSv/year (82% from radon), whereas the average dose in London is only 2.1 mSv because radon levels are low. The British government has set an 'action level' of 200 Bq. Building regulations will ensure that no new houses are built that will have radon concentrations above 100 Bq. This will give a dose of radiation in the air of 5 mSv/year.

The main evidence that exposure to radon increases mortality from lung cancer comes from miners working underground, where there are high concentrations of radon decay products. Figure 19.4 shows the increased risk in men and women at constant rates of annual exposure during their lifetime. (These risks are over and above the risk from cigarette smoking, which is the main cause of lung cancer.) The exposure rate is shown in terms of WLM per year: WLM is the so-called 'working level' for a month, which was appropriate for such miners, who received as much as 300 WLM per year in Czechoslovakia earlier in this century. As a consequence, there was a 50% incidence of lung cancer in such miners.

With improvements in the ventilation of mines, the average annual exposure has come down to not much more than 1 WLM. This would deliver an annual dose of 10 mSv of alpha radiation to localized regions in the bronchial epithelium. A value of 1 WLM/year corresponds to about 100 Bq/m^3, but the level in an ordinary home is much lower, of course, and on average this would be 0.2 WLM/year. The increased risk is small, therefore, but this is a stochastic effect (see next paragraph), i.e. there is no threshold dose shown in Figure 19.4. The National Radiological Protection Board (NRPB, 1993) estimates the lifetime risk of cancer as 5.9%/Sv for exposure to such low dose rate radiation. This means that even the small levels of radon in the average home will contribute to an increased incidence of lung cancer in the population as a whole. The best precaution is to ensure adequate ventilation, particularly in homes that are well insulated.

In this context the term *stochastic* is often used to describe detrimental effects for which there is no threshold dose and the severity is independent of dose. Stochastic effects are those for which only the probability of the occurrence of effect, and not its severity, is regarded as a function of dose, without threshold (ICRP, 1984). The principal stochastic effects are considered to be heritable and carcinogenic effects. By contrast, *non-stochastic* (or deterministic) effects are those types of damage that result from the collective injury of substantial numbers of cells in affected tissues. Examples of non-stochastic effects include cataract of the lens, cell depletion in the bone marrow leading to haematological deficiencies and gonadal cell damage leading to impairment of fertility. All these will appear after a latent period.

For non-stochastic effects there is a threshold dose below which no detrimental effects are seen, but thereafter the severity of the effect does depend on the size of the dose. In an ideal world the non-stochastic effects of radiation should be avoidable altogether if the general public keeps below the maximum permissible dose (discussed in Chapter 20). Stochastic effects cannot be avoided because of background radiation.

ULTRAVIOLET RADIATION

Just as radon increases the risk of one particular form of cancer – in the lung – so UV radiation is the main cause of another form in the skin, particularly melanoma; so, although UV is non-ionizing radiation, it deserves discussion in this chapter. Non-ionizing electromagnetic radiation varies in frequency from low-frequency radiowaves, through microwaves and infrared radiation to visible light, and finally to the ultraviolet (UV) part of the spectrum (Figure 19.5). The higher the frequency, the greater is the energy in each photon of radiation, which means that only UV radiation has enough energy to cause photochemical reactions, the lower frequencies merely heating the tissues where they are absorbed. These frequencies are

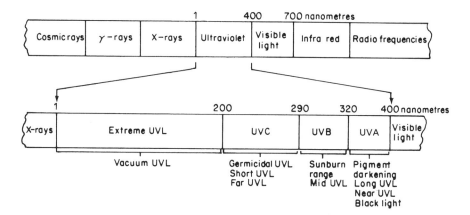

Figure 19.5. The ultraviolet portion of the electromagnetic spectrum. (Reproduced from Lawrence and Marks, 1983, by permission of Update.)

not sufficiently energetic to cause ionization, in contrast to X-rays and γ-rays.

All the UV radiation in the environment comes from the Sun, most of whose energy is in the visible band of the electromagnetic spectrum. Six per cent is radiated in the UV part of the spectrum at wavelengths shorter than 400 nm. Extreme UV light is absorbed by nitrogen and oxygen in the atmosphere and ozone is formed. The ozone absorbs far-UV light between 200 and 300 nm and then there is near-UV light in the band from 300 to 400 nm.

Radiation from 290 to 320 nm is biologically active and it is this UVB radiation that causes sunburn and skin cancer. If the ozone layer in the stratosphere is depleted there will be an increase in the amount of this UV radiation. The best precaution is to avoid excessive exposure to sunlight and avoid the use of 'sun-lamps'. A layer of clothing will always be more protective than a sun-cream.

RADIATION AND FOOD

Many countries in the world permit the sale of properly irradiated food under certain conditions (e.g. labelling to indicate that the food has been irradiated). Such irradiation kills most of the bacteria that occur naturally in food and can also slow down the natural development and ripening of plant material. A food irradiation apparatus incorporates a source of γ-rays from cobalt-60 (^{60}Co) or caesium-137 (^{137}Cs) and a conveyor belt that passes food under the source. Such apparatus has been used for many years to sterilize medical equipment. A dose of 25–50 kGy is needed for such bacterial sterilization: this would eradicate *Escherichia coli* infection but not the prions involved in bovine spongiform encephalopathy (BSE).

Much lower doses are used for food: 1 kGy will inhibit sprouting of potatoes and onions, delay ripening of some fruits (such as apples and strawberries), disinfest cereal grains of insects and eradicate trichinella in pork. Larger doses of 5–10 kGy will extend the shelf-life of foods by reducing microbial loads and eliminating non-sporing pathogens from spices, chicken and fish. Some foods cannot be irradiated without changing the taste and making them unpalatable, e.g. eggs, milk, cheese and other dairy products. The foods that are likely to be sold will taste no different from usual and it may be difficult to tell that they have been irradiated. They will certainly *not* be radioactive because they have been irradiated by γ-rays from an external source such as ^{137}Cs.

In contrast, some foodstuffs may contain radioactive isotopes such as ^{137}Cs because of pollution of the food chain from radioactive fallout, either from nuclear weapons tests or reactor accidents (e.g. Chernobyl in 1986). The other main pollutant is iodine-131 (^{131}I) which will concentrate in and irradiate the thyroid gland. Because the half-life of ^{131}I is only 8 days, the food chain is only contaminated for a short period of time and steps can be taken to block uptake into the thyroid by taking potassium iodide or, better

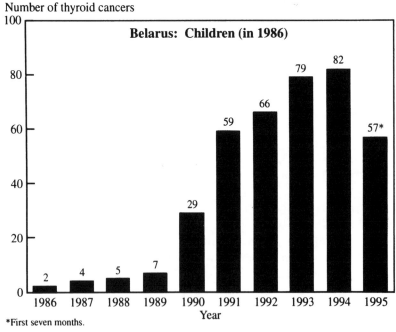

Figure 19.6. Thyroid cancers in children in Belarus. (Reproduced from Wachholz, 1996, by permission of Oxford University Press.)

still, avoiding such contaminated foods for a few weeks. Unfortunately, radioactive iodine from the Chernobyl fallout has caused an increasing number of cases of thyroid cancer in children of the locality (Figure 19.6).

By contrast, the half-life of ^{137}Cs is 30 years and there was prolonged contamination of the countryside, especially downwind from the source of the radioactive cloud, which travelled some distance before precipitation by rainfall. The regulatory authorities had to set 'safety' levels to guide farmers and fishermen as to when it would be permissible to sell their produce. These could only be arbitrary levels because, with natural background radiation, a zero level of radioactivity is unobtainable.

NUCLEAR POWER INDUSTRY

According to the official limits the general public should not receive more than 0.15% of their total radiation exposure from the nuclear industry. Those who choose to work in the industry are 'allowed' a higher dose but ALARA applies to them also (Chapter 20).

Most of the reactors in nuclear power stations are thermal reactors fuelled by a mixture of natural ^{238}U enriched with ^{235}U. This enrichment (from the normal 0.7% to 2.4%) needs to be done in order to increase the fuel's ability to sustain a chain reaction. The fission of uranium generates a large amount of heat, which is converted to steam and used to drive electricity generators. The amount of heat produced depends upon the position of the control rods around the fuel elements. Fission products are gradually formed within the fuel elements and some of these absorb neutrons.

Eventually, there are insufficient neutrons for further fission and the fuel elements have to be removed for reprocessing. Spent fuel is sent to a reprocessing plant (e.g. Sellafield) where valuable fission products such as plutonium are separated from waste products. Plutonium can be used as a substitute for ^{235}U in thermal reactors, as the fuel for fast-breeder reactors and for nuclear weapons.

The spent fuel elements are stored for 3 months in cooling ponds to allow the short-lived radioactive isotopes to decay before the reprocessing procedures are begun. Radioactive particles are filtered from gases before they are released from high chimneys. Low-activity liquid waste is released into rivers or the sea. This release of gases and liquid is carefully controlled and only amounts to 1% of the long-lived radioactivity produced by the nuclear power industry. Even so, the amount of ^{137}Cs released into the Irish Sea from Sellafield has reached significant levels, although still within the official limit. High-level liquid waste and solid waste has to be stored and this presents an increasing problem of space, security and safety. Nevertheless, the average dose to the general population from the discharge of radioactivity by the nuclear power industry is less than 1 μSv/year.

Shellfish, however, concentrate radioactive materials, so heavy consumers of seafoods in Cumbria can receive somewhat higher doses.

A possible association between paternal radiation exposure sustained by radiation workers and leukaemia in their children was raised by Gardner et al (1990). The view that mutations in the gonads of radiation workers might be passed on to their children as a malignancy led to much research. The current consensus is that there is no firm evidence for such an association (Doll et al, 1994).

OCCUPATIONAL DOSES

People who choose to work with ionizing radiation may be exposed to higher doses than the general public. Table 19.1 shows the doses received by fuel reprocessing workers at Sellafield in 1996. The average annual dose was 1.7 mSv and this gives a total collective dose of 11.6 man-Sv for all the workers added together. (In 1988 the figures were 5 mSv and 30 man-Sv, respectively.) In 1996 only one worker received more than the 20 mSv limit now recommended for occupational workers (Chapter 20). The average dose received by the 10 000 workers in all the establishments in the UK was 1.5 mSv.

As with medical exposure (Chapter 18), occupational exposure to radiation affects only a small number of people, i.e. 156 000 in the UK (NRPB, 1994). The overall doses received by such workers show that the most exposed were those who received their doses from natural sources (e.g. in radon areas). Very few workers received more than the 20 mSv dose limit (Chapter 20) in a year. Average annual doses are: 1 mSv for the nuclear industry, 0.5 mSv for general radiation workers and 0.1 mSv for medical radiation workers.

These doses should be compared with the 2.6 mSv annual background dose. Average doses in the nuclear industry in 1991 were half those in 1987.

Table 19.1. Distribution of dose for fuel reprocessing workers at Sellafield (1996)

Dose range (mSv)	Number of workers
0–5	6088
5–10	581
10–15	71
15–20	1
20–30	0
30–40	0
40–50	0
>50	1
Total workers	6742
Collective exposure man Sv	11.6
Average exposure mSv	11.7

Reproduced from BNFL, 1996, by permission of BNFL.

Most workers in nuclear power stations and medical radiation would be put in a low dose category. The higher dose group includes industrial radiographers (who have a poor safety record), uranium miners, the crews of jet aircraft and some of those who work in nuclear reactors, nuclear fuel reprocessing and the manufacture of radiation sources for industry and medicine. Except for medical exposures, the percentage contribution to the population from all the other sources amounts to less than 1% of the total.

RADIATION CARCINOGENESIS AND LEUKAEMOGENESIS

Much concern is expressed about the carcinogenic effects of ionizing radiations and yet, compared to many chemical agents, these radiations are not highly dangerous in this respect. The leukaemias are the most important neoplastic diseases induced by ionizing radiations. UNSCEAR (1988) predicted a lifetime fatal cancer risk of 5% in a population exposed to 1 Sv of whole-body radiation. Nowadays, the ICRP (1993) suggests a variable risk dependent on the dose rate and the age at exposure.

Table 19.2 shows the reason for this variation. At high dose and high dose rates (HDR) the percentage risk of death per sievert is twice as high as it is for low doses and low dose rates (LDR). In both cases the risk falls with age as the lifetime of exposure becomes shorter. For a general UK population the total risk of radiation-induced cancer is estimated from these figures as 11.8%/Sv for exposure to low linear energy transfer (LET) radiation at HDR and 5.9%/Sv at LDR. The total level of background radiation, including natural and other sources, in the UK is about 2.6 mSv/year and the number of cancers produced by this order of dose is very small indeed (approximately 2%) compared to the number of cases from other causes. In respect of leukaemia, however, it has been estimated that 10% of all cases may be due to radiation exposure and that perhaps over half of the other forms of cancer in humans are caused by chemicals.

Because the incidence of malignant change following irradiation is so small, large populations at risk have to be studied to allow reliable interpretation to be made of the observations. Because the latent period for the induction of cancer is so long, 5–8 years for leukaemia and perhaps 15 or more years for most other forms of cancer, these observations have to be made for very many years in most circumstances. There is uncertainty about the spontaneous incidence rates of cancer and leukaemia in particular populations. Deaths from intercurrent diseases also make comparative analysis of data from exposed populations a difficult statistical exercise. The incidence of both cancer and leukaemia naturally increases with age and this factor must be controlled carefully in assessing the risks of radiation.

Exposure to ionizing radiations certainly increases the natural rate of malignant transformations in some organs, but the amount by which the

Table 19.2. Estimates of radiation-induced fatal cancer risks in the UK

	Deaths (10^{-2}/Sv) Lifetime projection	
Age at exposure (years)	High dose rate	Low dose rate
0–9	22.3	11.1
10–19	19.8	9.9
20–29	13.1	6.6
30–39	8.9	4.5
40–49	8.4	4.2
50–59	8.0	4.0
60–69	6.2	3.1
70–79	3.3	1.6
80+	1.5	0.75

Reproduced from NRPB, 1993, by permission of NRPB/SO.

probability is increased in relation to the dose of radiation received is often uncertain and ill understood. It is still not possible to exclude the existence of a threshold dose below which there is no increased incidence of cancer, although this is thought to be unlikely. The evidence shown in Figure 19.4 certainly implied that there is no threshold for the effect of radon, so that radiation carcinogenesis is a stochastic effect.

If the incidence of cancer is a linear function of radiation dose, this implies a single-event transformation with dose. Such a hypothesis is not supported by most other evidence but some clinical data are consistent with this theory (see Chapter 18, Figure 18.5). A linear function would certainly be more convenient for risk assessment.

In 1980 the Biological Effects of Ionizing Radiations (BEIR) Committee offered the choice of three mathematical solutions. In Figure 19.7 the top-left diagram shows the general form of the dose–response data, including the relatively higher dose range. As dose increases, the incidence of cancer increases up to a point but then decreases at higher dose levels. The reason for this is illustrated by the experimental data shown in Figure 19.8. The upper part shows a survival curve for normal cells from a mouse embryo ($10\,T\frac{1}{2}$ cells), with the usual shoulder portion for doses up to 500 cGy; thereafter, the curve is exponential with $D_0 = 150$ cGy. The lower part of Figure 19.8 shows a curve for malignant transformation of these cells (see Chapter 12), which rises to a maximum at 500 cGy and then falls, with a final slope parallel to that of the cell survival curve. Thus, with higher doses, cell killing exceeds malignant transformation and so the relative incidence of malignant change is much lower.

The main problem arises over the low dose range. If we return to Figure 19.7, the other three diagrams provide a choice between a simple linear, a

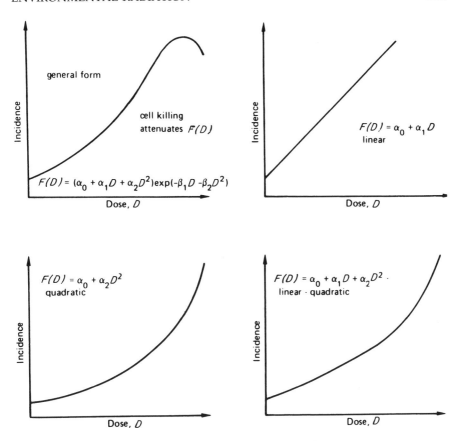

Figure 19.7. Alternative dose–response curves for radiation carcinogenesis. (Reproduced from BEIR Committee, 1980, by permission of National Academy of Sciences.)

pure quadratic and a linear-quadratic dose response. In 1980 the majority of the BEIR Committee chose the linear-quadratic version, but the subject remains controversial and a later BEIR Committee report (1990) did not resolve it. This is because very low doses can only produce such small effects. Statistically significant data might only be obtained from 'mega-mouse' experiments but 'mega-human' surveys are really needed to estimate the additional risk to human populations of exposure to such low-level radiation, bearing in mind the irreducible background level of natural radiation. None of the curves in Figure 19.7 start at zero because there is a natural level of cancer incidence.

A typical dose–response relationship for induction of cancer and leukaemia *in vivo* is illustrated by the curve of Figure 19.9. Like the *in vitro* curve in Figure 19.8, there is an initial ascending part rising to a

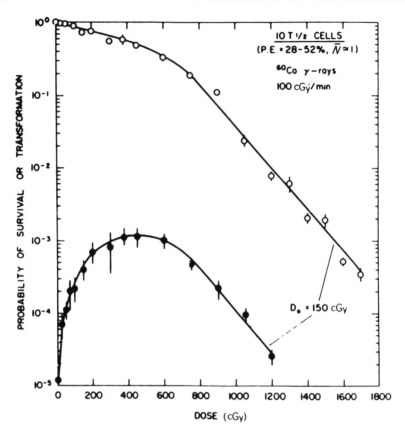

Figure 19.8. Survival and malignant transformation of 10 T½ cells exposed to ⁶⁰Co gamma rays. (Reproduced from Han et al, 1980, by permission of AACR.)

summit before a final descending part. It is the accurate measurement of the initial part of the curve that has proved to be difficult to determine with animal experiments because, in this very low dose range (under 100 cGy), unacceptably large numbers of animals would be required.

Not only is the total dose of radiation important in relation to cancer induction, but also the dose rate. The evidence seems to indicate that higher dose rates are more effective (Table 19.2). This is drawn schematically in Figure 19.10. The carcinogenic effect of low LET radiation is shown both as the usual bell-shaped curve (A) and as a linear interpolation (B), two of the choices in Figure 19.7. Curves C and D represent the effect of low-dose-rate radiation when it is of low LET. Curve D shows the limiting slope for very low doses and dose rates. Curve C shows the slope for intermediate dose rates (NRPB, 1995).

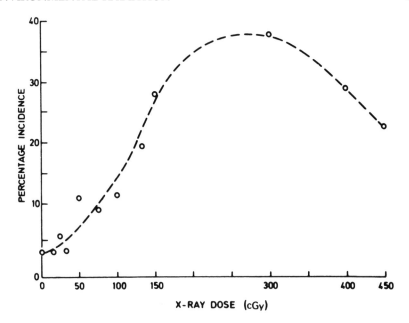

Figure 19.9. Incidence of myeloid leukaemia in mice following TBI. (Reproduced from Upton, 1961, by permission of AACR.)

The quality of radiation is also important and high-LET radiations, such as fast neutrons, are much more effective in producing transformation than low-LET radiations. For this reason the high-LET curve (H) in Figure 19.10 is steeper and also 'bends over' after a lower dose because cells are more sensitive to such radiation. Furthermore, there is no dose rate effect with high-LET radiation. On the other hand, the relative biological effectiveness (RBE) of high-LET radiations is dose dependent (Chapter 9) and some caution has to be exercised in assuming single values for carcinogenesis and leukaemogenesis, especially when the mechanisms involved may be different for different tissues. For example, an RBE of 20 for fast neutrons has been reported for the induction of thyroid cancer in a certain strain of rat, and more information is needed on these effects in other tissues and organs.

MECHANISMS OF CARCINOGENESIS

The nature of the essential injury that produces malignant transformation is still being worked out by molecular biological techniques. In the field of chemical carcinogenesis, three stages were believed to be required and these had to follow the correct sequence:

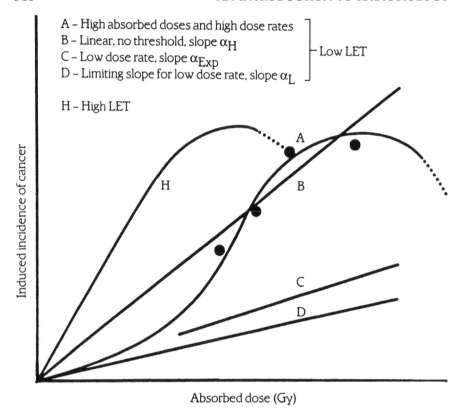

A - High absorbed doses and high dose rates ⎤
B - Linear, no threshold, slope α_H ⎥
C - Low dose rate, slope α_{Exp} ⎥─ Low LET
D - Limiting slope for low dose rate, slope α_L ⎦

H - High LET

Induced incidence of cancer (y-axis)

Absorbed dose (Gy) (x-axis)

Figure 19.10. Dose–response relationship for radiation-induced cancer. (Reproduced from NRPB, 1995, by permission of NRPB/SO.)

(1) initiation (e.g. by dimethyl benzanthracene);
(2) promotion (e.g. by croton oil);
(3) progression.

The third stage was necessary before frankly malignant tumour cells were produced.

In radiation carcinogenesis these initiation, promotion and progression stages may also apply but the random distribution of radiation lesions to the genome will fulfil these requirements from time to time according to the dose, dose rate and LET factors already described. Although carcinogenesis is a multi-step cellular process, it seems to have its origins in single gene mutations in single cells. As mentioned earlier, there is no evidence for a low dose threshold for radiation carcinogenesis.

In the view of the NRPB (1993): at low doses, radiation probably contributes to cancer risk by increasing the number of initiated cells rather than increasing the progress of pre-neoplastic cells towards full malignancy.

With respect to cellular DNA repair, this will not be totally error-free and the repair of tumour-initiating DNA lesions is also unlikely to lead to a low dose threshold for carcinogenesis. With ionizing radiation, tumour initiation due to gene loss mutations is likely to be more frequent than that involving DNA base-pair changes.

There is a normal baseline frequency at which errors occur in the genome but radiation will induce additional *genomic instability* (see Chapter 6 and Morgan et al, 1996). If there is already a genetic defect in a cell population, then further damage to the DNA structure will be that much easier to induce. This is shown by patients with xeroderma pigmentosum, who carry a high probability of developing skin cancer after exposure to UV radiation and have defective repair of DNA-induced radiation lesions. Patients with ataxia–telangiectasia have a similar repair deficiency but they are more sensitive to X-irradiation and have increased tendency to develop lymphoma.

ATOMIC BOMB EXPLOSIONS

The survivors of the atomic bomb explosions in Hiroshima and Nagasaki in 1945 provide the best evidence in humans of an increased incidence of both leukaemia and various forms of cancer following irradiation. It used to be thought that there was a difference in the incidence of leukaemia between the survivors of the Hiroshima and Nagasaki bombs because the two bombs emitted different proportions of gamma and neutron radiation. Modern dosimetry seems to suggest that there were virtually no neutrons at either city (Straume et al, 1996). This means that the data can now be fitted to a single dose–response curve that has a similar shape (over the first 2 Gy) to those in Figures 19.8 and 19.9 (for low-LET radiation) and fits the linear-quadratic model in Figure 19.7. There was obviously a problem of dosimetry at the time of the explosions: Figure 19.11 shows that the subsequent incidence of leukaemia in Hiroshima was 10–15 times higher in those living within 5000 m of the hypocentre of the bomb than in those who lived elsewhere (and are presumed not to have been irradiated).

THE LATENT PERIOD

There is always a long latent period of a number of years between the time of irradiation and the clinical appearance of the induced cancer. The processes that account for this delay are not known, but it may indicate that factors other than irradiation are involved in promotion of the neoplastic disease. The long latent period may simply be a reflection of the number of transformed cells and their cellular kinetics, which leads to the slow accumulation of such abnormal cells. The latent period is shorter for leukaemia than for other cancers, with a minimum of 4–5 years and a mean

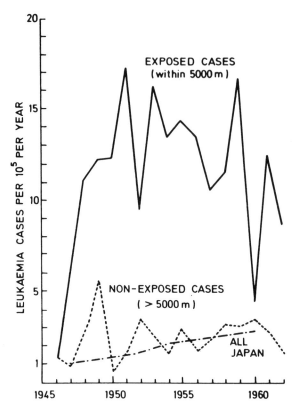

Figure 19.11. Incidence of leukaemia in Hiroshima. (Reproduced from UNSCEAR, 1964, by permission of United Nations.)

of 8 years. Figure 19.11 covers the first 25 years after the bombs were dropped. It shows that the leukaemia incidence at Hiroshima had peaked by 1950. Figure 19.12 covers the 30 years between 1950 and 1980 and shows that, after the peak in 1950, the incidence of leukaemia declined at a rate of 10.7% per year; but the period of risk continues.

The latent period for other types of cancer is much longer, with a minimum of 10 years and a mean of about 15 years. The period of risk continues for more than 25 years. This is shown in Figure 19.12, where, although the incidence of such cancers in Hiroshima was much lower than it was for leukaemia, the curve was still rising at a rate of 4.8% per year. These figures refer to the relative risk of leukaemogenesis and carcinogenesis at a dose level of 1 Gy. They refer to an increase in malignant disease over and above the 'natural' incidence due to other causes.

These studies on the mortality of atomic bomb survivors were extended up to 1990 by Pierce et al (1996): 86 572 people were analysed, 60% of whom

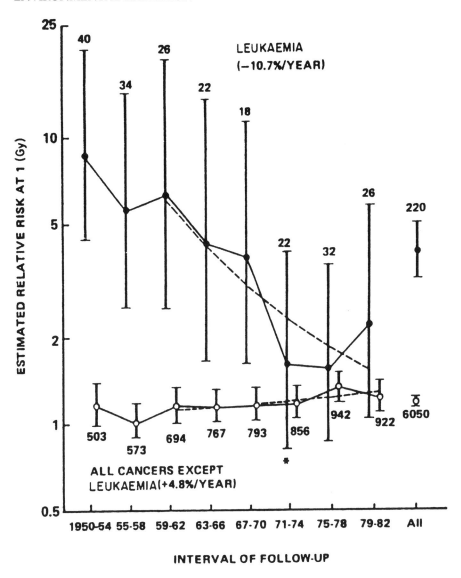

Figure 19.12. Relative risk of mortality from leukaemia or other cancers in atomic bomb survivors (the numbers of deaths are shown for each confidence interval). (Reproduced from Preston et al, 1987, by permission of Academic Press, Inc.)

had received a dose of at least 5 mSv. During the period 1950–1990 there were 420 excess cancer deaths, of which 85 were due to leukaemia. As already shown, most of the excess for leukaemia occurred in the first 15 years after exposure. For solid cancers the pattern of excess risk is more like a life-long elevation of the natural age-specific risk. The excess lifetime risk per sievert for solid cancers for those exposed at age 30 years was estimated to be 10% for males and 14% for females. The risk for leukaemia was estimated to be 1.5%/Sv for males and 0.8% for females.

The purpose of this chapter has been to describe the sources of radiation that occur in the environment and the dose levels that are involved. Some of these doses can be reduced if suitable precautions are taken, but the doses from natural background radiation cannot be avoided. Earlier chapters have described the various biological effects of radiation. Most of the responses abate but some of the late responses do not, and these detrimental effects are the risks of radiation.

Although the dosage varies in different parts of the country, radiation from the environment affects everybody. There is no such thing as a zero level of radiation dosage from natural background sources. By contrast, dosage from medical and other artificial sources of radiation can be avoided; only a small proportion of the population is exposed to such sources. When those doses are averaged out over the whole population they are very much lower than those from natural sources. In comparison with the 2.6 mSv from background radiation, the annual average dose from medical uses (Chapter 18) is 0.37 mSv and from all the other artificial sources it is less than 0.013 mSv.

The consequence of all this is that natural background radiation contributes only about 2% of all the cancers in the population, 1% of the genetic disorders and 0–0.5% of severe mental retardation. The risks from the medical uses of radiation are an order of magnitude smaller, while the contribution from the nuclear industry is a further order of magnitude smaller, i.e. only 1% of all the detrimental effects of background radiation (Coggle, 1990).

SUMMARY OF CONCLUSIONS

(1) About 85.5% of environmental radiation comes from natural sources and there is a total dose of 2.6 mSv per annum.
(2) Much of this is from ^{222}Rn in the air and this dosage can be reduced by adequate ventilation of buildings.
(3) Ultraviolet radiation is not iodizing but is biologically active, UVB causes sunburn and skin cancer.
(4) Some foodstuffs can be sterilized by irradiation.
(5) The nuclear power industry uses enriched uranium whose waste products need to be reprocessed safely. Reprocessing workers are exposed to higher doses of radiation than other radiation workers but the average annual dose is still only 1.5 mSv.

(6) Radiation is a known carcinogen and there is no dose threshold; this is a *stochastic effect*. The cancer risk is 12%/Sv at high doses and dose rates and 6%/Sv at low doses and dose rates.

(7) There is a latent period of about 5 years for leukaemia and 10 years for other cancers between irradiation and the incidence of the disease.

(8) Background radiation is responsible for only 2% of cancers and 1% of genetic disorders in the population.

REFERENCES

BEIR Committee, 1980. *The Effects on Population Exposure to Low Levels of Ionizing Radiation*. 1980 Committee on the Biological Effects of Ionizing Radiation of the National Research Council. National Academy Press, Washington, DC.

BEIR Committee, 1988. *Health Risks of Radon and Other Internally Deposited Alpha-emitters*. Committee on the Biological Effects of Ionizing Radiation of the National Research Council. National Academy Press, Washington, DC.

BEIR Committee, 1990. *Health Effects of Exposure to Low Levels of Ionizing Radiation. BEIR V*. Committee on the Biological Effects of Ionizing Radiations of the National Research Council. National Academy Press, Washington, DC.

BNFL, 1996. *Safety and Health. Annual Report 1996*. Safety, Health and Environment Directorate, British Nuclear Fuels, Risley, Cheshire.

Coggle, J. E., 1990. Medical effects of low doses of ionizing radiation. *Journal of Radiation Protection Dosimetry*, **30**, 5–12.

Doll, Evans and Darby, 1994. Paternal exposure is not to blame. *Nature*, **367**, 678–680.

Gardner, M. J., Snee, M. P., Hall, A. J., et al, 1990. Results of a case-control study of leukaemia and lymphoma among young people near Sellafield nuclear plant in West Cumbria. *British Medical Journal*, **300**, 423–429.

Han, A., Hill, C. K. and Elkind, M. M., 1980. Repair of cell killing and neoplastic transformation at reduced dose-rates of ^{60}Cobalt gamma rays. *Cancer Research*, **40**, 1–18.

Hughes, J. S. and O'Riordan, M. C., 1993. *Radiation Exposure of the UK Population – 1993 Review*. National Radiological Protection Board, HMSO, London.

ICRP, 1977. Recommendations of the International Commission on Radiological Protection. *ICRP Publications 26 and 27*. Pergamon Press, Oxford.

ICRP, 1984. Non-stochastic effects of ionizing radiation. *ICRP Publication 41*. Pergamon Press, Oxford.

Lawrence, C. and Marks, J., 1983. Psoriasis, aetiology and treatment. *Hospital Update*, **9**, 271–285.

Morgan, W. F., Day, J. P., Kaplan, M. I., McGhee, E. M. and Limoli, C. L., 1996. Genomic instability induced by radiation. *Radiation Research*, **146**, 247–258.

NRPB, 1993. Estimates of late radiation risks to the UK population. *Documents of the NRPB*, **4** (no. 4). National Radiological Protection Board, HMSO, London.

NRPB, 1994. *At-a-Glance Series: Radiation Doses – Maps and Magnitudes*, 2nd edn. National Radiological Protection Board, HMSO, London.

NRPB, 1995. Risk of radiation-induced cancer at low doses and low dose rates for radiation protection purposes. *Documents of the NRPB*, **6** (no. 1). National Radiological Protection Board, HMSO, London.

Pierce, D. A., Shimizu, Y., Preston, D. L., Vaeth, M. and Mabuchi, K., 1996. Studies of the mortality of atomic bomb survivors. Report 12, Part 1. Cancer: 1950–1990. *Radiation Research*, **146**, 1–27.

Preston, D. K., Kato, H., Kopecky, K. J. and Fugita, S., 1987. Studies of the mortality of A-bomb survivors. 8. Cancer mortality 1950–1982. *Radiation Research*, **111**, 151–178.

UNSCEAR, 1964. *Nineteenth Session, Suppl. 14 [A/5184]*. United Nations Scientific Committee on the Effects of Atomic Radiation. United Nations, New York.

UNSCEAR, 1988. *Sources, Effects and Risks of Ionizing Radiation*. United Nations Scientific Committee on the Effects of Atomic Radiation. United Nations, New York.

Upton, A. C., 1961. The dose–response relation in radiation induced cancer. *Cancer Research*, **21**, 717–729.

Wachholz, B. W., 1996. Thyroid cancers in children in Belarus. *Journal of the National Cancer Institute*, **88**, 946.

Wrixon, A. D., Green, B. M. R., Lomas, P. R., Miles, J. C. H., Cliff, K. D., Francis, E. A., Driscoll, C. M. H., James, A. C. and O'Riordan, M. C., 1988. *Natural Radiation Exposure in UK Dwellings*. National Radiological Protection Board, NRPB-R190, HMSO, London.

20 Radiation Protection

There is an unavoidable level of ionizing radiation in the environment. The dosage varies but it can always be measured in the atmosphere and in the ground. The guiding principle of radiation protection does not therefore strive for zero dosage, which is obviously unobtainable. Instead, the aim is to reduce all additional dosage from 'man-made' sources to a level that is as low as is reasonably achievable – ALARA. In the medical field, there are radiation procedures that can be beneficial to some patients. Such benefit has to be set against the detriment that has been shown by this book to follow all radiation dosage. A large benefit will obviously outweigh a small detriment. These are the considerations that guide the ICRP (International Commission on Radiological Protection) when it recommends 'safety limits' to guide users of radiation.

This chapter will describe the ICRP recommendations both for the general public and for those whose occupation involves ionizing radiation. Unlike many chemical hazards, radiation can be monitored with great accuracy; routine dosimetry will be discussed, with special emphasis on the sievert unit. It is sometimes possible for the equivalent dose of a chemical hazard to be measured in terms of a radiobiological parameter, and this will be illustrated. For the most part, however, the detrimental effects of radiation can be compared most easily with those from other hazards in terms of the deaths that they cause. This is because mortality is a definite fact for which there are firm statistics, in contrast to those for morbidity and social discomfort.

RISK COMPARISONS

Deaths from the peaceful uses of nuclear radiation are very uncommon. Up to now, the worst accident at a nuclear power station was the one at Chernobyl in 1986. By 1989 the only deaths were of the 31 people actually involved in the power station at the time (although there have since been increasing numbers of children suffering from thyroid cancer; see Figure 19.6). The Three Mile Island accident in 1979 did not lead to any deaths. By contrast, 167 workers died at the Piper Alpha oil rig fire in 1988 and 3300 people died at the Bophal chemical accident in 1984.

It has been estimated that, because the emissions from coal-fired power stations lead to premature deaths from lung and other diseases, there would actually be a saving of 72 lives for every 1000 MW if nuclear power was substituted for coal. Nuclear power stations emit radioactive materials but oil- and coal-fired power stations discharge sulphur dioxide. If one compares the lethal doses of such emissions, then the limits set for nuclear power stations are 100 times lower than those for fossil fuel stations.

The problem of disposing of radioactive waste from nuclear power stations is very real but at least the isotopes *decay* in radioactivity and, of course, the radiation dose can very easily be measured because of the physical nature of radiation. By contrast, some chemicals may never be made safe and are difficult to measure. The dioxin released from the chemical accident at Seveso in 1976 still remains unchanged as a toxic pollutant in that region of Italy.

The most objective method of measuring the risks of radiation is to compare the risks with those of other categories. Table 20.1 makes this comparison in terms of the average lifespan shortening associated with each factor. Radiation proves to be one of the safest and, not surprisingly, smoking one of the most dangerous. Radon has already been shown to be more dangerous than medical X-rays in Chapter 19. The modes of death will be different, however, because cancer is the fatal risk for radiation workers and physical injury is the usual cause of death with other categories.

The cancer risk of the radiation workers is based upon the fact that some of them receive an average dose of 1.7 mSv/year (Chapter 19, Table 19.1).

Table 20.1. Average lifespan shortening associated with various categories

Category	Days
Cigarette smoking (male)	2400
Heart disease	2100
30% overweight	1560
Cancer	980
Stroke	700
Accidents with small cars	290
Accidents at home	74
Accidents at work	60
AIDS	55
Jogging (for 30 years)	50
Radon in homes	29
Drowning	24
Natural radiation (excl. radon)	9
Medical X-rays	6
Reactor accidents	0.02–2
Smoke alarm at home	−9
Seat belts in cars	−69

Reproduced from Cohen, 1991, by permission of *Health Phys.*

Because the overall fatal cancer risk is 5.9%/Sv, the annual risk for the radiation workers will be 10^{-4}. It is this sort of risk estimate that is used by the ICRP (and the NRPB in the UK) when they set 'safe limits' for radiation, both for those working in the industry and for the general public.

DOSE LIMITS

The aim of all the recommended levels of radiation dose is to strike a working balance between the advantages to a population of a controlled level of radiation exposure and the detrimental effects. The medical use of X-rays has obvious advantages to those who are ill, but indiscriminate exposure to radiation is detrimental to the healthy. The recommended doses of radiation are expressed as yearly limits (Table 20.2). It is recommended that the general population should not normally receive an annual dose to the whole body that is greater than 1 mSv; this excludes both background radiation (Chapter 19) and any medical exposure they may come to receive (Chapter 18).

It is obvious why such a level has been set because it would be pointless to go much lower than the unavoidable minimum level in the background. The possible detriment of a small increase in radiation over and above that minimum is outweighed by the advantage to be gained by the careful use of diagnostic X-rays. For those who choose an occupation that involves exposure to radiation, the standards are less stringent. Their dose to the whole body must not exceed 20 mSv/year but some less important organs may receive considerably higher doses. In each case the dose is ten times higher than is permitted for the general population. In all circumstances, however, the guiding principle is to keep the dose as low as is reasonably achievable (ALARA).

The 20 mSv/year limit given in Table 20.2 for radiation workers amounts to nearly 12 times their present average of 1.7 mSv. If such a dose *was* received,

Table 20.2. Recommended dose limits

Application	Dose limit	
	Occupational	Public
Effective dose	20 mSv/year averaged over defined periods of 5 years	1 mSv/year
Annual equivalent dose in:		
Lens of the eye	150 mSv	15 mSv
Skin	500 mSv	50 mSv
Hands and feet	500 mSv	–

Reproduced from ICRP, 1991, by permission of ICRP.

then radiation would become a more dangerous category in Table 20.1. As a rule, however, the dose can usually be kept to no more than one-tenth of the recommended limit. The limits are higher for individual organs than for the whole body because of the 'weighting factors' (Chapter 18, Table 18.2) used by the ICRP for such organs and tissues. It is obviously more hazardous when radiation is delivered to the whole body (Chapter 14) but individual organs and tissues do vary in their susceptibility to the detrimental effects of radiation, and this applies especially to carcinogenesis.

Table 20.2 is mainly concerned with the limits for stochastic effects. These are different from those for deterministic (non-stochastic) effects because there is no threshold dose and the severity of the effect is independent of the size of the dose. Carcinogenesis is the main stochastic effect; very small doses may transform cells to malignancy and lead to cancer. For deterministic effects there *is* a threshold dose below which no detrimental effects are seen, but above that threshold the severity of the effect does depend on the size of the dose. Examples of deterministic effects include the sort of radiation pathology described in Chapter 13 (e.g. damage to blood vessels, the kidney, the nervous system and the eye, i.e. cataract) and genetic effects (Chapter 18).

Nowadays the objectives of radiation risk management are to prevent deterministic risks altogether and to restrict stochastic risk to acceptable levels. The obvious exception is radiotherapy, where a deterministic effect is intentional. Clarke (1997) listed three principles:

(1) Justification – should provide more benefit than detriment, i.e. do more good than harm.
(2) Optimization – ALARA economic and social factors are taken into account but individual doses are constrained.
(3) Dose limits – monitor with a film badge on the person for medium doses or in the workplace for lower doses.

Table 20.3 shows how radiation risk assessment can be categorized in terms of 'acceptability'. A dose in excess of 20 mSv/year is now unacceptable. One should bear in mind that the present risk of a car fatality is 1/10 000 per year, so the 'tolerable' risk of < 5/10 000 from a dose range of 10–20 mSv seems to strike the right balance.

DOSE MONITORING

The various methods of radiation dosimetry were described in Chapter 4. Some of these are suitable for routine monitoring of radiation personnel. Hospital staff who work with X-rays wear a film badge that is changed once a month. Calibration curves are produced by exposing films to a ^{137}Cs reference source at known dose levels. These are then used to convert the

Table 20.3. Risk assessment

	Unacceptable	Tolerable	Acceptable	Trivial
Dose	>20 mSv	10–20 mSv	Few mSv	<1 mSv
Risk	>1 in 1000	<5 in 10 000	<1 in 10 000	<1 in 100 000

Reproduced from Clarke, 1997, by permission of Royal Society of Medicine.

optical densities measured under the different filter areas of the badge holder to apparent doses, from which the true dose can be calculated. The film can detect a dose as low as 0.05 mSv if diagnostic X-rays are involved. With X-rays of higher energy (as used for radiotherapy) the badge is less sensitive and the minimum dose that it can detect is 0.2 mSv.

As an alternative, thermoluminescent dosimetry (TLD) can be used. Chips of lithium fluoride can detect 0.2 mSv of X-rays of any energy and the chips can be placed at some point of interest in the body and then 'read out' after whatever period of time is convenient. New TLDs are being developed with a sensitivity of >0.01 mSv. Staff at special risk can also carry a pocket monitor in the form of an integrating dosimeter with a digital read-out that can detect 1 μSv. The usual monitoring device is a Geiger dose-rate counter, which can read down to 1 μSv/h. It is also possible to get scintillation monitors that are 10 times more sensitive.

Biological dosimetry can be used in the case of an accidental exposure to radiation. Chromosomal aberrations can be detected in a blood sample taken some time after the event. The technique was described in Chapter 5 (see Figure 5.8), as is the FISH technique that can also be used for this purpose (Lucas et al, 1992).

Table 20.4 shows the range of lifetime doses received by about 95 000 workers in the UK National Registry for Radiation Workers (NRRW). Analysis of these data (Kendall et al, 1992) showed that the mean lifetime dose received was 33.6 mSv, but over 8000 workers received more than 100 mSv. The majority of such people work in the field of diagnostic radiology, where very low doses are the general rule. A small number work in that branch of radiotherapy that involves the use of radioactive sources, such as radium or [137]Cs. In 1981 this sort of work was often performed by a small group of more senior staff, and a survey of occupational exposure in NW England showed that 33 people received annual doses of 10 mSv or more

Table 20.4. Lifetime doses received by workers in the National Registry for Radiation Workers

Average dose (mSv)		2	14	32	71	140	278	594
Proportion of population (%)	62	10	12	7	5	3	1

Reproduced from NRPB, 1995, by permission of NRPB/SO.

(Pratt and Sweeney, 1989). Nowadays this work is shared amongst more staff in order to follow the ALARA principle, and only seven people received more than 10 mSv in 1986. Twice the percentage of staff received 5–10 mSv, however. Even so, these are mostly low doses in relation to the current ICRP limit of 20 mSv for staff, and 72% fell within that limit in 1986.

In this chapter (and the previous two) radiation doses have been quoted in sievert (Sv) units. The sievert is directly equivalent to the unit of absorbed radiation dose used for low linear energy transfer (LET) radiations, such as X-rays or γ-rays. For higher LET radiations, however, the doses have to be multiplied by a weighting factor to take into account the increased relative biological effectiveness (RBE) of these types of radiation (Chapter 9). Table 20.5 lists the weighting factors recommended by the ICRP. The highest factor is 20 for the most densely ionizing radiations, such as alpha particles and neutrons in the 100 keV–2 MeV range. Other neutrons have a lower factor, depending on their energy. These factors can be used to calculate the sievert units that are used in the present context of radiation protection.

RAD EQUIVALENCE

Rad equivalence refers to the idea of studying the effects of chemical mutagens and carcinogens in terms of the equivalent lesions produced by ionizing radiation. It often happens that the lesions produced in genetic material by chemical mutagens and radiation are very similar. In both cases they are either lesions in DNA (strand breaks, base lesions that produce a change in the shape of the double helix, interstrand cross-links) or changes in the bonds between this DNA and the proteins that surround it. The lesions are sufficiently similar to elicit, in both cases, the activity of the same repair systems. These act by resealing breaks, by opening cross-links, by

Table 20.5. Radiation weighting factors recommended by the ICRP

Type and energy range	Radiation weighting factor
Photons, all energies	1
Electrons and muons, all energies	1
Neutrons, energy <10 keV	5
>10–100 keV	10
>100 keV–2 MeV	20
>2 MeV–20 MeV	10
>20 MeV	5
Protons, energy >2 MeV	5
Alpha particles, fission fragments, heavy nuclei	20

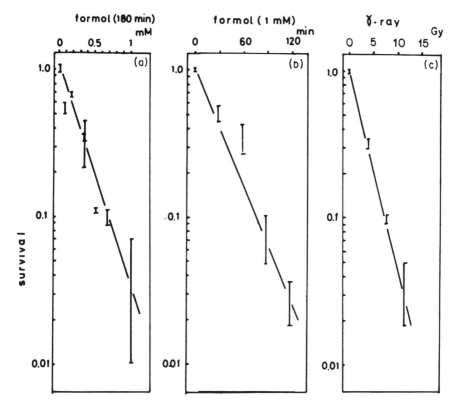

Figure 20.1. Survival of mouse kidney cells to treatment with: (a) formol at increasing concentrations for 180 min; (b) formol for increasing times at 1 mM concentration; (c) γ-irradiation. (Reproduced from Chanet et al, 1977, by permission of Commission of the European Communities.)

excision of the damaged bases, by genetic recombination or by an inducible repair mechanism. The similarity between chemical- and radiation-induced mutagenesis can be demonstrated by checking that a strain of cells that is hypersensitive to radiation because it lacks some repair system is also hypersensitive to most chemical mutagens.

It follows from this that one can establish an equivalence between the 'dose' of a chemical and a dose of radiation, on the basis of the effects produced on some biological systems of reference. This has been done for formaldehyde, which has many industrial uses; formaldehyde is also used for sterilization purposes in agriculture and is found in fuel and cigarette smoke. Figure 20.1 shows the data for a study of rad equivalence, where mouse kidney cells were exposed to formol or to γ-irradiation. The formol treatment was either for a fixed time at increasing concentrations or with a fixed concentration for increasing times. This enabled the rad equivalence for formaldehyde to be calculated within the range 5.5–9.1 cGy for 1 mM/min formaldehyde. In terms of continuous exposure to formaldehyde in the environment for 1 year, 20 μg/m^3 is equivalent to 5.25 cGy, which is about the same dose (50 mSv) that radiation workers used to be permitted to receive in 1 year.

This represents a very precise level of rad equivalence for a particular chemical hazard. It shows an example of what might be achieved by toxicologists if they made use of some of the radiobiological parameters described in this book. As long as the 'dose' of the chemical toxin can be measured with reasonable precision, the assays should reveal biological effects in a quantitative manner. Some drugs are 'radiomimetic' for some parameters (Barot et al, 1985) but there will obviously be examples where different mechanisms of toxicity make it necessary to use other parameters.

There may also be circumstances where both radiation and chemical hazards exist together. For example, the food chain may be contaminated both by a chemical that is carcinogenic and a radioactive isotope. The question will arise as to whether the two types of hazard are additive in their effect upon the consumer. The types of bioassays described in this book may help to answer such questions.

GENERAL GUIDELINES

The radiation exposure limits set by the ICRP are intended to be maximum values that must not be exceeded. In accepting the ICRP's recommendations, it is common practice for organizations to aim for limits lower than those given in the recommendations, in line with the principle of ALARA (as low as is reasonably achievable). Most workers in the nuclear industry achieve doses that are well within these regulated limits (see Tables 19.1 and 20.3).

The ICRP also makes the prudent assumption that there are health effects, varying directly with the dose received, right down to zero dose (even though zero dose is an ideal that cannot be reached because we can never avoid all natural radiation). The ICRP recommendations do not apply to radiation doses received from natural background radiation or from medical uses, but they do cover those from all other sources.

With proper precautions, most radiation workers need not receive any more dose than a member of the public. Radiotherapists have largely ceased to implant radium and other unshielded sources by hand and now use afterloading techniques. Beam therapy is always conducted under fully shielded conditions, as is nearly all diagnostic radiology. Image intensifiers reduce radiological exposures of staff to a minimum during screening. Therapeutic doses of radioactive isotopes *may* present a hazard in the field of nuclear medicine. The most hazardous branch of radiology is in the industrial field, largely because precautions are not always followed. This leaves only the nuclear power industry. Radiation accidents will continue to happen but the vast majority involve relatively small doses to small groups of the people employed at nuclear installations. The Chernobyl accident was the worst example to date.

The dosimetry of radiation is very sensitive compared to the dosimetry of chemical and viral carcinogens, because the units are physical. The ICRP has made a recommendation that the public should not receive an additional dosage of more than 1 mSv/year over a lifetime, but they already receive more than twice that from the background of 2.6 mSv/year.

SUMMARY OF CONCLUSIONS

(1) The basis of radiation protection is to reduce additional doses from 'man-made' sources to as low as is reasonably achievable (ALARA). The benefit should exceed the detriment.
(2) The risks of radiation exposure can be compared with those from other walks of life. The Chernobyl radiation accident killed 31 people at the time. The Bophal chemical accident killed 3300.
(3) The present ICRP recommendations set yearly levels of 20 mSv for radiation workers.
(4) Over a lifetime, the ICRP recommends that the general public should not receive an additional dosage of more than 1 mSv/year. Everyone receives 2.6 mSv/year from natural background radiation anyway.
(5) The present average dose received by radiation workers is 1.7 mSv/year. Because the cancer risk is estimated to be 5.9%/Sv, the annual risk for radiation workers is 10^{-4}. The risk for the general public will be very much lower.
(6) Chemical hazards can be compared with those of radiation in terms of rad equivalence.

REFERENCES

Barot, H. A., Laverick, M. and Nias, A. H. W., 1985. The radiomimetic properties of a platinum drug. *British Journal of Radiology*, **58**, 51–62.
Chanet, R., Magana-Schwencke, N., Yoshikura, H. and Moustacchi, E., 1977. An attempt to apply the rad-equivalence notion to the biological effects of formaldehyde. In *First European Symposium on Rad-Equivalence*. Commission of the European Communities, Brussels, pp. 171–191.
Cohen, B. L., 1991. Catalog of risks extended and updated. *Health Physics*, **61**, 317–335.
Clarke, R. H., 1997. Managing radiation risks. *Journal of the Royal Society of Medicine*, **90**, 88–92.

ICRP, 1991. 1990 Recommendations of the International Commission on Radiological Protection. ICRP Publication 60. *Annals of the ICRP*, **21** (nos 1–3).

Kendall, G. M., Muirhead, C. R., MacGibbon, B. H., et al, 1992. Mortality and occupational exposure to radiation: first analysis of the National Registry for Radiation Workers. *British Medical Journal*, **304**, 220–225.

Lucas, J. N., Awa, A., Straume, T., Poggensee, M., Kodama, Y., Nakano, M., Ohtaki, K., Weier, H. U., Pinkel, D., Gray, J. and Littlefield, G., 1992. Rapid translocation frequency analysis in humans decades after exposure to ionizing radiation. *International Journal of Radiation Biology*, **62**, 53–63.

NRPB, 1989. *Living with Radiation*. National Radiological Protection Board. HMSO, London.

NRPB, 1995. Risk of radiation-induced cancer at low doses and low dose rates for radiation protection purposes. *Documents of the NRPB*, **6** (no. 1). National Radiological Protection Board, HMSO, London.

Pratt, T. A. and Sweeney, J. K., 1989. A review of occupational exposure in the North-Western Region. *British Journal of Radiology*, **62**, 734–738.

Further Reading

Alper, T., 1979. Cellular Radiobiology. Cambridge University Press, Cambridge

Awwad, H. K., 1990. Radiation Oncology: Radiobiological and Physiological Perspectives. Kluwer Academic Publishers, Dordrecht, The Netherlands.

Bond, V. P., Fliedner, T. M. and Archambeau, J. O., 1965. Mammalian Radiation Lethality. A Disturbance in Cellular Kinetics. Academic Press, New York.

Coggle, J. E., 1983. Biological Effects of Radiation, 2nd edn. Taylor & Francis, London.

Elkind, M. M. and Whitmore, G. F., 1967. Radiobiology of Cultured Mammalian Cells. Gordon and Breach, New York.

Hall, E. J., 1997. Radiobiology for Radiologists, 4th edn. Lippincott-Raven, Philadelphia.

ICRP, 1977. Recommendations of the International Commission on Radiation Protection. ICRP Publications 26 and 27, Pergamon Press, Oxford.

Mererdith, W. J. and Massey, J. B., 1978. Fundamental Physics of Radiology. Wright, Bristol.

Meyn, R. E. and Withers, H. R. (eds), 1980. Radiation Biology in Cancer Research. Raven Press, New York.

Nias, A. H. W., 1989. Clinical Radiobiology, 2nd edn. Churchill Livingstone, Edinburgh.

NRPB, 1989. Living with Radiation, 4th edn. National Radiological Protection Board, HMSO, London, 62pp.

Potten, C. S. and Hendry, J. H., 1983. Cytotoxic Insult to Tissue. Churchill Livingstone, Edinburgh.

Sonntag, C. Von, 1987. The Chemical Basis of Radiation Biology. Taylor and Francis, London.

Steel, G. G. (ed), 1997. Basic Clinical Radiobiology, 2nd edn. Edward Arnold, London.

Tannock, I. F. and Hill, R. P., 1992. The Basic Science of Oncology, 2nd edn. McGraw-Hill, New York.

Thames, H. D. and Hendry, J. H., 1987. Fractionation in Radiotherapy. Taylor and Francis, London.

UNSCEAR, 1977. Sources and Effects of Ionising Radiation. United Nations Scientific Committee on the Effects of Atomic Radiation. United Nations, New York, Publication E.77.ix.1.

Yarnold, J. R., Stratton, M. and McMillan, T. J., 1996. Molecular Biology for Oncologists, 2nd edn. Elsevier Science, Amsterdam.

Glossary

α/β ratio   The ratio of the parameters α and β in the equation describing the shape of the survival curve or the iso-effect plot.

Cell cycle time (t_C)   The time between one mitosis and the next.

Cell loss (CL)   The proportional loss of extra cells added by division.

D_0   Dose that reduces survival to e^{-1} (0.37 or 37%) of its previous value on the exponential portion of the survival curve.

Direct action   Ionization or excitation of a molecule by direct interaction with radiation.

Dose equivalent   Quantity obtained by multiplying the absorbed dose (Gy) by a quality factor to allow for the degree of effectiveness of particular types of radiation. The unit is the sievert (Sv).

Doubling time (t_D)   Time for a cell population to double its size.

Effective dose equivalent   Quantity obtained by multiplying the dose equivalent to a tissue by the appropriate risk weighting factor for that tissue. Expressed in sieverts.

Extrapolation number   Point of extrapolation of the exponential portion of a multi-target survival curve to the y-axis.

Flexible tissues   Cell populations capable of both division and function.

Free radical   A chemical species containing an unpaired electron.

Genetically significant dose (GSD)   The dose that, if given to every member of a population, should produce the same hereditary damage as the actual doses received by the gonads of the particular individuals that receive radiation. Expressed in sieverts, this dose takes into account the child-bearing potential of those receiving the dose.

Growth fraction (GF)   The proportion of cells in cycle in a population.

Hierarchical tissues   Cell populations comprising a lineage of stem cells, proliferative cells, and mature cells. The mature cells do not divide.

Indirect action   Transfer of energy to biological molecules through intermediary free radicals.

Interphase death   Cell death in the absence of mitosis.

LD$_{50/30}$ Dose to produce lethality in 50% of subjects by 30 days.

Linear energy transfer (LET)   The rate of energy loss along the track of an ionizing particle, imparted by charged particles of specified energy. Usually expressed in keV/μm.

Mitotic death   Cell death caused by failure to complete mitotis correctly and produce two viable daughter cells.

Non-stochastic effect An effect where the severity increases with increasing dose after a threshold region.

Oxygen enhancement ratio (OER) The ratio of dose given under anoxic conditions to the dose resulting in the same effect when given under oxic conditions.

Potential doubling time (t_{pot}) The volume doubling time that would be measured in the absence of cell loss.

Potentially lethal damage Injury that can be repaired in the interval between irradiation and assay.

Quality factor A multiplication factor to take into account the increased RBE of radiations that have a higher LET.

Quasi-threshold dose (D_q) Point of extrapolation of the exponential portion of a multi-target survival curve to the level of zero cell kill.

Relative biological effectiveness (RBE) Ratio of doses of a reference radiation quality and the test radiation type that produce equal effect.

Stem cells Cells capable of self-renewal and of differentiation to produce all the various types of cells in a lineage.

Stochastic effect An effect where the incidence, but not the severity, increases with increasing dose.

Sublethal damage Injury that can be repaired or will accumulate with further dose to become lethal.

Tumour bed effect (TBE) Slower rate of tumour growth after irradiation due to stromal injury in the irradiated connective-tissue 'bed'.

Index

Note: index entries referring to Figures and Tables are indicating by *italic page numbers*; alphabetization is letter-by-letter (ignoring spaces).

Index compiled by Paul Nash